Pediatric Allergy

Nima Rezaei
Editor

Pediatric Allergy

A Case-Based Collection with MCQs, Volume 1

Springer

Editor
Nima Rezaei
Department of Immunology, School of Medicine
Research Center for Immunodeficiencies (RCID)
Children's Medical Center
Tehran University of Medical Sciences (TUMS)
Tehran
Iran

Network of Immunity in Infection, Malignancy
and Autoimmunity (NIIMA)
Universal Scientific Education and Research
Network (USERN)
Tehran
Iran

ISBN 978-3-030-18281-6 ISBN 978-3-030-18282-3 (eBook)
https://doi.org/10.1007/978-3-030-18282-3

This Springer imprint is published by the registered company Springer Nature Switzerland AG
The registered company address is: Gewerbestrasse 11, 6330 Cham, Switzerland

Preface

Immunology has found its way well into the practice of pediatrics. Years after publication of the first pediatric text books, footprints of immunology can be found in diagnosis and practice of almost all pediatric disorders. Delivering a magnificent contribution is the advent of novel diagnostic methods of molecular genetics in pediatric practice. Genetic diagnosis is now an indispensable part of the routine practice of primary immunodeficiency diseases, inborn metabolic errors, and monogenic malformations, making its way into diagnostic criteria of some as well. It wont go far wrong to state that the science of pediatrics has entered an era of interdisciplinary practice with genetics and immunology. The rapid flow of discovery of biological drugs during the last decade, availability of whole exome (and genome) sequencing methods, and the outstanding boost in the rate of success of hematopoietic and solid organ transplantation are all affirmative to this notion. Thanks to molecular genetic methods, an increasing number of the newly introduced monogenic diseases are being characterized, donors and recipients are being cross-matched using intricate genotype:phenotype cross matching, and immunotherapy for allergy benefits from state-of-the-art characterization of culprit epitopes in peptide scale. This book series tries to strike a balance between cutting-edge science of immunology and clinical practice of pediatrics, through a series of meticulously chosen case discussions, presented by pediatric practitioners and immunology experts.

This three-volume book series is a collection of well-presented case discussions in the field of pediatric immunology and allergy. Volume I, *Pediatric Allergy*, is focused on diagnosis and practice of allergy, asthma, atopy, and relevant disorders. Volume II, *Pediatric Immunology*, thoroughly addresses primary immunodeficiency disorders, and finally, Volume III, *Pediatric Autoimmunity and Transplantation*, is a constellation of cases in autoimmune and rheumatologic disorders of childhood, secondary immunodeficiency conditions, and real cases with hematopoietic and solid organ transplantation.

Volume I of this series is dedicated to represent some of the many faces of hypersensitivity disorders, from food and drug allergy to allergic rhinitis, atopic dermatitis, to asthma, and finally anaphylaxis as a fatal outcome of all hypersensitivity reactions. Starting by Chapters 2–12, with allergic rhinitis as the prototype of allergic disorders, we move onto Chapters 13–25, focused on case discussions on food allergy, and Chapters 26–36 presenting case discussions on urticaria and atopic dermatitis. Completing the picture of atopy triad, Chapters 37–44 give a glimpse over state-of-the art guidelines for asthma diagnosis and management. In Chapters 45–53, the reader is introduced to drug hypersensitivity reactions, as second most common cause of allergic reactions in the pediatric population. The final chapters of this volume, from Chapters 54–60, are dedicated to anaphylaxis, a potentially lethal systemic hypersensitivity reaction, and a must-know for every physician practicing in pediatric care.

The *Pediatric Immunology and Allergy Series* is the result of a multinational collaboration of more than 350 scientists from more than 100 well-known universities/institutes worldwide. I would like to hereby acknowledge the expertise of all contributors and their generous devotion of time and effort in preparing each of the 290 chapters of the series. I would like to extend my gratitude to the Springer publication for providing me the opportunity to publish the book.

Hopeful I remain that this book provides an exemplary touch to the fast-growing intersection of pediatric medicine and basic immunology, and a useful guide for pediatric practitioners worldwide.

Tehran, Iran Nima Rezaei

Acknowledgment

I would like to express my sincere gratitude for the tremendous efforts of my Editorial Assistant, Dr. Farzaneh Rahmani. I would like to gratefully acknowledge her fine work, without which completion of this book would not have been possible.

Nima Rezaei

Contents

Contributors

Carmo Abreu, MD Centro Hospitalar do Porto, Porto, Portugal

Stefania Arasi, MD Allergy Unit, Department of Pediatrics, University of Messina, Messina, Italy

Sonia de Arriba-Méndez, MD, PhD Pediatric Service, University Hospital Salamanca, Salamanca, Spain

Suna Asilsoy, MD Department of Pediatric Allergy and Immunology, Dokuz Eylul University, İzmir, Turkey

Ryan H. Avery, BS Department of Pathobiological Sciences, Louisiana State University School of Veterinary Medicine, Baton Rouge, LA, USA

Annamaria Bagnato Unit of Pediatric, Department of Pediatrics, University of Messina, Messina, Italy

Wojciech Baran, MD, PhD Department of Dermatology, Venereology and Allergology, Wroclaw Medical University, Wroclaw, Poland

Andrea Barbalace, MD Unit of Pediatric, Department of Pediatrics, University of Messina, Messina, Italy

Mohammad Hassan Bemanian, MD Department of Allergy and Clinical Immunology, Rasoul Akram Hospital, Iran University of Medical Sciences, Tehran, Iran

Elena Camelia Berghea, MD Emergency Clinical Hospital for Children M.S. Curie, Bucharest, Romania

University of Medicine and Pharmacy Carol Davila, Bucharest, Romania

Terri F. Brown-Whitehorn, MD Division of Allergy and Immunology, Children's Hospital of Philadelphia, Philadelphia, PA, USA

Department of Pediatrics, Perelman School of Medicine at the University of Pennsylvania, Philadelphia, PA, USA

Lucia Caminiti, MD Allergy Unit, Department of Pediatrics, University of Messina, Messina, Italy

Álvaro Carrillo, MD Unidad de Rinología y Cirugía de Base de Cráneo, Servicio de Otorrinolaringología, Hospital Universitario Ramón y Cajal, Madrid, Spain

Taher Cheraghi, MD Department of Pediatrics, 17th Shahrivar Children's Hospital, School of Medicine, Guilan University of Medical Sciences, Rasht, Iran

Brian K. Y. Chia, MBBS, MRCP National Skin Centre, Singapore, Singapore

Kok Wee Chong, MBBS, MRCPCH (UK) Allergy Service, Department of Paediatric Medicine, KK Women's and Children's Hospital, Singapore, Singapore

Martin Cuk, MD Nephrology Department, Children's Hospital Zagreb, Zagreb, Croatia

Caterina Cuppari, MD Unit of Pediatric, Department of Pediatrics, University of Messina, Messina, Italy

Renato Cutrera, MD Respiratory Unit, Academic Department of Pediatrics, Bambino Gesù Children's Hospital, IRCCS, Rome, Italy

Ignacio Dávila, MD, PhD Allergy Department, University Hospital of Salamanca, Salamanca, Spain

Allergy Service, Department of Biomedical and Diagnostic Sciences, Biosanitary Institute of Investigation, University Hospital of Salamanca, Salamanca, Spain

Purificacion Gonzalez-Delgado, MD Allergy Section, Alicante University General Hospital-ISABIAL, Alicante, Spain

Jaime M. Del-Rio-Chivardi, MD Hospital Infantil de México Federico Gómez, Ciudad de México, Mexico

Antonella Diamanti Artificial Nutrition Unit-Gastroenterology, Hepatology and Nutrition Unit, Bambino Gesù Children's Hospital, Rome, Italy

Valeria Dipasquale, MD Unit of Pediatric, Department of Pediatrics, University of Messina, Messina, Italy

Michael E. Dunham, MD Pediatric Otolaryngology, Children's Hospital, Louisiana State University School of Medicine, New Orleans, LA, USA

Hossein Esmaeilzadeh, MD Allergy Research Center, Namazi Hospital, Shiraz University of Medical Sciences, Shiraz, Iran

Bianca Faraci Unit of Pediatric, Department of Pediatrics, University of Messina, Messina, Italy

Javier Fernandez, MD Allergy Section, Alicante University General Hospital-ISABIAL, Alicante, Spain

Department of Clinical Medicine, Miguel Hernandez University, Alicante, Spain

Emily Y. Gan, MBBS, MRCP, MD Department of Dermatology, KK Women's and Children's Hospital, Singapore, Singapore

Javad Ghaffari, MD Department of Allergy and Clinical Immunology, Mazandaran University of Medical Sciences, Sari, Iran

Kevin S. Gipson, MD, MS Division of Pediatric Pulmonology, Department of Pediatrics, Massachusetts General Hospital, Harvard Medical School, Boston, MA, USA

Eva Rebelo Gomes, MD Basic and Clinical Immunology Unit, Laboratory of Immunology, Faculty of Medicine, University of Porto, Porto, Portugal

Allergy and Clinical Immunology Service, Centro Hospitalar Universitario do Porto, Porto, Portugal

Michihiro Hide, MD, PhD Department of Dermatology, Institute of Biomedical and Health Sciences, Hiroshima University, Hiroshima, Japan

David A. Hill, MD, PhD Division of Allergy and Immunology, Department of Pediatrics, Children's Hospital of Philadelphia, Philadelphia, PA, USA

Makiko Hiragun, MD Department of Dermatology, Institute of Biomedical and Health Sciences, Hiroshima University, Hiroshima, Japan

Sakine Işık, MD Department of Pediatric Allergy and Immunology, Süreyyapaşa Chest Diseases and Thoracic Surgery Training Hospital, Istanbul, Turkey

Irena Ivkovic-Jurekovic, MD, PhD Children's Hospital Zagreb, Zagreb, Croatia

Faculty of Medicine, University of Osijek, Osijek, Croatia

Faculty of Dental Medicine and Healthcare, University of Osijek, Osijek, Croatia

Nikolaos A. Karantaglis, MD, MSc Pediatric Pulmonology Unit, 3rd Pediatric Department, Hippokrateion Hospital, Aristotle University of Thessaloniki, Thessaloniki, Greece

Mojgan Kianiamin, MD Chamran Medical Hospital, Tehran, Iran

Alexandra Langlois, MD Division of Pediatric Allergy, Dermatology and Clinical Immunology, Department of Pediatrics, Montreal Children's Hospital, McGill University Health Centre, Montreal, QC, Canada

Milagros Lázaro, MD, PhD Allergy Department, University Hospital of Salamanca, Salamanca, Spain

Jan Hau Lee, MBBS, MRCPCH (UK), MCI Children's Intensive Care Unit, KK Women's and Children's Hospital, Singapore, Singapore

Wenyin Loh, MBBS, MRCPCH (UK) Allergy Service, Department of Paediatric Medicine, KK Women's and Children's Hospital, Singapore, Singapore

Eva Macías, MD, PhD Allergy Department, University Hospital of Salamanca, Salamanca, Spain

Mahboubeh Mansouri, MD Department of Immunology and Allergy, Mofid Children's Hospital, Shahid Beheshti University of Medical Sciences, Tehran, Iran

Sara Manti, MD Unit of Pediatric, Department of Pediatrics, University of Messina, Messina, Italy

Franklin Mariño-Sánchez, MD, PhD Unidad de Rinologia y Cirugia de Base de Craneo, Servicio de Otorrinolaringologia, Hospital Universitario Ramon y Cajal, Madrid, Spain

INGENIO, Immunoal.lèrgia Respiratòria Clínica i Experimental (IRCE), Institut d'Investigacions Biomèdiques August Pi i Sunyer (IDIBAPS), Barcelona, Catalunya, Spain

CIBER de Enfermedades Respiratorias (CIBERES), Barcelona, Catalunya, Spain

Iraj Mohammadzadeh, MD Non-Communicable Pediatric Diseases Research Center, Babol University of Medical Sciences, Babol, Iran

Joaquim Mullol, MD, PhD INGENIO, Immunoal.lèrgia Respiratòria Clínica i Experimental (IRCE), Institut d'Investigacions Biomèdiques August Pi i Sunyer (IDIBAPS), Barcelona, Catalunya, Spain

CIBER de Enfermedades Respiratorias (CIBERES), Barcelona, Catalunya, Spain

Unitat de Rinologia i Clinica de l'Olfacte, Servei d'Otorinolaringologia, Hospital Clínic i Universitari, Barcelona, Catalunya, Spain

Gordon Myers, MD Section of Allergy Immunology, Department of Pediatrics, Children's Hospital, Louisiana State University School of Medicine, New Orleans, LA, USA

Mohammad Nabavi, MD Department of Allergy and Clinical Immunology, Rasoul Akram Hospital, Iran University of Medical Sciences, Tehran, Iran

Elsy M. Navarrete-Rodríguez, PhD Hospital Infantil de México Federico Gómez, Ciudad de México, Mexico

Marta Navratil, MD, PhD Children's Hospital Zagreb, Zagreb, Croatia

Faculty of Dental Medicine and Healthcare, University of Osijek, Osijek, Croatia

Plamena Ivanova Novakova, MD Clinic of Clinical Allergy, Medical University, Sofia, Bulgaria

Silviya Mihaylova Novakova, MD, PhD Allergy Unit, Internal Consulting Department, University Hospital "St. George", Plovdiv, Bulgaria

Ivan Petkov Novakov, MD, PhD, MSc Department of Special Surgery, Medical University, Plovdiv, Bulgaria

Maria Giovanna Paglietti, MD Respiratory Unit, Academic Department of Pediatrics, Bambino Gesù Children's Hospital, IRCCS, Rome, Italy

Giovanni Battista Pajno, MD Allergy Unit, Department of Pediatrics, University of Messina, Messina, Italy

Charmi Patel, MD Division of Allergy and Immunology, Department of Medicine, Albany Medical Center, Albany Medical College, Albany, NY, USA

Punita Ponda, MD Division of Allergy and Immunology, Cohen Children's Hospital of New York, Donald and Barbara Zucker School of Medicine at Hofstra/Northwell, Great Neck, NY, USA

Federica Porcaro, MD Respiratory Unit, Academic Department of Pediatrics, Bambino Gesù Children's Hospital, IRCCS, Rome, Italy

Farzaneh Rahmani, MD, MPH Network of Immunity in Infection, Malignancy and Autoimmunity (NIIMA), Universal Scientific Education and Research Network (USERN), Tehran, Iran

NeuroImaging Network (NIN), Universal Scientific Education and Research Network (USERN), Tehran, Iran

Maryam Rahmani, MD Shahid Beheshti University of Medical Sciences (SBMU), Tehran, Iran

Nima Rezaei, MD, PhD Department of Immunology, School of Medicine, Research Center for Immunodeficiencies (RCID), Children's Medical Center, Tehran University of Medical Sciences (TUMS), Tehran, Iran

Network of Immunity in Infection, Malignancy and Autoimmunity (NIIMA), Universal Scientific Education and Research Network (USERN), Tehran, Iran

Darko Richter, MD, PhD Outpatient and Emergency Service, Department of Pediatrics, University Hospital Center, Zagreb, Croatia

Melanie A. Ruffner, MD, PhD Division of Allergy and Immunology, Children's Hospital of Philadelphia, Philadelphia, PA, USA

Department of Pediatrics, Perelman School of Medicine at University of Pennsylvania, Philadelphia, PA, USA

Carmelo Damiano Salpietro, MD Unit of Pediatric, Department of Pediatrics, University of Messina, Messina, Italy

Omar J. Saucedo-Ramirez, MD Hospital Infantil de México Federico Gómez, Ciudad de México, Mexico

Alireza Shafiei, MD Department of Allergy and Clinical Immunology, Bahrami Hospital, School of Medicine, Tehran University of Medical Sciences, Tehran, Iran

Samin Sharafian, MD Department of Allergy and Clinical Immunology, Bushehr University of Medical Sciences, School of Medicine, Bushehr, Iran

Sima Shokri, MD Department of Allergy and Clinical Immunology, Rasoul Akram Hospital, Iran University of Medical Sciences, Tehran, Iran

Moshe Ben Shoshan, MD, MSc Division of Pediatric Allergy, Dermatology and Clinical Immunology, Department of Pediatrics, Montreal Children's Hospital, McGill University Health Centre, Montreal, QC, Canada

Juan J. L. Sienra-Monge, MD Hospital Infantil de México Federico Gómez, Ciudad de México, Mexico

Maria Toncheva Staevska, MD, PhD Clinic of Clinical Allergy, Medical University, Sofia, Bulgaria

Jacek Szepietowski, MD, PhD Department of Dermatology, Venereology and Allergology, Wroclaw Medical University, Wroclaw, Poland

Shunsuke Takahagi, MD Department of Dermatology, Institute of Biomedical and Health Sciences, Hiroshima University, Hiroshima, Japan

Iva Topalusic, MD Children's Hospital Zagreb, Zagreb, Croatia

Meritxell Valls-Mateus, MD, PhD Unitat de Rinologia i Clinica de l'Olfacte, Servei d'Otorinolaringologia, Hospital Clínic i Universitari, Barcelona, Catalunya, Spain

Luke A. Wall, MD Section of Allergy Immunology, Children's Hospital, Louisiana State University School of Medicine, New Orleans, LA, USA

Manuela Dimitrova Yoncheva, MD Internal Consulting Department, University Hospital "St. George", Plovdiv, Bulgaria

Abbreviations

6-FED	6 most common food-allergens, milk, soy, egg, wheat, peanuts, tree nuts, and shellfish, fish
aAEDS	Atopic AEDS
ABPA	Allergic bronchopulmonary aspergillosis
ABPM	Allergic bronchopulmonary mycosis
ACE	Angiotensin-converting enzyme
AD	Atopic dermatitis
ADHD	Attention deficit hyperactivity disorder
ADR	Adverse drug reactions
AEDS	Atopic eczema/dermatitis syndrome
AERD	Aspirin exacerbated respiratory disease
AFRS	Allergic fungal rhinosinusitis
AFS	Allergic fungal sinusitis
AIT	Allergen immunotherapy
ANA	Anti-nuclear antibody
ANC	Absolute neutrophil count
ANCA	Anti-neutrophil cytoplasmic antibodies
Anti-TG	Anti-thyroglobulin
Anti-TPO	Anti-thyroid peroxidase
Anti-tTG	Tissue transglutaminase antibody
APK	Aquagenic palmar keratoderma
AR	Autosomal recessive
ASST	Autologous serum skin test
A-T	Ataxia-telangiectasia
BAL	Bronchoalveolar lavage
BANS	Budesonide aqueous nasal spray
BCG	Bacillus Calmette–Guérin (BCG)
BDP	Beclomethasone dipropionate
BMZ	Basement membrane zone
BP	Blood pressure
bpm	Beats per minute

BSA	Body surface area
c-ANCA	Cytosolic anti-neutrophil cytoplasmic antibodies
CBC	Complete blood count
CD	Cluster of differentiation
CF	Cystic fibrosis
CFTR	Cystic fibrosis transmembrane conductance regulator
CIndUs	Chronic inducible urticaria
CLR	Clarithromycin
CM	Cutaneous mastocytosis
CNIs	Calcineurin inhibitors
COPD	Chronic obstructive pulmonary disease
CRP	C-reactive protein
CRS	Chronic rhinosinusitis
CRSsNP	CRS without nasal polyposis
CRSwNP	CRS with nasal polyposis
CsA	Cyclosporine A
CSU	Chronic spontaneous urticaria
CT	Computed tomography
CTL	Cytotoxic T-lymphocytes
CTMs	Chinese topical medications
CXR	Chest X-ray
DAO	Diamine oxidase
DCM	Diffuse cutaneous mastocytosis
DHR	Drug-induced hypersensitivity reactions
DIA	Drug-induced anaphylaxis
DIF	Direct immunofluorescence
DNA	Deoxyribonucleic acid
DOCK8	Dedicator of cytokinesis 8
DPT	Drug provocation test
DT	Diphteria and tetanus toxoids full strength
dT	Diphtheria-tetanus toxoids with reduced content of diphtheria
DtaP	Diphtheria-tetanus acellular pertussis vaccine
DTaP3	Diphtheria-tetanus-3-component acellular pertussis vaccine
DTaP5-IPV-Hib	Diphtheria-tetanus-3-component acellular pertussis-inactivated polio haemophilus influenzae type b"
DTaP-IPV-HBV+Hib	Hexavalent diphteria-tetanus-acellular pertussis-inactivated polio-hepatitis B vccine
EAACI	European academy of allergy and clinical immunology
EBV	Epstein-Barr virus
EGD	Esophagogastroduodenal endoscopy
EGIDs	Eosinophilic gastrointestinal disorders
EGPA	Eosinophilic granulomatosis with polyangiitis
ELISA	Enzyme-linked immunosorbent assay

EM	Erythma multiformis
EMM	Erythema multiform major
ESR	Erythrocyte sedimentation rate
FcεRIα	Fc subunit of high-affinity IgE receptor
FDA	Food and drug administration
FDEIA	Food-dependent exercise-induced anaphylaxis
FEF25%–FEF75%	Forced expiratory flow at 25–75%
FESS	Functional endoscopic sinus surgery
FEV1	Forced expiratory volume in 1 second
FF	Fluticasone furoate
FFP	Fresh frozen plasma
FiO_2	Fraction of inspired oxygen
FPIES	Food-protein induced enterocolitis syndrome
FPNS	Fluticasone propionate nasal spray
FTU	Finger-tip unit
FVC	Forced vital capacity
GI	Gastrointestinal
GINA	Global initiative for asthma
GOS	Galacto-oligosaccharide
GU	Genitourinary
HAE	Hereditary angioedema
HAV	Hepatitis A vaccine
Hb	Hemoglobin
HBV	Hepatitis B virus
HCV	Hepatitis C virus
HDM	House dust mite
HFP	Histamine fish poisoning
HFS	Hyaline fibromatosis syndrome
Hib	Haemophilus influenza type b vaccine
HIES	Hyper-IgE syndrome
HIV	Human immunodeficiency virus
HLA	Human leukocyte antigens
HP	Hypersensitivity pneumonitis
HPA	Hereditary papulotranslucent acrokeratoderma
HPLC	High-performance liquid chromatography
HPV	Human papilloma virus
HRCT	High-resolution computed tomography
HR-test	Histamine release test
HSV	Herpes simplex virus
IA	Idiopathic anaphylaxis
ICD	Irritant contact dermatitis
ICS	Inhaled corticosteroids
ICU	Intensive care unit
IFN	Interferon
IFN-γ	Interferon-γ

IgA	Immunoglobulin A
IgE	Immunoglobulin E
IgG	Immunoglobulin G
IgM	Immunoglobulin M
IIF	Indirect immunofluorescence
IIV	Inactivated influenza vaccine
IL	Interleukin
IL-12	Interleukin-12
IM	Intramuscular
INCs	Intranasal corticosteroids
Inf	Influenza vaccine
INH	Isoniazide
IPEX	Immune dysregulation, polyendocrinopathy, enteropathy, X-linked syndrome
IPV	Inactivated polio vaccine
IV	Intravenous
kg	Kilogram
LABA	Long-acting beta-agonists
LDL	Low-density lipoprotein
LE	Lupus erythematosus
LFT	Liver function test
LP	Lumbar puncture
LTRAs	Leukotriene receptor antagonists
LTs	Leukotrienes
MAOIs	Monoamine oxidase inhibitors
MBL	Mannose-binding lectin
MCV	Mean corpuscular volume
Men	Meningococcal vaccine
MenCV4	4-Valent (A,C,W-135,Y) conjugate meningococcal vaccine
MFNS	Mometasone furoate nasal spray
MIS	Mastocytosis in the skin
mmHg	Millimetre of mercury
MMR	Measles-mumps-rubella
MRI	Magnetic resonance imaging
naAEDS	Non-atopic AEDS
NEC	Necrotizing enterocolitis
NECD	NSAID-exacerbated cutaneous disease
NERD	NSAID-exacerbated respiratory disease
NFAT	Nuclear factor of activated T cells
NIH	National institute of health
NIUA	NSAID-induced urticaria/angioedema
NK cell	Natural killer cell
NMBAs	Neuromuscular blocking agents
NOMID	Neonatal-onset multisystem inflammatory disease

NRS	Numeric rating scale
NSAIDs	Non-steroidal anti-inflammatory drugs
NUV	Normocomplementemic urticarial vasculitis
OAS	Oral allergy syndrome
OCS	Oral corticosteroid
OFC	Oral food challenge
OPV	Oral polio vaccine
ORS	Oral rehydration serum
OS	Omenn's syndrome
PAF	Platelet-activating factor
p-ANCA	Perinuclear anti-neutrophil cytoplasmic antibodies
PCD	Primary ciliary dyskinesia
PCR	Polymerase chain reaction
PCV	Pneumococcal conjugate vaccine
PEF	Peak expiratory flow rate
PER	Persistent allergic rhinitis
PFS	Pollen-food syndrome
PFT	Pulmonary function test
PIDs	Primary immunodeficiencies
PLE	Protein losing enteropathy
pMDI	Pressurized metered-dose inhalers
PO	Per os/oral
PPI	Proton pump inhibitor
PPSV	Pneumococcal polysaccharide vaccine
RAST	Radioallergosorbent test
RBC	Red blood cell
ROS	Reactive oxygen species
RSV	Respiratory syncytial virus
RV	Rotavirus vaccine
SABA	Short-acting beta-2 agonists
SBS	Short bowel syndrome
SCORAD	SCORing Atopic Dermatitis
SCUAD	Severe chronic upper airway disease
SI	Stimulation index
sIgE	Specific IgE
SLIT	Sublingual immunotherapy
SNIUAA	Single-NSAID-induced urticaria/angioedema or anaphylaxis
SPT	Skin prick test
STAT3	Signal transducer and activator of transcription 3
SU	Solar urticaria
T	Tetanus toxoid
TANS	Triamcinolone aqueous nasal spray
TBHT	Temporary black henna tattoo
TBI	Total body irradiation

TCD	Total cumulative dose
TCIs	Topical calcineurin inhibitors
TCS	Topical corticosteroids
Tdpa	Tetanus-diphtheria-acellular pertussis with reduced content of diphtheria an pertussis antigens
TG	Triglyceride
Th1	T helper 1
Th17	T helper 17
Th2	T helper 2
TIV	Trivalent influenza vaccine
TnT	Troponin T
TPO	Thyroid peroxidase
TPO-Ab	Thyroid peroxidase antibody level
TSH	Thyroid stimulating hormone
UA	Urinary analysis
URI	Upper respiratory tract infection
UV	Ultraviolet
Var	Varicella vaccine
VIT	Venom immunotherapy
VLM	Visceral larva migrans
VZIG	Varicella-zoster immune globulin
VZV	Varicella zoster virus
WAS	Wiskott-Aldrich syndrome
WBC	White blood cell
WBE	Whole-body extract
WDEIA	Wheat-associated FDEIA

Chapter 1
Introduction to Allergy

Luke A. Wall, Maryam Rahmani, Farzaneh Rahmani, Iva Topalusic, Hossein Esmaeilzadeh, Sara Manti, Samin Sharafian, Carmelo Damiano Salpietro, Caterina Cuppari, Kevin S. Gipson, and Nima Rezaei

L. A. Wall
Section of Allergy Immunology, Children's Hospital,
Louisiana State University School of Medicine, New Orleans, LA, USA

M. Rahmani
Shahid Beheshti University of Medical Sciences (SBMU), Tehran, Iran

F. Rahmani
Network of Immunity in Infection, Malignancy and Autoimmunity (NIIMA),
Universal Scientific Education and Research Network (USERN), Tehran, Iran

Students Scientific Research Center, Tehran University of Medical Sciences, Tehran, Iran
e-mail: f-rahmani@alumnus.tums.ac.ir

I. Topalusic
Children's Hospital Zagreb, Zagreb, Croatia

H. Esmaeilzadeh
Allergy Research Center, Namazi Hospital, Shiraz University of Medical Sciences,
Shiraz, Iran

S. Manti · C. D. Salpietro · C. Cuppari
Unit of Pediatric, Department of Pediatrics, University of Messina, Messina, Italy

S. Sharafian
Department of Allergy and Clinical Immunology, Tehran University of Medical Sciences,
Tehran, Iran

K. S. Gipson
Division of Pediatric Pulmonology, Department of Pediatrics,
Massachusetts General Hospital, Harvard Medical School, Boston, MA, USA

N. Rezaei (ed.), *Pediatric Allergy*, https://doi.org/10.1007/978-3-030-18282-3_1

N. Rezaei (✉)
Department of Immunology, School of Medicine, Research Center for Immunodeficiencies (RCID), Children's Medical Center, Tehran University of Medical Sciences (TUMS), Tehran, Iran

Network of Immunity in Infection, Malignancy and Autoimmunity (NIIMA), Universal Scientific Education and Research Network (USERN), Tehran, Iran
e-mail: rezaei_nima@tums.ac.ir

Allergic diseases are one of the most common disorders worldwide. One in five Americans experiences **Allergic rhinitis** in lifetime. Prevalence of allergic rhinitis is even higher in pediatric population, estimated up to 40% [1]. Children bear the greatest burden of the increasing trends in global rates of allergic disorders. School drop-outs, decreased learning ability and increased risk for metabolic syndromes, obesity, and cardiovascular disorders, all comprise to the increase in global burden of allergic disorders. With the upsloping figures of allergic rhinitis in middle and low income countries, allergic rhinitis is now considered a global health issue. Real life cases of patients with allergic rhinitis, state-of-art care and immunotherapy of allergic rhinitis are presented in the first few chapters this volume (Chaps. 2–12).

Food allergy affects between 5–10% of people in all age groups in the Western world, emerging as an important public health problem [2]. Food allergies may develop at any age, commonly starting in early childhood. Overall, about 90% of food allergies in children are induced by cow's milk, eggs, soybean, wheat, peanut, tree nuts, fish, and shellfish.

Food hypersensitivity/allergy disorders are classified into three subtypes: (1) those primarily involving IgE-mediated reactions, (2) those involving non-IgE-mediated mechanisms, and finally (3) those that involve both IgE- and non-IgE-mediated mechanisms. Symptoms of an allergic reaction to food are not confined to the tegumental system, as in hives, itching, eczema, or angioedema, but may involve the gastrointestinal tract (abdominal pain, diarrhea, nausea or vomiting), the cardiovascular system (dizziness, lightheadedness or fainting), or the respiratory tract (wheezing, nasal congestion or trouble breathing), as well.

Non-allergic adverse reactions to foods are also common and might result from either food intolerances or adverse physiologic reactions the ingredients. Food intolerances are indeed the most common cause of adverse reactions to food and might rise as a result of interaction between inherent characteristics of the food such as toxic contaminants or additives with the host through idiosyncratic responses. Physicians might frequently face patients who think they are "allergic" to a certain food item but are actually "intolerant" to it (Fig. 1.1).

Diagnose of food allergy starts with a comprehensive medical history that frequently reveals the culprit food. Laboratory investigations such as skin prick test (SPT), serum antibody testing using ImmunoCAP, double-blinded, placebo-controlled oral food challenge (OFC), which is considered to be the gold standard for food allergy diagnosis and finally, trial elimination diet are the next diagnostic strategies. Food aversions may mimic adverse food reactions, but are not typically reproduced when the patient is evaluated with double-blind placebo-controlled food

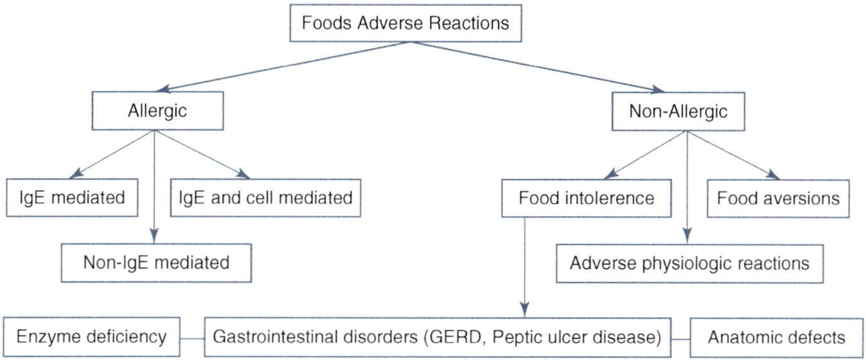

Fig. 1.1 Classification of adverse food reactions (GERD: gastroesophageal reflux disease)

challenge test. Unfortunately OFC carries a risk for anaphylaxis and is not readily available in all diagnostic settings [3].

The primary step to prevent food allergies, is to avoid consuming troublesome foods. This might not always be possible, especially in children during the growing ages. In this case a dietitian should be able to help. Careful checking of ingredient labels of food products is of utmost importance. Fatal or near-fatal food allergy reactions can occur at school or other places outside the home. Hence, parents of a child with food allergies need to make sure that their child's school has a written emergency action plan. Allergen immunotherapy is routinely used in the treatment of IgE-mediated food allergy to common items such as wheat, milk, egg and peanut. The mechanisms underlying effectiveness of food allergen immunotherapy have only begun to be fully understood. Chapters 13–25 of this volume are dedicated to present case discussion on real patients with different types of food allergy and associated conditions.

Urticaria is a term coined to refer to a group of diseases characterized by the development of wheals (hives), angioedema, or both. Urticaria is featured by itchy, pink-to-red edematous, recurrent lesions that are variable in size, from a few millimeters to several centimeters, with pale centers. Chapters 26–36 of this volume will present several case discussions on atopic dermatitis and urticaria.

Mast cells are the primary effectors in urticaria. Mast cells are widely distributed in the skin. Binding of antigen to IgE induces mast cells degranulation and release of chemical mediators such as histamine, platelet-activating factor (PAF), leukotrienes and prostaglandins. This culminates in vasodilation and leakage of plasma into the dermis and below the epidermis, and formation of the so called "hives".

The spectrum of clinical manifestations of urticaria is very wide. Depending on the duration of symptoms and the presence or absence of triggering stimuli, urticaria is classified into acute, with lesions beings present for less than 6 weeks or chronic, i.e. persistence of lesions for more than 6 weeks.

Foods, viral or parasitic infections, medications, insect venom, and contact allergens are the most common triggers of acute urticaria. In the remaining 50% of patients the cause of acute urticaria can not be identified, designated as acute idiopathic urticaria. Acute urticaria typically has a good prognosis [4].

Chronic urticaria is later classified as chronic spontaneous urticaria (CSU) or chronic inducible urticaria (CIndUs), based on the presumed/identified cause. This latter is also subclassified as physical urticaria which later includes symptomatic dermographism, urticaria factitia, cold- and heat-induced urticaria, delayed pressure urticaria, solar urticaria, and vibratory angioedema. Cholinergic urticaria, contact urticaria, and aquagenic urticaria are the remaining other, "non-physical" types of CIndUs. Figure 1.2 summarizes urticaria classification for clinical use.

When a physical stimulus e.g. mechanical (friction, vibration, pressure), thermal (changes in body temperature; exposure to cold or heat) or electromagnetic (ultra-violet light), triggers the onset of urticaria the diagnosis of "physical urticaria" is made. Symptomatic dermographism is one simple example of this group with an exaggerated local response to a minor physical trigger [4]. In cold- and heat-induced urticaria the wheals develop immediately after local exposure of the skin to cold or heat. Pressure urticaria is characterized by painful angioedema-like swellings, itching, and burning features after exposure to vertical pressure (e.g. carrying heavy backpacks or bags, sitting on hard chairs, tight shoes). Symptoms of pressure urticaria usually persist for as long as 24 h. Solar urticaria develops after exposure to UV-A and, less frequently, to UV-B. Wheals and angioedema that develop after exposure to local vibration, such as snoring or dental procedures, feature the clinical picture of vibratory angioedema [4]. Finally, cholinergic urticaria, contact urticaria, and aquagenic urticaria are triggered by non-physical stimuli, such as sudden increase of body temperature, contact with the provoking substance, and contact to water, sweat, or tears, respectively.

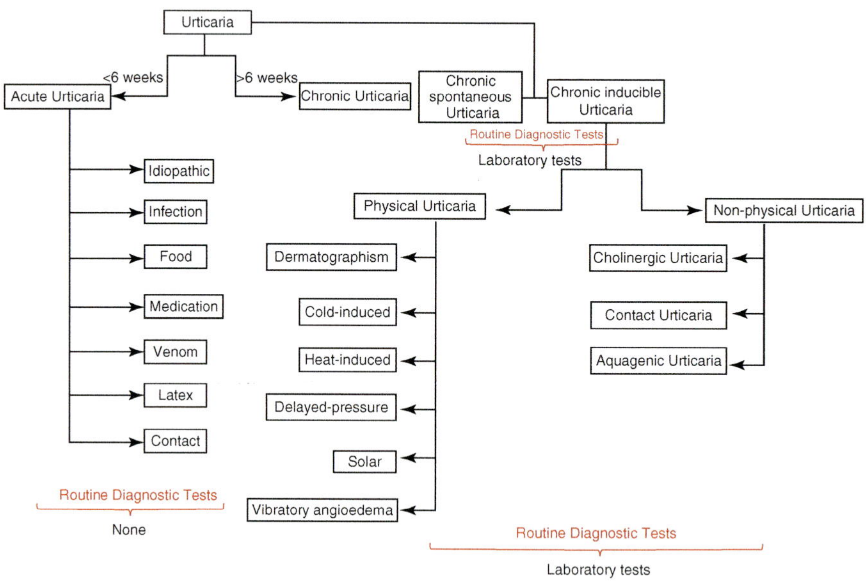

Fig. 1.2 Urticaria classification and diagnostic approach

CSU is a diagnostic challenge for many physicians. Association of CSU with systemic and autoimmune disorders is not rare and patients are recommended to undergo assessment for autoimmune thyroid disorder, glucose intolerance, and liver and kidney function tests. Infectious diseases, particularly *Helicobacter pylori* infection, obesity, anxiety, and malignancies are also associated with an increased risk of CSU. The autologous serum skin test (ASST) is used as screening for autoimmune CSU. Basophil activation test is further recommended in patients with positive anti-IgE receptor autoantibodies, to assess the functionality of these autoantibodies [4].

The diagnosis of urticaria is primarily based on clinical history including personal or family history of atopy, frequency, timing, duration and pattern of recurrence of lesions, habits and/or hobbies, stress, previous therapies, and physical examination entailing the shape, size, site and distribution of lesions. Due to its self-limiting nature, acute urticaria does not require routine diagnostic workup. However, SPT, and total and specific IgE (sIgE) levels may help confirm a diagnosis of allergic or IgE-mediated acute urticaria. Specific laboratory tests should be carried out on the basis of the individualized and suspected cause to make diagnosis of chronic autoimmune or idiopathic/spontaneous urticaria. An appropriate challenge testing, aimed to reproduce symptoms can confirm the diagnosis of induced forms of urticaria [4].

Management of urticaria is based on avoidance measures when a specific trigger has been identified, and use of second-generation, non-sedating, H1-receptor antihistamines for symptomatic control. If symptoms are not controlled with standard antihistamine doses, it is reasonable to continue treatment for several months and occasionally stop therapy for brief periods. It is common practice to increase the antihistamine dose to up to fourfold of standard, in patients who do not achieve adequate symptom control on standard treatment after 2 weeks. If symptoms persist for 1–4 further weeks, a trial of omalizumab, cyclosporine A (CsA) or montelukast as add on to standard therapies should be considered. A brief course of systemic corticosteroids is warranted only during severe exacerbations.

Atopic eczema/dermatitis syndrome (AEDS) is a chronic relapsing-remitting inflammatory skin disorder, affecting 15–30% of children and 2–10% of the adult population. AEDS happens due to a skin barrier dysfunction resulting in epidermal damage as well as an altered permeability to allergens and microbes. AEDS is characterized by a biphasic T cell polarization: in acute phase the lesions are infiltrated by Th2 cells producing IL-4, IL-5, and IL-13, while in chronic phase there is a switch towards a Th1 phenotype producing IFN-γ. Depending on the association with IgE sensitization, AEDS may be defined as atopic (aAEDS) or non-atopic (naAEDS). The aAEDS is the most prevalent form of the disease accounting for about 70–85% of the patients. These patients have high serum IgE levels, positive SPT reaction to common environmental allergens, such as foods and aeroallergens, and sometimes concomitant atopic diseases such as asthma and/or rhinitis. The naAEDS is associated with absence of sensitization to foods or aeroallergens, normal serum IgE values, negative SPT and no associated atopic diseases. Clinically, AEDS is featured by a chronic, pruritic, relapsing dermatitis occurring in a characteristic age-dependent distribution areas: with facial, scalp, and extensor involvement in infants and young children, and predominant flexural involvement in older children. Acute lesions are characterized by erythematous pruritic papules and excoriations with serous exudate. Chronic lesions instead show additional areas of lichenification and fibrotic nodules, with little erythema.

The major diagnostic criteria for AEDS, based on "Hanifin and Rajka" clinical guide are: (1) family or personal history of atopy, (2) onset before 2 years of age, (3) pruritus, (4) typical distribution, and (5) relapsing course. SCORing Atopic Dermatitis (SCORAD) is another clinical tool to assess the severity of AEDS. SCORAD consists of: (a) the interpretation of the extent of the disorder according to the rule of nines, which consists 20% of the total score, (b) the intensity of disease composed of six items: erythema, oedema/papules, effect of scratching, oozing/crust formation, lichenification and dryness, altogether consisting 60% of the total score, and (c) subjective symptoms such as itching and sleeplessness, which comprise 20% of the total score. The SCORAD permits distinction between mild, moderate and severe AEDS and helps with follow up of patients. On special occasions, skin biopsy specimens or lab tests may be helpful to rule out other or associated skin conditions.

The goal of AEDS management is both to improve quality of life and prevent infectious complications. Optimal control of all aspects of AEDS morbidity is achieved through hydration with emollients and ointments, restoration of the skin barrier, e.g. through ceramide-containing creams, and control of skin inflammation. Topical corticosteroids (TCS) are the most effective treatment to downregulate cutaneous inflammatory status. TCSs are available in a wide range of potencies, from the least potent Group 1 (e.g. hydrocortisone 1% ointment) to the most potent Group 7 preparations (e.g. clobetasol propionate 0.05% ointment). The long-term use of TCSs is often associated with atrophy, striae, acne, telangiectasias, and secondary infections. As steroid-sparing agents specially in patients requiring long-term anti-inflammatory treatment, topical calcineurin inhibitors are also administered. Systemic immunosuppressants such as cyclosporine, mycophenolate mofetil, azathioprine, and methotrexate are a treatment option for patients with severe, refractory AEDS, although a direct effect to restore the barrier function is not reported.

Asthma has been known to mankind since at least the time of Greek antiquity, and was first given its name in Homer's *Iliad* where it was described as a panting breathlessness which accompanied the rigors of battle [5]. It was not until the late 1800s that physicians began to understand the broad pathophysiologic mechanism of the acute asthma exacerbation, specifically, reversible constriction of the bronchioles. Henry Salter described this in his 1868 treatise on asthma as "inflammation or congestion of the mucous surface [which]… excites the muscular wall to contract." Sir William Osler later followed with his own description of the "spasmodic afflictions of the bronchial tubes" in 1901 [6–8]. In 1916, physicians Frances Rackemann of the Massachusetts General Hospital and Isaac Chandler Walker of what is now Brigham and Women's Hospital further disentangled the "extrinsic" causes of asthma and its acute exacerbation, laying the foundation for the current paradigm of allergic asthma [6].

In the modern age, allergic asthma remains a significant burden to public health and is a leading driver of hospitalization and illness in childhood. The United States' Centers for Disease Control and Prevention estimates that asthma impacts the lives of nearly 1 in 10 children in the United States, where it disproportionately affects ethnic minorities and those of disadvantaged socioeconomic backgrounds. Allergic asthma represents a significant burden in the US, where the prevalence of atopic disease and its attendant sequel appear to be on the rise.

As the complexities of asthma pathology and its relation to allergy and immune pathogenesis become increasingly apparent, a new and exciting field of asthma therapeutics has come to the forefront. Emerging therapies in allergic asthma, including the nascent and rapidly-expanding category of asthma biologics (e.g. monoclonal antibodies) and allergen immunotherapy, promise to significantly bolster the current mainstays of therapy, namely inhaled corticosteroids (ICS) and bronchodilators. Further, it is now clear that asthma is best cared for in a multidisciplinary team including primary care physicians and practitioners, pulmonologists, allergologists, nutritionists, and social workers. Only in such a setting can the full intricacies of the disease and its antecedents be addressed. Careful attention to the home environment and psychosocial dynamics are examples of such complexities.

Allergic asthma, like some fearsome beast of Greek mythology, is indeed protean in its presentation and pulmonary manifestations. Chapters 37–44 of this volume will familiarize the clinician with the tremendous breadth of this disease through a number of engaging patient cases and will review the most up-to-date asthma diagnosis and management strategies.

Drug-induced hypersensitivity reactions are immune-mediated reactions to drugs. These are also named as type B or "off-target" adverse drug reactions (ADR). Drug-induced hypersensitivity reactions are and have been a major concern for health-care systems due to their potentially severe nature and lethal outcomes.

Nonetheless, all four types of hypersensitivity reactions described by Coombs and Gell, i.e. type I (IgE mediated reactions), type II (antibody mediated cytotoxicity reactions), type III (immune complex-mediated reactions) and type IV (T-cell-mediated) hypersensitivity, are seen in immunological mechanisms underlying drug-induced hypersensitivity. Type I hypersensitivity reactions yield to the conventional acute mucocutaneous manifestation and occasionally multisystem reactions in form of anaphylaxis. Type III reactions, historically identified by serum sickness or serum sickness-like reactions, have also recently regained attention following widespread prescription of biological agents and emerging case of ADR to these agents.

Clinical phenotypes of drug-induced hypersensitivity reactions tend to be characterized by the time between exposure to the drug and onset of symptoms. Immediate reactions occur within an hour after re-exposure to a previously sensitized drug, and are often mediated by sIgE antibodies binding to high sensitivity IgE receptors on mast cells, i.e. type I hypersensitivity reaction. Clinical presentation can involve urticaria with or without angioedema or more severe systemic reactions including anaphylaxis or anaphylactic shock. Beta lactams are the most common drugs inducing this type of reactions. Nonetheless, a variety of other nonspecific immune mechanisms can cause immediate reactions, even after the first contact with the drug. These mechanisms include cross-reactivity, activation of alternative pathway of the complement system, direct activation of mast cells and basophils through G-protein and inhibition of cyclooxygenase-1, as seen in hypersensitivity to NSAIDs. It is possible that more than one mechanism is involved in drug-induced hypersensitivity reaction to a certain drug, as in NSAID-induced hypersensitivity, which can also be mediated by IgE-dependent mechanism in up to 30% of cases. Interestingly, a genetic predisposition based on certain human leukocyte antigen (HLA) loci have been demonstrated as risk factors for adverse reactions to anticonvulsants, sulfonamides and to anti-retroviral agent, abacavir.

On the other side of the spectrum, delayed drug-induced hypersensitivity reactions in type II, III and IV, occur within hours, days or even weeks after exposure to the drug. These types of reactions have a heterogeneous presentation and symptoms can range from maculopapular rash or delayed urticaria to a single or systemic organ involvement. Some of the most severe delayed-type reactions include acute generalized exanthematous pustulosis (AGEP), drug reaction with eosinophilia and systemic symptoms (DRESS), Stevens-Johnson syndrome (SJS), and toxic epidermal necrolysis (TEN). Finally, it is worth mentioning that there are drug-induced hypersensitivity reactions that occur within 1–6 h after drug exposure, called accelerated reactions, to which a certain immunological mechanism cannot be attributed.

Diagnostic algorithm of drug-induced hypersensitivity reactions is complex and includes both a detailed medical history and paraclinics. Both *in vitro* and *in vivo* tests should preferably be done after 4–6 weeks and no longer that 6 months after suspected reaction. *In vitro* methods have an overall higher specificity compared to *in vivo* tests. For example, measurement of serum levels of the basophil and mast cell mediators, such as leukotrienes (LTs) has a low sensitivity, as only trace amount of these substances are released into the blood stream with relatively short half-lives. Serum sIgE level assay is useful in diagnosis of IgE mediated reactions, but is available only for penicillin and drugs with large molecules, like insulin and streptokinase. Nonetheless, the basophil activation test, based on the measurement of CD63 and CD203 molecules on the cell surface of basophils after exposure to the drug, is an emerging and promising diagnostic test showing good results with quinolones, contrast media, dipyrone, anaesthetics, omeprazole and cyclosporine. Finally, lymphocyte proliferation test can be used for *in vitro* assay of delayed-type reactions, especially DRESS.

In vivo tests to confirm immediate-type reactions include SPT and early reaction in intradermal test. This is while late intradermal test reaction and epicutaneous tests are used to confirm delayed-type drug-induced hypersensitivity reactions. Drug provocation test (DPT) is the gold standard to confirm or exclude drug hypersensitivity reaction, proving most useful when previous investigations are inconclusive in the context of high clinical suspicion. DPT should only be performed in appropriate clinical setting and under surveillance of trained personnel. It is important to mention that DPT is contraindicated in patients with a history of anaphylaxis, vasculitis that is triggered or exacerbated by a certain drug, DRESS, APEG or SJS/TEN.

Patients with proven drug hypersensitivity should get an identification card with the recommendation of strict avoidance of the culprit drug(s). Desensitization is recommended if there is no alternative drug for the patient (e.g. enzyme replacement therapy in mucopolysaccharidosis). Chapters 45–53 of this volume are dedicated to case presentations of patients with drug hypersensitivity reactions.

Anaphylaxis is a severe life-threatening systemic hypersensitivity reaction. Anaphylaxis is commonly, but not always, mediated by an allergic mechanism usually through IgE. This sentence implicates that allergic/immunologic, but non-IgE-mediated forms of anaphylaxis and even non-allergic, anaphylactic reactions—formerly called anaphylactoid or pseudo-allergic reactions—can also occur. Surprisingly, all four types of hypersensitivity reactions can underlie an anaphylactic reaction, except for delayed-type T-cell-mediated reaction which appears to have minor role in anaphylaxis. Anaphylaxis is almost always a result of release of primary and secondary mediators from activated mast cell and eosinophils. These mediators induce a multi-organ involvement secondary to vasodilation and vascular leakage and smooth muscle spasm, to form the clinical picture of anaphylaxis.

Foods like peanut, tree nuts, seafood, and milk, are the most common causes of anaphylaxis. Other common triggers are medications, like β-lactam antibiotics, venoms, latex, allergen immunotherapy, and even exercise. Exercise can also act as a co-trigger in anaphylaxis to food or medication.

Diagnosis of anaphylaxis is based on clinical grounds and there is no gold standard laboratory diagnostic test. History and prick test are two usual diagnostics to find the cause of anaphylaxis, so to avoid exposure in future. There still remain 20–30% of all anaphylactic reactions that remain idiopathic.

Cutaneous symptoms, such as flushing, itching, urticaria, and angioedema are most common and occur in more than 90% of patients, and often the first symptom noted. Respiratory signs and symptoms, e.g. dysphonia, cough, stridor, wheezing, dyspnea, and chest tightness, and gastrointestinal manifestations such as nausea, vomiting, bloating, cramping, and diarrhea, happen in 40–70% of patients and cardiovascular manifestations are fortunately the least prevalent. Signs and symptoms of anaphylaxis usually appear within 5–30 min. This means that late-onset anaphylaxis is quite rare. Late-onset anaphylaxis should not be confused with the "late-phase" of biphasic anaphylactic reactions.

Emergency treatment in anaphylaxis is based on maintaining proper oxygenation, supine positioning of the patient and injecting epinephrine. Antihistamines and glucocorticoids are commonly used adjuvant drugs. It is important for the practicing clinician to know that the more rapid the onset of anaphylaxis, the more serious the reaction is. The main prophylactic point for anaphylaxis is to find the trigger and to avoid it. Final chapters of this series, Chaps. 54–60, focus on real cases based on patients presenting with anaphylactic reactions.

References

1. Pawankar R. Allergic diseases and asthma: a global public health concern and a call to action. World Allergy Organ J. 2014;7(1):1–3.
2. Tang ML, Mullins RJ. Food allergy: is prevalence increasing? Intern Med J. 2017;47(3):256–61.
3. Boyce JA, Assa'ad A, Burks AW, Jones SM, Sampson HA, Wood RA, Plaut M, Cooper SF, Fenton MJ, Arshad SH, Bahna SL, Beck LA, Byrd-Bredbenner C, Camargo CA Jr, Eichenfield L, Furuta GT, Hanifin JM, Jones C, Kraft M, Levy BD, Lieberman P, Luccioli S, McCall KM, Schneider LC, Simon RA, Simons FE, Teach SJ, Yawn BP, Schwaninger JM. Guidelines for the diagnosis and management of food allergy in the United States: summary of the NIAID-sponsored expert panel report. J Allergy Clin Immunol. 2010;126(6):1105–18.
4. Radonjic-Hoesli S, Hofmeier KS, Micaletto S, Schmid-Grendelmeier P, Bircher A, Simon D. Urticaria and angioedema: an update on classification and pathogenesis. Clin Rev Allergy Immunol. 2018;54(1):88–101.
5. Marketos SG, Ballas CN. Bronchial asthma in the medical literature of Greek antiquity. J Asthma. 1982;19(4):263–9.
6. ER MF Jr. A century of asthma. Am J Respir Crit Care Med. 2004;170(3):215–21.
7. Jackson M. Asthma, illness, and identity. Lancet. 372(9643):1030–1.
8. Jackson M. Asthma: the biography. Oxford: Oxford University Press; 2009.

Chapter 2
Sneezing and Rhinorrhea

Maryam Rahmani

A 10-year-old girl presented to immunologists office complaining about clear rhinorrhea, nasal obstruction, itching of the inner ear and clearing her throat several times through the day. She has had similar symptoms throughout the year for about 3 years. Her symptoms exacerbated about 3 weeks ago after she returned school from spring vacations. Her parents deny any prior respiratory infection and she did not have a fever, although she has occasionally developed fever and headaches along with other symptoms and received antibiotic therapy. The family does not own any pets and the girl does not take any drugs, except for cetirizine tablets she takes occasionally to alleviate the symptoms.

Q1. What is the most probable diagnosis?

A. Allergic rhinitis
B. Acute infectious rhinitis
C. Chronic rhinosinusitis
D. Chronic non-allergic rhinitis
E. Sinusitis

Answer*: The correct answer is* **A**.

Diagnosis of allergic rhinitis can be made on clinical grounds in the presence of characteristic clinical symptoms including paroxysms of sneezing rhinorrhea, nasal obstruction, nasal itching, postnasal drip cough, irritability and fatigue along with clinical signs like infraorbital edema and darkening (i.e. allergic shiners) and allergic salute (i.e. transvers nasal crease caused by repeated rubbing). Routine laboratory tests are usually normal. Allergy skin test can confirm whether the patient is sensitized to certain aeroallergens, but is not necessary for the diagnosis.

M. Rahmani (✉)
Shahid Beheshti University of Medical Sciences (SBMU), Tehran, Iran

N. Rezaei (ed.), *Pediatric Allergy*, https://doi.org/10.1007/978-3-030-18282-3_2

The culprit allergens might be identified by history alone. Allergic rhinitis in spring is often caused by tree and grass pollens while patients sensitized to ragweed pollen are often symptomatic in fall. On the contrary, the culprit allergen in perennial/persistent allergic rhinitis is usually indoors, such as dust mites, cockroaches or animal dander. The clinician would be lucky if there is an obvious connection between exposure to a certain allergen like an animal or onset of symptoms following house dusting.

Sinusitis frequently accompanies allergic rhinitis, as nasal mucosal inflammation associated with allergic rhinitis can cause obstruction of the sinuses ostiomeatal complex predisposing to sinusitis. Up to 30% of acute and 80% of episodes of chronic bacterial sinusitis can be attributed to underlying allergic rhinitis [1]. Importantly, clinical symptoms are not sensitive or specific enough to discriminate between bacterial sinusitis and allergic or viral rhinitis. This, added to shared/closed etiology of the two conditions, often mandates a joint approach to fully alleviate patients symptoms. Nonetheless, bacterial sinusitis symptoms might include purulent rhinorrhea, post nasal drip, facial or dental pain and cough that are usually absent in allergic rhinitis. Other disorders associated with allergic rhinitis include: allergic conjunctivitis, asthma, and atopic dermatitis.

Q2. The patient mentions difficulty in sleeping due to nasal congestion and thus had difficulty concentrating. What is the first-line recommendation for her?

A. Intra nasal corticosteroids
B. Antihistamine nasal sprays
C. Nasal decongestant sprays
D. Cromolyn sodium

Answer: *The correct answer is* ***A***.

Intranasal corticosteroids (INCs) are by far the first line and most effective single maintenance therapy for allergic rhinitis [2]. They are be divided into first and second generations with no significant difference in efficacy:

- First generation: beclomethasone dipropionate (BDP), flunisolide and budesonide
- Second generation: fluticasone propionate, mometasone furoate (MFNS) and fluticasone furoate

Onset of action for most INCs is within a few hours, while reaching maximal effect takes longer for days to weeks. Treatment can be initiated with maximal dose for age and stepped down gradually to the lowest effective dose. Patients who have a good compliance in avoiding the potential culprit allergen(s), might even achieve symptom control with every other day or "as need" use.

INCs combination with decongestant sprays is only approved in adults with disturbing and voluminous rhinorrhea. Instead, combination with antihistamine sprays are generally approved for symptom relief of children over 12 years old.

Q3. The patient's parents are worried about the potential side effects of nasal inhalers from previous personal experience. Which of the following conditions is an indication for discontinuation of the drug?

A. Traces of blood in the nasal mucus following the use of INC
B. Patients' parent are worried about glucocorticoids affecting their child's growth
C. Dry and burning sensation of nasal mucosa following the use of INC
D. None of the above

Answer: *The correct answer is* ***D***.

Good technique in use of INCs ensures maximum efficacy and avoiding side effects like nasal musical ulcerations or atrophy (Chapter 12). A single report has provided results in favor of intranasal BDP adversely affecting children's growth [3], but not other glucocorticoids, while the results were not supported by subsequent controlled trials.

Nasal decongestant sprays such as phenylephrine, oxymetazoline or naphazoline should not be used as a prolonged single therapy in allergic rhinitis. Emergence of rapid rebound of symptoms after discontinuation of the drug have been reported even with 3–7 days of persistent use.

Oral antihistamines are available under three main generations: first, second and third generation. First generation of oral antihistamines include diphenhydramine, chlorpheniramine, hydroxyzine and brompheniramine, all causing significant sedation owing to their lipophilic nature and anti-muscarinic traits in the central nervous system. Because of these numerous side effects, first generation antihistamines have a limited use in treatment of allergic rhinitis. Second generation antihistamines include loratadine, cetirizine, azelastine and olopatadine, while levocetirizine and desloratadine are referred to as third generation antihistamines. Third generation antihistamines are regarded as having minimal antimuscarinic side-effects. Slight subjective eye dryness that occurs with the use of cetirizine often resolves rapidly when the patient stops the medication. Using medication at bed time and wearing sunglasses would help resolve symptoms. It is useful to know that antihistamines are less effective in symptomatic relieve of allergic rhinitis compared to INCs and are equally or slightly more efficacious than cromolyn [2].

Cromolyn sodium is a mast cell stabilizer and inhibits release of histamines and other inflammatory mediators from mast cells, reducing allergic symptoms in a preventive manner. Even when used shortly before inhalation of the allergen, cromolyn sodium effectively prevents onset of allergic symptoms, proving most effective for treatment of episodic allergic rhinitis when taken at least 30 min before exposure to animal dander or days before the "pollen season" [2]. Montelukast, an anti-leukotriene agent, has been approved for treatment of concomitant allergic rhinitis and asthma.

Nasal irrigation with normal saline should be recommended to all patients just before other medications are applied so that the mucosa is freshly clean. Even when used as a single therapy, nasal irrigation effectively alleviates mild symptoms of nasal congestion and itching.

Q4. Patient's parents express a desire to lower the dose of medication by avoiding the allergens she is sensitized to. The girl is now a candidate for a skin testing. Which of the following is a contraindication in skin testing for allergy diseases or may affect the results?

A. History of using cetirizine 10 days ago
B. Using fluticasone nasal spray the just before testing
C. History of atopic dermatitis affecting extensor side of arms and elbows
D. Using a beta 2-antagonist the day before testing

Answer*: The correct answer is* ***D****.*

Skin testing, including skin prick testing (SPT) or intradermal method, is the most rapid, sensitive, and cost effective testing modality for the detection of IgE-mediated disease. In the absence of contraindications, skin prick/puncture is often the most appropriate initial test. Patients with allergic asthma or allergic rhinitis are often tested for the following aeroallergens:

- Tree, grass, and weed pollens, with choices added, reflecting regional flora.
- Molds, including *Alternaria alternata*, *Penicillium notatum*, *Aspergillus fumigatus*, and *Cladosporium* spp.
- Dust mites, including *Dermatophagoides pteronyssinus* and *Dermatophagoides farinae*, and cockroach.
- Animal danders, including cat pelt and dog epithelium.

SPT is generally considered a safe diagnostic test. Yet, there are some important contraindications for SPT including:

- Patients high risk for anaphylaxis reaction, including those with poorly controlled asthma and reduced lung function, or history of severe reactions to even minute amounts of allergen.
- Recent anaphylaxis episodes, i.e. within the last 4 weeks, as it may cause a false negative result.
- Skin condition such as dermographism, urticaria, and cutaneous mastocytosis which can yield to false positive results. Importantly, patients with atopic dermatitis can be skin tested normally if the test is applied to unaffected areas.
- Using Beta-2 antagonists and angiotensin-converting enzyme antagonists is a contraindication for allergy skin testing as they can interfere with management of possible anaphylaxis reaction. In this group *in vitro* antigen testing should be initial diagnostic modality.

Drug interference should be strongly considered if a negative or week response is seen in histamine control. H1 blocking antihistamines can blunt skin reaction ingested up to 7 days prior testing and should be suspended. Systemic glucocorticoids even in large doses and chronic use, intranasal or inhaled glucocorticoid do not affect skin test results. Meanwhile, use of topical glucocorticoids can suppress skin reaction by reducing number of mast cells in the area. SPT should therefore be performed on non-inflamed skin which have not been treated by topical glucocorticoids. Omalizumab and anti-IgE antibodies may blunt skin reactions for up to 6 months.

The overall positive predictive value of SPT is less than 50%. Hence, every positive result should be confirmed by a convincing history or allergen challenge test. Negative predictive value of SPT is on the other hand high and a negative result confirms the absence of an IgE-mediated reaction with greater than 95% accuracy. Inversely, intradermal method is more sensitive, but yields more false positive results and has a greater risk for systemic reactions compared to SPT. Intradermal skin test should only be performed following a negative prick/puncture test and a high suspicion for IgE/allergen mediated reaction.

In a standard SPT, the volar surface of the arm or upper back is cleaned with 70% alcohol solution. Droplets of 1:10 or 1:20 diluted allergens are then applied epicutaneously, two centimeters apart each. To verify the normal responses of patients' skin, a positive control of histamine dichloride and a negative control of diluting agent (usually saline) should also be applied.

A positive reaction contains a weal surrounded by erythema and is recorded by measuring the greatest diameter of wheal and erythema separately at 10 min for histamine control, and 10–20 min for allergen extracts. A positive result is defined as a wheal equal or larger in size than histamine control which usually produces a wheal of at least 3 mm in diameter. Alternatively, a wheal with a diameter greater than 3 mm may be considered positive.

Intradermal method consists of injecting of 0.02–0.05 mL of a 1:500 to 1:1000 weight/volume allergen extract into the skin. Injection is performed at a 45° angle by a 26 or 27 gauge needle. If a prick/puncture test were performed before, there will be no need to histamine control but a negative control is included in order to control for reactions rising in response to the injection method. Our patient had positive skin test results for *Dermatophagoides pteronyssinus* and *Dermatophagoides farina*.

Q5. Which of the following measures is true regarding effective allergen avoidance in treatment of allergic rhinitis?

A. Outdoor allergens like pollens are the easiest allergens to avoid
B. Air filtration is an important measure to control exposures to dust mites
C. In case of animal danders allergy, restraining the animal to a specific part of the house can be an effective measure
D. If the animal remains in the house, extensive vacuum cleaning with HEPA filters and air filter will help reduce the allergen burden and hence exposure
E. Using dust mite impermeable bedding covers is an essential component of any strategy to reduce dust mite exposure

Answer*: The correct answer is* ***E****.*

Practical Points

- Intranasal corticosteroids are first line and most effective single maintenance therapy for allergic rhinitis
- Use of topical decongestants should be limited to a maximum of 7 days due to a risk of rebound rhinitis
- Skin prick testing and intradermal methods are the most sensitive and cost effective modalities IgE-mediated allergic rhinitis
- Patients with a high risk for anaphylaxis or those with recent anaphylactic attack within the last 4 weeks should not undergo skin prick or intradermal allergen testing
- Atopic dermatitis is not a contraindication for skin prick testing and does not affect test results if performed on unaffected areas

References

1. Fokkens WJ, Lund VJ, Mullol J, Bachert C, Alobid I, Baroody F, Cohen N, Cervin A, Douglas R, Gevaert P, Georgalas C, Goossens H, Harvey R, Hellings P, Hopkins C, Jones N, Joos G, Kalogjera L, Kern B, Kowalski M, Price D, Riechelmann H, Schlosser R, Senior B, Thomas M, Toskala E, Voegels R, Wang de Y, Wormald PJ. EPOS 2012: European position paper on rhinosinusitis and nasal polyps 2012. A summary for otorhinolaryngologists. Rhinology. 2012;50(1):1–12.
2. Brozek JL, Bousquet J, Agache I, Agarwal A, Bachert C, Bosnic-Anticevich S, Brignardello-Petersen R, Canonica GW, Casale T, Chavannes NH, Correia de Sousa J, Cruz AA, Cuello-Garcia CA, Demoly P, Dykewicz M, Etxeandia-Ikobaltzeta I, Florez ID, Fokkens W, Fonseca J, Hellings PW, Klimek L, Kowalski S, Kuna P, Laisaar KT, Larenas-Linnemann DE, Lodrup Carlsen KC, Manning PJ, Meltzer E, Mullol J, Muraro A, O'Hehir R, Ohta K, Panzner P, Papadopoulos N, Park HS, Passalacqua G, Pawankar R, Price D, Riva JJ, Roldan Y, Ryan D, Sadeghirad B, Samolinski B, Schmid-Grendelmeier P, Sheikh A, Togias A, Valero A, Valiulis A, Valovirta E, Ventresca M, Wallace D, Waserman S, Wickman M, Wiercioch W, Yepes-Nunez JJ, Zhang L, Zhang Y, Zidarn M, Zuberbier T, Schunemann HJ. Allergic Rhinitis and its Impact on Asthma (ARIA) guidelines-2016 revision. J Allergy Clin Immunol. 2017;140(4):950–8.
3. Skoner DP, Rachelefsky GS, Meltzer EO, Chervinsky P, Morris RM, Seltzer JM, Storms WW, Wood RA. Detection of growth suppression in children during treatment with intranasal beclomethasone dipropionate. Pediatrics. 2000;105(2):E23.

Chapter 3
Persistent Rhinitis

Juan J. L. Sienra-Monge, Omar J. Saucedo-Ramirez, and Elsy M. Navarrete-Rodríguez

A 6-year-old boy with a history of atopic dermatitis, presents to our clinic with symptoms of rhinorrhea, persistent nasal congestion, and watery eyes since a year ago. His symptoms are associated with productive cough, but his parents deny wheezing or shortness of breath. His parents have recently noticed his snoring at night. He has had poor school performance. When asking about family history, his father reveals he is asthmatic. At the physical exploration he has oral breathing, posterior hyaline rhinorrhea and normal size tonsils.

Q1. Which of the following condition is the most likely diagnosis?

A. Chronic sinusitis
B. Allergic rhinitis
C. Asthma
D. Postnasal drip syndrome
E. Alpha 1 antitrypsin deficiency

Answer: *The correct answer is **B**.*

Allergic rhinitis is the most common form of non-infectious rhinitis. In the United States, surveys that require a physician-confirmed diagnosis for allergic rhinitis report prevalence rates of 14% in US adults and 13% in US children [1]. The diagnosis must be suspected with symptoms like itchy nose, palate or eyes, sneezing, nasal congestion, sniffling, clear rhinorrhea, and postnasal drip, often associated with a cough. Children may only complain of malaise or fatigue [2, 3].

Q2. Which of the following test should be the initial laboratory test to evaluate this patient's presenting symptoms?

A. Plain radiographic profile of paranasal sinuses
B. Spirometry

J. J. L. Sienra-Monge · O. J. Saucedo-Ramirez · E. M. Navarrete-Rodríguez (✉)
Hospital Infantil de México Federico Gómez, Ciudad de México, Mexico

N. Rezaei (ed.), *Pediatric Allergy*, https://doi.org/10.1007/978-3-030-18282-3_3

C. Skin prick test
D. Oscillometry
E. Nasal endoscopy

***Answer**: The correct answer is **C**.*

The diagnosis of allergic rhinitis is based upon the coordination between a typical history of allergic symptoms and diagnostic tests. *In vivo* and *in vitro* tests used to diagnose allergic diseases are directed towards the detection of free or cell-bound IgE [3]. Skin prick test should be carried our routinely to determine if the rhinitis is allergic or non-allergic. This test has a high negative predictive value [4].

Q3. Which of the following is the most likely the etiology of chronic cough in this patient?

A. Asthma
B. Postnasal drip
C. Acute pharyngitis
D. Chronic cough
E. Foreign body

***Answer**: The correct answer is **B**.*

This patient has no history of wheezing. The productive cough is most likely a result of rhinitis associated with postnasal drip.

Q4. Which one of the following would be the best treatment option at this time?

A. Topic nasal steroid
B. Inhaled steroid with spacer chamber
C. Empiric antibiotic therapy
D. Allergen specific immunotherapy
E. Omalizumab

***Answer**: The correct answer is **A**.*

Inhaled corticosteroids are the most efficacious medications available for the treatment of allergic and non-allergic rhinitis. These medications are effective in improving almost all symptoms of allergic rhinitis including ocular symptoms [3].

Q5. Which of the following is the only treatment that can modify the course of allergic rhinitis?

A. Topic nasal steroid
B. Inhaled steroid with spacer chamber
C. Empiric antibiotic therapy
D. Allergen-specific immunotherapy
E. Omalizumab

***Answer**: The correct answer is **D**.*

Allergen-specific immunotherapy induces clinical and immunologic tolerance, has long-term efficacy and may prevent the progression of allergic disease [2, 3]. Allergen-specific immunotherapy has been shown to improve comorbid conditions such as asthma, allergic conjunctivitis, as well as disease-specific quality of life. Randomized controlled trials have shown that specific immunotherapy may even prevent the development of asthma and new allergic sensitivities in the future [2].

Practical Points

- Allergen-specific immunotherapy is the only disease modifying treatment in allergic rhinitis
- Immunotherapy improves comorbid conditions, such as asthma and conjunctivitis
- Skin prick test is the primary test to determine whether rhinitis is allergic or non-allergic
- Skin prick test has a high negative predictive value

References

1. Meltzer EO, Blaiss MS, Naclerio RM, Stoloff SW, Derebery MJ, Nelson HS, Boyle JM, Wingertzahn MA. Burden of allergic rhinitis: allergies in America, Latin America, and Asia-Pacific adult surveys. Allergy Asthma Proc. 2012;33(Suppl 1):S113–41.
2. Seidman MD, Gurgel RK, Lin SY, Schwartz SR, Baroody FM, Bonner JR, Dawson DE, Dykewicz MS, Hackell JM, Han JK, Ishman SL, Krouse HJ, Malekzadeh S, Mims JW, Omole FS, Reddy WD, Wallace DV, Walsh SA, Warren BE, Wilson MN, Nnacheta LC. Guideline Otolaryngology Development Group A-H. Clinical practice guideline: allergic rhinitis. Otolaryngol Head Neck Surg. 2015;152(1 Suppl):S1–43.
3. Bousquet J, Khaltaev N, Cruz AA, Denburg J, Fokkens WJ, Togias A, Zuberbier T, Baena-Cagnani CE, Canonica GW, van Weel C, Agache I, Ait-Khaled N, Bachert C, Blaiss MS, Bonini S, Boulet LP, Bousquet PJ, Camargos P, Carlsen KH, Chen Y, Custovic A, Dahl R, Demoly P, Douagui H, Durham SR, van Wijk RG, Kalayci O, Kaliner MA, Kim YY, Kowalski ML, Kuna P, Le LT, Lemiere C, Li J, Lockey RF, Mavale-Manuel S, Meltzer EO, Mohammad Y, Mullol J, Naclerio R, O'Hehir RE, Ohta K, Ouedraogo S, Palkonen S, Papadopoulos N, Passalacqua G, Pawankar R, Popov TA, Rabe KF, Rosado-Pinto J, Scadding GK, Simons FE, Toskala E, Valovirta E, van Cauwenberge P, Wang DY, Wickman M, Yawn BP, Yorgancioglu A, Yusuf OM, Zar H, Annesi-Maesano I, Bateman ED, Ben Kheder A, Boakye DA, Bouchard J, Burney P, Busse WW, Chan-Yeung M, Chavannes NH, Chuchalin A, Dolen WK, Emuzyte R, Grouse L, Humbert M, Jackson C, Johnston SL, Keith PK, Kemp JP, Klossek JM, Larenas-Linnemann D, Lipworth B, Malo JL, Marshall GD, Naspitz C, Nekam K, Niggemann B, Nizankowska-Mogilnicka E, Okamoto Y, Orru MP, Potter P, Price D, Stoloff SW, Vandenplas O, Viegi G, Williams D, World Health Organization; GA(2)LEN; AllerGen. Allergic Rhinitis and its Impact on Asthma (ARIA) 2008 update (in collaboration with the World Health Organization, GA(2)LEN and AllerGen). Allergy. 2008;(63 Suppl 86):8–160.
4. Scadding GK, Kariyawasam HH, Scadding G, Mirakian R, Buckley RJ, Dixon T, Durham SR, Farooque S, Jones N, Leech S, Nasser SM, Powell R, Roberts G, Rotiroti G, Simpson A, Smith H, Clark AT. BSACI guideline for the diagnosis and management of allergic and non-allergic rhinitis (Revised Edition 2017; First edition 2007). Clin Exp Allergy. 2017;47:856–89.

Chapter 4
Itchy and Blocked Nose

Juan J. L. Sienra-Monge, Jaime M. Del-Rio-Chivardi, and Elsy M. Navarrete-Rodríguez

An 8-year-old boy presented with itchy and blocked nose. For the last 2 years, he has had runny nose, itchy, red eye and blocked nose, which worsen when he catches cold, and often during autumn and winter. A physician has once told his parents about the possibility of hay fever, but they have not complied with his recommendations.

On physical examination, you identify a boy with oral breathing, Dennie Morgan lines, purulent postnasal drip and hypertrophied pale turbinates. The thorax auscultation has slight wheezing, but no evidence of dyspnea. Pulse oximetry shows saturation of over 95%. The rest of the physical exam is normal. You ask the mother about other symptoms to establish the severity. The patient is unable to sleep for more than 6 hours a night due to blocked nose, wakes up several times to clean his nose, and looks sleepy all day.

Q1. Which is the best diagnosis based of symptoms?

A. Persistent asthma
B. Nasal polyps
C. Allergic rhinitis
D. Allergic rhinoconjunctivitis
E. Upper air ways infection

Answer*: The correct answer is* ***D****.*

For the last 15 or 20 years, rhinitis and conjunctivitis have been described as one entity, as they share the same epithelium, anatomical structures and symptoms.

J. J. L. Sienra-Monge · J. M. Del-Rio-Chivardi · E. M. Navarrete-Rodríguez (✉)
Hospital Infantil de México Federico Gómez, Ciudad de México, Mexico

N. Rezaei (ed.), *Pediatric Allergy*, https://doi.org/10.1007/978-3-030-18282-3_4

Q2. You suspect sinusitis as a comorbidity associated with this condition. Which of the following symptoms below potentiates you impression?

A. Frontal headache
B. Purulent postnasal drip
C. Adenoid inflammation
D. Persistent runny nose
E. Fever and sore throat

Answer: *The correct answer is* ***B***.

Patients with allergic rhino-conjunctivitis often have other comorbidities like otitis media, upper respiratory tract infections and sinusitis. The first two are in a way easy to diagnose as the symptoms are specific, with the local pain and presence or absence of otorrhea. Adult patients with sinusitis often report facial pain and sometimes fever, which are characteristic. Presence of a purulent postnasal drip and halitosis could be the only signs that guides to sinusitis in children.

Q3. Is asthma associated with allergic rhino sinusitis?

A. No, asthma and allergic rhino-sinusitis never been associated
B. Yes, but only in a few cases this condition is present
C. Yes, all the asthmatic cases are associated with rhino-sinusitis
D. Yes, most cases of rhino-sinusitis are associated with asthma

Answer: *The correct answer is* ***D***.

When asthma appears first place, only 50% of patients will develop rhinosinusitis. Alternatively, when rhinosinusitis is the first presenting condition, asthma appears in eventually in up to 80% of the patients.

Q4. According to allergic rhinitis and its impact on asthma ARIA 2017 classification [1], how do you classify the disease in this patient?

A. Mild persistent
B. Moderate persistent
C. Mild intermittent
D. Moderate intermittent
E. Perennial

Answer: *The correct answer is* ***B***.

Classification before 2008 was based on seasonal or perennial duration of symptoms, not considering persistence or quality of life of the patients. In this new classification, patients who are symptomatic for more than 4 days of more than 4 weeks, are considered to have persistent allergic rhinitis. If patient's lifestyle is affected allergic rhinitis will be considered be moderate/severe and if not, as mild.

Q5. You prescribe topical steroid and montelukast for the next three months. The patient does continues this medication for over a year until he presents with epistaxis. You suspend the medication knowing that the cause of the epistaxis is:

A. Due to pollen exposition
B. Due to the alcohol used as a propellant
C. Due to nasal trauma
D. Due to a sun exposition
E. Due to extended time using topical steroids

Answer*: The correct answer is* ***B****.*

The use of propellants such as alcohol or fragrances on topical nasal steroids is the most frequent cause of nasal irritation or epistaxis. The treatment only consists of suspending the medication, using lubricants and changing for a steroid complex that is based on water [2–5].

Practical Points

- Asthma and allergic rhinitis frequently appear together
- Otitis media, upper respiratory tract infections and sinusitis are frequent comorbidities of allergic rhinoconjunctivitis
- Persistent allergic rhinitis is defined as having symptoms for more than 4 days a week and for over 4 weeks

References

1. Brozek JL, Bousquet J, Agache I, Agarwal A, Bachert C, Bosnic-Anticevich S, Brignardello-Petersen R, Canonica GW, Casale T, Chavannes NH, Correia de Sousa J, Cruz AA, Cuello-Garcia CA, Demoly P, Dykewicz M, Etxeandia-Ikobaltzeta I, Florez ID, Fokkens W, Fonseca J, Hellings PW, Klimek L, Kowalski S, Kuna P, Laisaar KT, Larenas-Linnemann DE, Lodrup Carlsen KC, Manning PJ, Meltzer E, Mullol J, Muraro A, O'Hehir R, Ohta K, Panzner P, Papadopoulos N, Park HS, Passalacqua G, Pawankar R, Price D, Riva JJ, Roldan Y, Ryan D, Sadeghirad B, Samolinski B, Schmid-Grendelmeier P, Sheikh A, Togias A, Valero A, Valiulis A, Valovirta E, Ventresca M, Wallace D, Waserman S, Wickman M, Wiercioch W, Yepes-Nunez JJ, Zhang L, Zhang Y, Zidarn M, Zuberbier T, Schunemann HJ. Allergic Rhinitis and its Impact on Asthma (ARIA) guidelines-2016 revision. J Allergy Clin Immunol. 2017;140(4):950–8.
2. Adkinson NF, Middleton E. Middleton's allergy: principles and practice. 8th ed.
3. Bousquet J, Hellings PW, Agache I, Bedbrook A, Bachert C, Bergmann KC, Bewick M, Bindslev-Jensen C, Bosnic-Anticevitch S, Bucca C, Caimmi DP, Camargos PA, Canonica GW, Casale T, Chavannes NH, Cruz AA, De Carlo G, Dahl R, Demoly P, Devillier P, Fonseca J, Fokkens WJ, Guldemond NA, Haahtela T, Illario M, Just J, Keil T, Klimek L, Kuna P,

Larenas-Linnemann D, Morais-Almeida M, Mullol J, Murray R, Naclerio R, O'Hehir RE, Papadopoulos NG, Pawankar R, Potter P, Ryan D, Samolinski B, Schunemann HJ, Sheikh A, Simons FE, Stellato C, Todo-Bom A, Tomazic PV, Valiulis A, Valovirta E, Ventura MT, Wickman M, Young I, Yorgancioglu A, Zuberbier T, Aberer W, Akdis CA, Akdis M, Annesi-Maesano I, Ankri J, Ansotegui IJ, Anto JM, Arnavielhe S, Asarnoj A, Arshad H, Avolio F, Baiardini I, Barbara C, Barbagallo M, Bateman ED, Beghe B, Bel EH, Bennoor KS, Benson M, Bialoszewski AZ, Bieber T, Bjermer L, Blain H, Blasi F, Boner AL, Bonini M, Bonini S, Bosse I, Bouchard J, Boulet LP, Bourret R, Bousquet PJ, Braido F, Briggs AH, Brightling CE, Brozek J, Buhl R, Bunu C, Burte E, Bush A, Caballero-Fonseca F, Calderon MA, Camuzat T, Cardona V, Carreiro-Martins P, Carriazo AM, Carlsen KH, Carr W, Cepeda Sarabia AM, Cesari M, Chatzi L, Chiron R, Chivato T, Chkhartishvili E, Chuchalin AG, Chung KF, Ciprandi G, de Sousa JC, Cox L, Crooks G, Custovic A, Dahlen SE, Darsow U, Dedeu T, Deleanu D, Denburg JA, De Vries G, Didier A, Dinh-Xuan AT, Dokic D, Douagui H, Dray G, Dubakiene R, Durham SR, Du Toit G, Dykewicz MS, Eklund P, El-Gamal Y, Ellers E, Emuzyte R, Farrell J, Fink Wagner A, Fiocchi A, Fletcher M, Forastiere F, Gaga M, Gamkrelidze A, Gemicioglu B, Gereda JE, van Wick RG, Gonzalez Diaz S, Grisle I, Grouse L, Gutter Z, Guzman MA, Hellquist-Dahl B, Heinrich J, Horak F, Hourihane JO, Humbert M, Hyland M, Iaccarino G, Jares EJ, Jeandel C, Johnston SL, Joos G, Jonquet O, Jung KS, Jutel M, Kaidashev I, Khaitov M, Kalayci O, Kalyoncu AF, Kardas P, Keith PK, Kerkhof M, Kerstjens HA, Khaltaev N, Kogevinas M, Kolek V, Koppelman GH, Kowalski ML, Kuitunen M, Kull I, Kvedariene V, Lambrecht B, Lau S, Laune D, Le LT, Lieberman P, Lipworth B, Li J, Lodrup Carlsen KC, Louis R, Lupinek C, MacNee W, Magar Y, Magnan A, Mahboub B, Maier D, Majer I, Malva J, Manning P, De Manuel Keenoy E, Marshall GD, Masjedi MR, Mathieu-Dupas E, Maurer M, Mavale-Manuel S, Melen E, Melo-Gomes E, Meltzer EO, Mercier J, Merk H, Miculinic N, Mihaltan F, Milenkovic B, Millot-Keurinck J, Mohammad Y, Momas I, Mosges R, Muraro A, Namazova-Baranova L, Nadif R, Neffen H, Nekam K, Nieto A, Niggemann B, Nogueira-Silva L, Nogues M, Nyembue TD, Ohta K, Okamoto Y, Okubo K, Olive-Elias M, Ouedraogo S, Paggiaro P, Pali-Scholl I, Palkonen S, Panzner P, Papi A, Park HS, Passalacqua G, Pedersen S, Pereira AM, Pfaar O, Picard R, Pigearias B, Pin I, Plavec D, Pohl W, Popov TA, Portejoie F, Postma D, Poulsen LK, Price D, Rabe KF, Raciborski F, Roberts G, Robalo-Cordeiro C, Rodenas F, Rodriguez-Manas L, Rolland C, Roman Rodriguez M, Romano A, Rosado-Pinto J, Rosario N, Rottem M, Sanchez-Borges M, Sastre-Dominguez J, Scadding GK, Scichilone N, Schmid-Grendelmeier P, Serrano E, Shields M, Siroux V, Sisul JC, Skrindo I, Smit HA, Sole D, Sooronbaev T, Spranger O, Stelmach R, Sterk PJ, Strandberg T, Sunyer J, Thijs C, Triggiani M, Valenta R, Valero A, van Eerd M, van Ganse E, van Hague M, Vandenplas O, Varona LL, Vellas B, Vezzani G, Vazankari T, Viegi G, Vontetsianos T, Wagenmann M, Walker S, Wang DY, Wahn U, Werfel T, Whalley B, Williams DM, Williams S, Wilson N, Wright J, Yawn BP, Yiallouros PK, Yusuf OM, Zaidi A, Zar HJ, Zernotti ME, Zhang L, Zhong N, Zidarn M. ARIA 2016: care pathways implementing emerging technologies for predictive medicine in rhinitis and asthma across the life cycle. Clin Transl Allergy. 2016;6:47.

4. Bousquet J, Van Cauwenberge P, Khaltaev N, Aria Workshop G, World Health O. Allergic rhinitis and its impact on asthma. J Allergy Clin Immunol. 2001;108(5 Suppl):S147–334.
5. Scadding GK, Kariyawasam HH, Scadding G, Mirakian R, Buckley RJ, Dixon T, Durham SR, Farooque S, Jones N, Leech S, Nasser SM, Powell R, Roberts G, Rotiroti G, Simpson A, Smith H, Clark AT. BSACI guideline for the diagnosis and management of allergic and non-allergic rhinitis (Revised Edition 2017; First edition 2007). Clin Exp Allergy. 2017;47:856–89.

Chapter 5
History of Paranasal Sinus Surgery and Recurrent Rhinitis

Juan J. L. Sienra-Monge, Omar J. Saucedo-Ramirez, and Elsy M. Navarrete-Rodríguez

A 16-year-old girl with a history of paranasal sinus surgery a year ago, presented to our clinic with recurrent symptoms of congestion, nasal itching and pruritus of the oral mucosa with some fruits. The surgery note, describes a turbinoplasty without any other procedure. The patient mentions having oral mucosa pruritus without any systemic symptom when she eats fresh apples or peaches and complains of low quality in night sleep. Physical examination revealed severe swelling of the inferior turbinate with pale color mucosa.

Q1. Which one of the following is the most likely diagnosis?

A. Chronic sinusitis
B. Acute sinusitis
C. Allergic rhinitis
D. Food allergy
E. Asthma

Answer: *The correct answer is **C**.*

Rhinitis is defined as an inflammation of the lining of the nose and is characterized by nasal symptoms including anterior or posterior rhinorrhea, nasal blockage and itching of the nose. Allergic rhinitis is the most common form of non-infectious rhinitis and is associated with an IgE-mediated immune response against allergens [1]. In this case, the oral allergy syndrome confirms that the patient has an IgE-mediated pathology [1].

In the Unites States, allergic rhinitis is the 16th most common primary diagnosis for outpatient office visits and affects one in six persons. The clinical diagnosis must be suspected with symptoms like itchy nose, palate or eyes, sneezing, nasal congestion, sniffing, clear rhinorrhea, or postnasal drip [1, 2].

J. J. L. Sienra-Monge · O. J. Saucedo-Ramirez · E. M. Navarrete-Rodríguez (✉)
Hospital Infantil de México Federico Gómez, Ciudad de México, Mexico

N. Rezaei (ed.), *Pediatric Allergy*, https://doi.org/10.1007/978-3-030-18282-3_5

Q2. Which one of the following statements is true regarding of the oral allergy syndrome in this patient?

A. The oral allergy syndrome in this patient results from primary sensitization to inhalant allergens that cross react with food allergens
B. The oral allergy syndrome results from primary sensitization to food allergens that cross react with inhalant allergens
C. The oral allergy syndrome never produces anaphylaxis
D. The oral allergy syndrome always produces anaphylaxis
E. The oral allergy syndrome is only present with allergic rhinitis

Answer*: The correct answer is* ***A****.*

IgE cross-reactivity between pollen and food allergens is the molecular basis for oral allergy syndrome [1].

Q3. Which of the following would be the best treatment option at this time?

A. Oral antihistamines
B. Intramuscular adrenaline
C. Antibiotic empiric therapy
D. Topical nasal steroids
E. Topical nasal antihistamines

Answer*: The correct answer is* ***D****.*

Topical corticosteroids are the mainstay of anti-inflammatory intervention in allergic rhinitis. Intranasal corticosteroids (INCs) reduce almost all symptoms of rhinitis [3]. Meta-analysis shows that INCs are superior to oral antihistamines or leukotriene receptor antagonists alone in all aspects of allergic rhinitis [4, 5].

Q4. Which one of the following laboratory tests would confirm the diagnosis of this patient?

A. Plain paranasal sinus radiographs
B. Spirometry with reversibility test
C. Prick test or IgE specific serum test
D. Double-blind placebo-controlled food challenge
E. Single-blind placebo-controlled food challenge

Answer*: The correct answer is* ***C****.*

Skin tests are the first diagnostic method in patients with a suggestive history of allergic rhinitis and/or asthma [6].

Q5. Which one of the following is the most frequent associated co-morbid condition?

A. Asthma
B. Acute sinusitis
C. Chronic sinusitis

D. Otitis media with effusion
E. Sleep disorders

***Answer**: The correct answer is **A**.*

Approximately, one half of patients with chronic rhinitis have asthma, and more than three fourth of patients with asthma suffer with rhinitis. Allergic rhinitis is a strong risk factor for asthma [1].

Practical Points
- Allergic rhinitis is the most common form of non-infectious rhinitis
- Intranasal corticosteroids are superior to oral antihistamines or leukotriene receptor antagonists to control all aspects of allergic rhinitis
- Asthma is the most frequent comorbid condition with allergic rhinitis

References

1. Bousquet J, Khaltaev N, Cruz AA, Denburg J, Fokkens WJ, Togias A, Zuberbier T, Baena-Cagnani CE, Canonica GW, van Weel C, Agache I, Ait-Khaled N, Bachert C, Blaiss MS, Bonini S, Boulet LP, Bousquet PJ, Camargos P, Carlsen KH, Chen Y, Custovic A, Dahl R, Demoly P, Douagui H, Durham SR, van Wijk RG, Kalayci O, Kaliner MA, Kim YY, Kowalski ML, Kuna P, Le LT, Lemiere C, Li J, Lockey RF, Mavale-Manuel S, Meltzer EO, Mohammad Y, Mullol J, Naclerio R, O'Hehir RE, Ohta K, Ouedraogo S, Palkonen S, Papadopoulos N, Passalacqua G, Pawankar R, Popov TA, Rabe KF, Rosado-Pinto J, Scadding GK, Simons FE, Toskala E, Valovirta E, van Cauwenberge P, Wang DY, Wickman M, Yawn BP, Yorgancioglu A, Yusuf OM, Zar H, Annesi-Maesano I, Bateman ED, Ben Kheder A, Boakye DA, Bouchard J, Burney P, Busse WW, Chan-Yeung M, Chavannes NH, Chuchalin A, Dolen WK, Emuzyte R, Grouse L, Humbert M, Jackson C, Johnston SL, Keith PK, Kemp JP, Klossek JM, Larenas-Linnemann D, Lipworth B, Malo JL, Marshall GD, Naspitz C, Nekam K, Niggemann B, Nizankowska-Mogilnicka E, Okamoto Y, Orru MP, Potter P, Price D, Stoloff SW, Vandenplas O, Viegi G, Williams D, World Health O, Galen, AllerGen. Allergic Rhinitis and its Impact on Asthma (ARIA) 2008 update (in collaboration with the World Health Organization, GA(2)LEN and AllerGen). Allergy. 2008;63 Suppl 86:8–160.
2. Seidman MD, Gurgel RK, Lin SY, Schwartz SR, Baroody FM, Bonner JR, Dawson DE, Dykewicz MS, Hackell JM, Han JK, Ishman SL, Krouse HJ, Malekzadeh S, Mims JW, Omole FS, Reddy WD, Wallace DV, Walsh SA, Warren BE, Wilson MN, Nnacheta LC, Guideline Otolaryngology Development Group A-H. Clinical practice guideline: allergic rhinitis. Otolaryngol Head Neck Surg. 2015;152(1 Suppl):S1–43.
3. Scadding GK, Kariyawasam HH, Scadding G, Mirakian R, Buckley RJ, Dixon T, Durham SR, Farooque S, Jones N, Leech S, Nasser SM, Powell R, Roberts G, Rotiroti G, Simpson A, Smith H, Clark AT. BSACI guideline for the diagnosis and management of allergic and non-allergic rhinitis (Revised Edition 2017; First edition 2007). Clin Exp Allergy. 2017;47:856–89.
4. Weiner JM, Abramson MJ, Puy RM. Intranasal corticosteroids versus oral H1 receptor antagonists in allergic rhinitis: systematic review of randomised controlled trials. BMJ. 1998;317(7173):1624–9.

5. Wilson AM, O'Byrne PM, Parameswaran K. Leukotriene receptor antagonists for allergic rhinitis: a systematic review and meta-analysis. Am J Med. 2004;116(5):338–44.
6. Bousquet J, Heinzerling L, Bachert C, Papadopoulos NG, Bousquet PJ, Burney PG, Canonica GW, Carlsen KH, Cox L, Haahtela T, Lodrup Carlsen KC, Price D, Samolinski B, Simons FE, Wickman M, Annesi-Maesano I, Baena-Cagnani CE, Bergmann KC, Bindslev-Jensen C, Casale TB, Chiriac A, Cruz AA, Dubakiene R, Durham SR, Fokkens WJ, Gerth-van-Wijk R, Kalayci O, Kowalski ML, Mari A, Mullol J, Nazamova-Baranova L, O'Hehir RE, Ohta K, Panzner P, Passalacqua G, Ring J, Rogala B, Romano A, Ryan D, Schmid-Grendelmeier P, Todo-Bom A, Valenta R, Woehrl S, Yusuf OM, Zuberbier T, Demoly P, Global A, Asthma European N, Allergic R, its Impact on A. Practical guide to skin prick tests in allergy to aeroallergens. Allergy 2012;67(1):18–24.

Chapter 6
Copious Nasal Secretions Since Early Childhood

Mohammad Nabavi, Mohammad Hassan Bemanian, and Sima Shokri

A 14-year-old boy presented to our clinic with copious nasal secretions since early childhood. He has suffered from nasal stuffiness, frequent need to clear secretions, nasal speech, and difficulty sleeping throughout the year. There is no exacerbation with seasonal changes and any change following environmental exposures. He also had suffered from atopic eczema during infancy. He had no history of recurrent wheezing or airway hyper reactivity. Evidence of food allergy was not detected. He was well nourished and had no history of recurrent infections.

Q1. What is the least possible diagnosis in this patient?

A. Chronic rhinosinusitis
B. Intermittent allergic rhinitis
C. Persistent allergic rhinitis
D. Sino-nasal polyposis

Answer: *The correct answer is* ***B***.

Chronic rhinosinusitis (CRS) is a common condition that is almost always associated with involvement of all paranasal sinuses. CRS is characterized by pansinusitis for more than 12 weeks despite optimum medical management and includes three different categories: (1) CRS with nasal polyposis (CRSwNP), (2) CRS without nasal polyposis (CRSsNP), and (3) allergic fungal sinusitis (AFS) [1].

Intermittent allergic rhinitis is a type of allergic rhinitis, formerly known as seasonal allergic rhinitis. Intermittent versus persistent allergic rhinitis can be differentiated based on frequency of syndromes. Presence of rhinitis for less than 4 days per week or less than 4 consecutive weeks, indicates an intermittent nature of the aller-

M. Nabavi (✉) · M. H. Bemanian · S. Shokri
Department of Allergy and Clinical Immunology, Rasoul Akram Hospital,
Iran University of Medical Sciences, Tehran, Iran

N. Rezaei (ed.), *Pediatric Allergy*, https://doi.org/10.1007/978-3-030-18282-3_6

gic rhinitis. Persistent allergic rhinitis is another type of allergic rhinitis in which the signs and symptoms must be present for more than 4 days per week and also for more than 4 weeks [2].

Nasal polyps are edematous semi-translucent masses in the nasal and paranasal cavities. Nasal polyps are classified into: (1) antrochoanal polyp, mostly arising from the maxillary sinus and prolapsing into the choana, (2) idiopathic unilateral or bilateral, commonly eosinophilic polyps without involvement of the lower airways, (3) bilateral eosinophilic polyposis with concomitant asthma and/or aspirin sensitivity, and (4) polyposis with underlying systemic disease such as cystic fibrosis, primary ciliary dyskinesia, Churg-Strauss syndrome, or Kartagener syndrome [1].

The boy complained of foul smelling secretions draining mostly from right nostril which were sometimes blood-tinged. He also had intermittent facial pain which exaggerated while bending forward and coughing and also a postnasal drip which sometimes accompanied fever.

Q2. What is the least possible underlying problem in this patient?

A. Primary immunodeficiency
B. Anatomical disorder
C. Allergic disorder
D. Primary ciliary dyskinesia
E. Cystic fibrosis

Answer*: The correct answer is* ***C****.*

Having no history of airway hyperreactivity and changing of symptoms with exposure to environmental factors in addition to unilateral symptoms are all findings which lead to diagnoses other than pure allergic etiology. Immunodeficiency diseases are relatively uncommon in the general population. Nevertheless, evaluation of a patient with frequent infections requires a careful history and physical examination directed at finding clues that may help to categorize the nature of the underlying immunodeficiency [1].

Ciliary dyskinesia refers to a syndrome of otosinopulmonary disease with other accompanying phenotypic features. It is often referred to as primary ciliary dyskinesia (PCD) and sometimes referred to as immotile cilia syndrome or Kartagener syndrome, or occasionally the motile ciliopathies. Establishing a definitive diagnosis requires a compatible phenotype and presence of functional and/or ultra-structural defects, besides newer screening tools such as nasal nitric oxide and genetics testing [3]. Besides chronic respiratory infections PCD can cause fertility problems and disorders of organ laterality, which were absent in our patient. Cystic fibrosis (CF) is one of the most common inherited life shortening diseases and presents with chronic sinopulmonary disease, exocrine pancreatic insufficiency and increased sweat electrolytes levels. Chronic sinusitis, multiple nasal polyps and hypertrophy of inferior turbinates with nasal airway obstruction are typical signs of CF. Sweat chloride levels are invariably above 60 mmol/L [4, 5].

Having symptoms of chronic rhinosinusitis and an atopic basis, he had been treated with a diagnosis of allergic rhinitis but without any persistent significant relief.

Q3. What is the best diagnostic tool in this patient?

A. Paranasal sinus computed tomography scan
B. Immunologic evaluation
C. Nasal nitric oxide testing
D. Smear and culture of nasal secretions
E. Allergy skin prick testing

Answer: *The correct answer is* ***A***.

A paranasal sinus computed tomography (CT) scan is necessary to confirm the diagnosis of CRS and to identify any anatomical or structural abnormalities such as nasal septal deviation, mass or foreign body [6].

Evaluation for primary or secondary immunodeficiency disorders, performing sweat chloride test for cystic fibrosis, nasal nitric oxide or saccharin blue test—to screen for primary ciliary dyskinesia—are second step evaluation to be performed, after confirming the diagnosis of CRS with paranasal sinus imaging or endoscopy. Due to the patients history of atopic dermatitis and allergic rhinitis, skin prick test (SPT) could be ordered to identify the suspected allergen. Unilateral symptoms alarmed us about an anatomic or localized problem in this patient. Paranasal sinus CT scan is as below (Fig. 6.1).

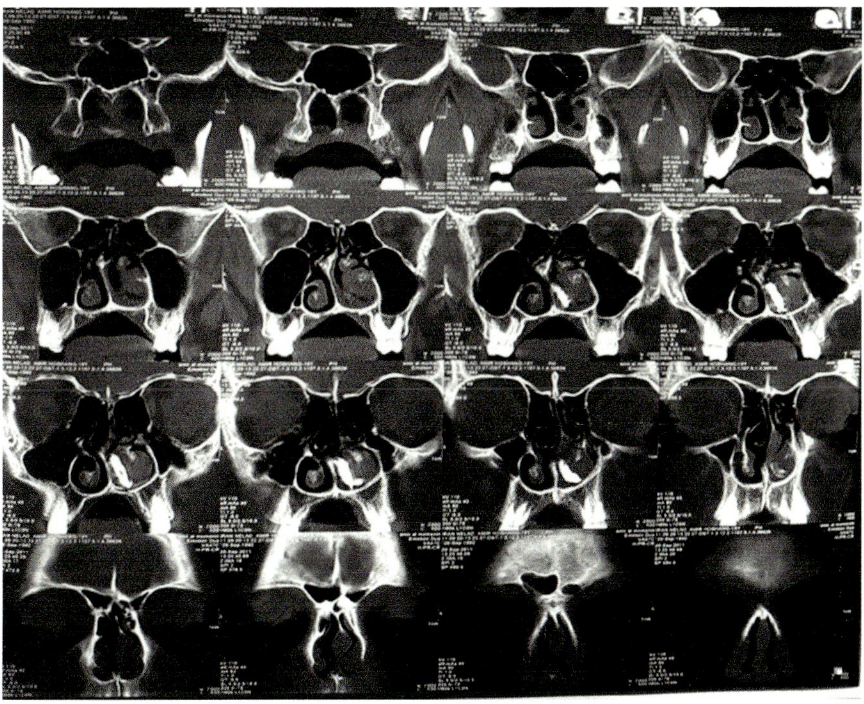

Fig. 6.1 Paranasal sinus computed tomography scan of a patient with copious nasal secretions. Foreign body with radiodense surrounding rhinolithiasis can be seen in right maxillary sinus in cuts 7 to 11

Q4. What is the most likely diagnosis?

A. Nasal foreign body leading to rhinolithiasis
B. Nasopharynx tumor
C. Nasal polyposis
D. Nasal mucocele

Answer*: The correct answer is* ***A****.*

Practical Points

- Consider a diagnosis of intermittent allergic rhinitis when symptoms are present for less than 4 days per week or less than 4 consecutive weeks in a year
- Paranasal sinus computed tomography scan is necessary to confirm the diagnosis of chronic rhinosinusitis or rule out the presence of anatomical or structural abnormalities such as nasal septal deviation, mass or foreign body
- Evaluation for primary or secondary immunodeficiency disorders, such as performing sweat chloride test for cystic fibrosis, nasal nitric oxide or saccharin blue test to screen for primary ciliary dyskinesia should be considered based on clinical grounds

References

1. O'Hollaren MT. A review of middleton's allergy: principles and practice, 6th edition, with online updates. MedGenMed. 2005;7(4):1.
2. Brozek JL, Bousquet J, Agache I, Agarwal A, Bachert C, Bosnic-Anticevich S, Brignardello-Petersen R, Canonica GW, Casale T, Chavannes NH, Correia de Sousa J, Cruz AA, Cuello-Garcia CA, Demoly P, Dykewicz M, Etxeandia-Ikobaltzeta I, Florez ID, Fokkens W, Fonseca J, Hellings PW, Klimek L, Kowalski S, Kuna P, Laisaar KT, Larenas-Linnemann DE, Lodrup Carlsen KC, Manning PJ, Meltzer E, Mullol J, Muraro A, O'Hehir R, Ohta K, Panzner P, Papadopoulos N, Park HS, Passalacqua G, Pawankar R, Price D, Riva JJ, Roldan Y, Ryan D, Sadeghirad B, Samolinski B, Schmid-Grendelmeier P, Sheikh A, Togias A, Valero A, Valiulis A, Valovirta E, Ventresca M, Wallace D, Waserman S, Wickman M, Wiercioch W, Yepes-Nunez JJ, Zhang L, Zhang Y, Zidarn M, Zuberbier T, Schunemann HJ. Allergic Rhinitis and its Impact on Asthma (ARIA) guidelines-2016 revision. J Allergy Clin Immunol. 2017;140(4):950–8.
3. Lobo LJ, Zariwala MA, Noone PG. Primary ciliary dyskinesia. QJM. 2014;107(9):691–9.
4. Smyth RL. Diagnosis and management of cystic fibrosis. Arch Dis Child Ed Pract. 2005;90(1):ep1.
5. Balfour-Lynn IM. Asthma in cystic fibrosis. J R Soc Med. 2003;96(Suppl 43):30–4.
6. Fokkens WJ, Lund VJ, Mullol J, Bachert C, Alobid I, Baroody F, Cohen N, Cervin A, Douglas R, Gevaert P, Georgalas C, Goossens H, Harvey R, Hellings P, Hopkins C, Jones N, Joos G, Kalogjera L, Kern B, Kowalski M, Price D, Riechelmann H, Schlosser R, Senior B, Thomas M, Toskala E, Voegels R, Wang de Y, Wormald PJ. EPOS 2012: European position paper on rhinosinusitis and nasal polyps 2012. A summary for otorhinolaryngologists. Rhinology. 2012;50(1):1–12.

Chapter 7
Perennial Rhinitis and Post Nasal Drip

Charmi Patel and Punita Ponda

An 8-year-old obese male seeks medical help for "a sense of drip in the back of the throat". He states that his symptoms of nasal congestion, sneezing and post nasal drip have been present for the last few years. Symptoms are worse during the summer season, but are present all year long. He denies any triggers such as animals. He states he has not tried antihistamines, but has tried a steroid nasal spray without much improvement. He denies any ocular symptoms.

Other pertinent medical history includes valvular heart disease with dilated cardiomyopathy, hypertension, and a new diagnosis of attention deficit hyperactivity disorder (ADHD). Family history is remarkable for a sister with allergic rhinitis and asthma requiring immunotherapy. His current medications include metoprolol and furosemide.

Vital examination showed a blood pressure of 140/82 mmHg. On physical examination, obese body habitus, boggy, pale and edematous inferior nasal turbinates, posterior pharyngeal cobblestoning and clear rhinorrhea was noted. Skin prick test (SPT) for environmental allergens was positive for tree, grass and weed pollens.

Q1. What is the most appropriate diagnosis in this patient?

A. Mixed rhinitis
B. Vasomotor rhinitis
C. Atrophic rhinitis
D. Cerebrospinal fluid rhinorrhea

C. Patel
Division of Allergy and Immunology, Department of Medicine, Albany Medical Center, Albany Medical College, Albany, NY, USA

P. Ponda (✉)
Division of Allergy and Immunology, Cohen Children's Hospital of New York, Donald and Barbara Zucker School of Medicine at Hofstra/Northwell, Great Neck, NY, USA
e-mail: pponda@northwell.edu

N. Rezaei (ed.), *Pediatric Allergy*, https://doi.org/10.1007/978-3-030-18282-3_7

Answer: *The correct answer is* ***A***.

Mixed rhinitis is defined as both allergic and non-allergic rhinitis and is more common than isolated allergic rhinitis or nonallergic rhinitis [1, 2]. Mixed rhinitis can be found in approximately 44% to 87% of patients previously diagnosed with allergic rhinitis [1, 2]. Many patients with perennial symptoms with only seasonal triggers are thought to have mixed rhinitis. Vasomotor rhinitis is a type of nonallergic rhinitis with predominant nasal congestion and triggers including heightened sensitivity to temperature change, airborne irritants, foods (spicy foods), alcoholic beverages, cold dry air and exercise [3]. Atrophic rhinitis is a chronic condition referred to as the "empty nose syndrome" [3]. Classic characteristics include atrophy of nasal mucosa, nasal crusting and dryness due to atrophy of glandular cells and foul smelling nasal secretions [3]. Saline irrigation with topical or systemic antibiotics are the mainstay of treatment [3]. Cerebrospinal fluid rhinorrhea is typically due to clear rhinorrhea in a patient with recent trauma or cranial surgery [3]. Testing nasal secretions for the presence of β-2-transferrin is a sensitive method of diagnosing CSF rhinorrhea [3].

Q2. Which of the following is <u>not</u> a risk factor for allergic rhinitis?

A. Family history of atopy
B. Serum IgE above 100 IU/mL before age 6 years
C. Lower socioeconomic class
D. Presence of a positive allergy skin prick test

Answer: *The correct answer is* ***C***.

The risk factors for developing allergic rhinitis include a family history of atopy, serum IgE above 100 IU/mL age below 6, higher socioeconomic class and presence of a positive SPT which is defined as a wheal greater than 3 mm compared to saline [3].

Q3. Which of the following medications would <u>not</u> contribute to the patient's rhinitis?

A. Prazosin
B. Metoprolol
C. Amlodipine
D. Furosemide
E. Hydralazine

Answer: *The correct answer is* ***D***.

Antihypertensive drugs are the most commonly implicated medications with rhinitis as a side-effect. Alpha-blockers (e.g. prazosin), vasodilators (e.g. hydralazine), calcium channel blockers (e.g. amlodipine), and phosphodiesterase inhibitors are among other medications commonly associated with rhinitis. Less common culprits are angiotensin-converting enzyme inhibitors (e.g. losartan) and beta blockers (e.g. metoprolol) [4]. Furosemide has not been associated with rhinitis.

Q4. Which of the following statements is correct regarding early and late-phase nasal allergic response?

A. Preformed mast cell's mediators such as histamine, tryptase and chymase are involved in both early and late-phase response.
B. In response to allergen, LTC4 increases both during early and late-phase response.
C. Mast cell mediators such as cytokines primarily play a role in early-phase response.
D. IL-1β, IL-4, IL-5 and IL-13 are significantly elevated during the early-phase response.

***Answer**: The correct answer is **B**.*

Early-phase responses are mediated by immediate release of mast cell's preformed mediators such as histamine, tryptase, chymase, kininogenase, and heparin [3]. Prostaglandin D_2 and cys leukotriene (cysLTs) (LTC_4, LTD_4, and LTE_4) are newly-formed mediators involved in early-phase response. LTC_4 is an exception which increases during both early and late-phase responses. In the late-phase response, initiated within 4–8 h of exposure, cytokines including IL-1β, IL-4, IL-5 and IL-13 are the primary mediators [3]. Major basic protein, eosinophilic cationic protein, hypohalides, leukotrienes, and products of eosinophils, are also among mediators in the late-phase response [3].

Q5. Which of the following treatments is most effective in reducing eosinophils and the release of cytokines during the late-phase response?

A. Nasal glucocorticoids
B. Nasal antihistamines
C. Nasal anticholinergic
D. Nasal mast cell stabilizer

***Answer**: The correct answer is **A**.*

Reduction in eosinophils and cytokine secretion can be most effectively achieved with nasal glucocorticoid pretreatment [3].

Q6. Which of the following is the best treatment of choice for mixed rhinitis?

A. Pseudoephedrine
B. Chlorpheniramine
C. Fexofenadine
D. Oxymetazoline

***Answer**: The correct answer is **C**.*

Intranasal glucocorticoids, second generation antihistamines and intranasal antihistamines are the safest and most effective in this patient population in treatment of allergic rhinitis. First generation antihistamines are typically short-acting, cross the blood brain barrier and cause excessive sedation and therefore are not considered first-line in pediatric patients [5]. Case reports describe a paradoxical response to first generation antihistamine (i.e. diphenhydramine, chlorpheniramine) with paradoxical induction of hyperactivity which would need to be considered when using this class of medication in patients with ADHD [6]. Anticholinergic and cardiac adverse effects such as QT prolongation, are other restraining factors in use of first generation antihistamines [5]. Oxymetazoline and pseudoephedrine should only be used for short-term intervals due to possible adverse hypertensive effects and rebound rhinitis [7, 8].

Practical Points

- Risk factors for developing allergic rhinitis include: (1) family history of atopy, (2) serum IgE >100 IU/mL before age 6, (3) higher socioeconomic class and (4) presence of a positive skin prick test
- Early-phase responses include mast cell preformed mediators such as histamine, tryptase, chymase, kininogenase, heparin and newly formed mediators such as prostaglandin D_2 and cys leukotrienes
- Late-phase response mediators include cytokines IL-1β, IL-4, IL-5, IL-13 and products of eosinophils such as major basic protein, eosinophilic cationic protein, hypohalides and leukotrienes
- Nasal corticosteroids, oral and nasal antihistamines are typically well tolerated and efficacious in pediatric patients with allergic rhinitis
- Centrally-acting, first-generation antihistamines should be avoided due to sedation or in children, paradoxical excitation

References

1. Settipane RA. Rhinitis: a dose of epidemiological reality. Allergy Asthma Proc. 2003;24(3):147–54.
2. Settipane RA, Charnock DR. Epidemiology of rhinitis: allergic and nonallergic. Clin Allergy Immunol. 2007;19:23–34.
3. Wallace DV, Dykewicz MS, Bernstein DI, Blessing-Moore J, Cox L, Khan DA, Lang DM, Nicklas RA, Oppenheimer J, Portnoy JM, Randolph CC, Schuller D, Spector SL, Tilles SA. The diagnosis and management of rhinitis: an updated practice parameter. J Allergy Clin Immunol. 2008;122(2):S1–S84.
4. Varghese M, Glaum MC, Lockey RF. Drug-induced rhinitis. Clin Exp Allergy. 2010;40(3):381–4.
5. Anagnostou K, Swan KE, Brough H. The use of antihistamines in children. Paediatr Child Health. 2016;26(7):310–3.
6. de Leon J, Michele Nikoloff D. Paradoxical excitation on diphenhydramine may be associated with being a CYP2D6 ultrarapid metabolizer: three case reports. CNS Spectr. 2008;13(2):133–5.
7. Salerno SM, Jackson JL, Berbano EP. Effect of oral pseudoephedrine on blood pressure and heart rate: a meta-analysis. Arch Intern Med. 2005;165(15):1686–94.
8. Mortuaire G, de Gabory L, François M, Massé G, Bloch F, Brion N, Jankowski R, Serrano E. Rebound congestion and rhinitis medicamentosa: nasal decongestants in clinical practice. Critical review of the literature by a medical panel. Eur Ann Otorhinolaryngol Head Neck Dis. 2013;130(3):137–44.

Chapter 8
Nasal Congestion Since Childhood

Charmi Patel and Punita Ponda

A 16-year-old female with atopic dermatitis and asthma presents with complaint of a nasal congestion that is present throughout the year. She also reports runny nose and postnasal discharge associated with a cough. She has noted red, itchy and puffy eyes with expiratory wheezing, during the spring and when around dogs or cats. She has tried nasal fluticasone and budesonide spray with partial improvement. In addition to the nasal sprays, she has tried cetirizine, loratadine and fexofenadine tablets without significant improvement in symptoms. She has also tried over the counter eye drops, natural tears and cold compresses to overcome puffiness and itching associated with symptoms without improvement. She has also been frequently prescribed with ophthalmic steroids during spring time and albuterol metered dose inhaler as needed.

In addition to her seasonal ophthalmic symptoms and perennial nasal symptoms, she reports eczema on her neck, arms and back of her legs. Despite application of emollients three times a day with twice daily alclometasone, significant improvement is not reported.

She reports a family history of atopic dermatitis, allergic rhinitis and asthma in first degree relatives. Her vital signs are within normal limits. Her physical examination is remarkable for allergic shiners, conjunctival injection without tarsal cobblestoning, and pale edematous boggy turbinates with posterior pharyngeal cobblestoning. Eczematous erythematous lesions on the posterior cervical area,

C. Patel
Division of Allergy and Immunology, Department of Medicine, Albany Medical Center, Albany Medical College, Albany, NY, USA

P. Ponda (✉)
Division of Allergy and Immunology, Cohen Children's Hospital of New York, Donald and Barbara Zucker School of Medicine at Hofstra/Northwell, Great Neck, NY, USA
e-mail: pponda@northwell.edu

N. Rezaei (ed.), *Pediatric Allergy*, https://doi.org/10.1007/978-3-030-18282-3_8

bilateral antecubital fossae and posterior patellar area are also noted. There is lichenification on the back of the hands with excoriating marks. Skin prick test (SPT) was positive for dust mites, cockroach, cat, dog, molds, tree, weed and grass pollen extracts.

Q1. The patient requests starting allergen immunotherapy (AIT), which of the following is an indication for AIT in this patient?

A. Allergic rhinoconjunctivitis
B. Allergic asthma
C. Atopic dermatitis in patients with sensitization to inhalant allergens
D. All of the above

Answer: *The correct answer is **D**.*

Diagnostic indications for allergen immunotherapy include allergic rhinoconjunctivitis (seasonal or perennial), allergic asthma or both [1]. AIT is considered beneficial in patients with severe atopic dermatitis refractory to conventional therapy and relevant environmental sensitization with allergic rhinoconjunctivitis symptoms [2].

Q2. In addition to the diagnosis of allergic rhino-conjunctivitis or allergic asthma and sensitization to inhalant allergens, one must have at least which one of the following to qualify for AIT?

A. Response to pharmacotherapy, environmental measures or both
B. No significant side effects to the medications
C. Desire to avoid long-term pharmacotherapy
D. None of the above

Answer: *The correct answer is **C**.*

Lack of response to medications or allergen avoidance, adverse effects of medications, poor compliance with medications, patient's preference to avoid long-term pharmacotherapy or cost of long-term medications, and attempt to prevent asthma in patients with allergic rhinitis are among other qualification factor for AIT [1].

Q3. All of the following immunological changes are seen after initiation of immunotherapy, except:

A. Decreases in mast cell and basophil activity and degranulation
B. Early increase in allergen-specific IgE levels, which later decreases
C. Increase in allergen-specific IgG4 levels
D. Increase in allergen-specific regulatory T cells with increase in secretion of IL-10 and TGF-β
E. Transition from Th1 to Th2 cytokine response

Answer: *The correct answer is **E**.*

Mast cell, basophil activity and mast cell degranulation reduce with initiation of immunotherapy [1]. Tissue mast cells and eosinophils also decreased, leading to a decline in skin test reactivity over months after initiation of immunotherapy [1]. Changes in antibody isotypes with AIT include an initial increase in allergen-specific IgE and a subsequent decrease. This is concurrent with an increase in allergen-specific IgG1, IgG4, and IgA with time [1]. Regulatory allergen-specific T cells increase along with an increase in IL-10 and TGF-β. With sustained AIT, there is a predominant skewing from Th2 to Th1 cytokine responses [1].

Q4. Which of the following is not a standardized extract in the United States?

A. Fel d 1
B. Can f 1
C. Der p 1 / Der f 1
D. Hymenoptera venoms
E. Amb a 1

Answer*: The correct answer is* ***B****.*

Not all extracts in the United States are standardized. Cat hair and cat pelt (Fel d 1), Dust mites i.e. *Dermatophagoides pteronyssinus* (Der p 1) and *Dermatophagoides farinae* (Der f 1), short ragweed (Amb a 1), Bermuda grass, Kentucky bluegrass, perennial rye grass orchard grass, timothy grass, meadow fescue, red top, sweet vernal grass and hymenoptera venoms (yellow, jacket, honeybee, wasp, yellow hornet and white-faced hornet) are standardized extracts available in the United States [1].

Q5. Which of the following extracts contain high proteolytic enzymes in form of proteases?

A. Molds
B. Cockroach
C. Cat
D. Answers A and B
E. Answers A and C

Answer*: The correct answer is* ***D****.*

Proteolytic enzymes from one extract can degrade other allergenic proteins in other extracts, causing incompatibility of extracts [1]. For example, molds and cockroach have high levels of proteolytic activity while tree, grass and weed pollen and animal dander have low proteolytic activity [1, 3]. When extracts with high proteolytic activity (molds or cockroach) are mixed with extracts with low proteolytic activity, allergenic potency of the extract with low proteolytic activity is attenuated [4–6].

Q6. Which of the following extract doses fall within the effective dose range?

A. Cat hair/pelt 5000–10,000 BAU
B. Dust mites 1000–5000 AU
C. Grass 1000–4000 BAU
D. Ragweed 500–2000 AU

***Answer**: The correct answer is **C**.*

Probable effective dose range for standardized and nonstandardized US-licensed allergen extracts are summarized by Cox and colleagues [1].

Practical Points

- Allergic rhinitis and allergic asthma are common primary indications for allergen immunotherapy
- Immunological changes from immunotherapy include a decrease in mast cell and basophil degranulation, early increase and later decrease in allergen-specific IgE levels, increase in allergen-specific IgG, IgG4 and IgA levels, increase in regulatory T cells with an increase in IL-10 and TGF-β, and an immunological skewing from Th2 to Th1
- Cat, dust mites, ragweed and grass extracts are the only standardized environmental allergen extracts in the United States

References

1. Cox L, Nelson H, Lockey R, Calabria C, Chacko T, Finegold I, Nelson M, Weber R, Bernstein DI, Blessing-Moore J, Khan DA, Lang DM, Nicklas RA, Oppenheimer J, Portnoy JM, Randolph C, Schuller DE, Spector SL, Tilles S, Wallace D. Allergen immunotherapy: a practice parameter third update. J Allergy Clin Immunol. 127(1):S1–S55.
2. Darsow U. Allergen-specific immunotherapy for atopic eczema: updated. Curr Opin Allergy Clin Immunol. 2012;12(6):665–9.
3. Grier TJ, LeFevre DM, Duncan EA, Esch RE. Stability and mixing compatibility of dog epithelia and dog dander allergens. Ann Allergy Asthma Immunol. 2009;103(5):411–7.
4. Grier TJ, LeFevre DM, Duncan EA, Esch RE. Stability of standardized grass, dust mite, cat, and short ragweed allergens after mixing with mold or cockroach extracts. Ann Allergy Asthma Immunol. 2007;99(2):151–60.
5. Nelson HS, Ikle D, Buchmeier A. Studies of allergen extract stability: the effects of dilution and mixing. J Allergy Clin Immunol. 1996;98(2):382–8.
6. Kordash TR, Amend MJ, Williamson SL, Jones JK, Plunkett GA. Effect of mixing allergenic extracts containing Helminthosporium, D. farinae, and cockroach with perennial ryegrass. Ann Allergy. 1993;71(3):240–6.

Chapter 9
Nasal Congestion and Headache

Franklin Mariño-Sánchez, Álvaro Carrillo, Meritxell Valls-Mateus, and Joaquim Mullol

A 10-year-old boy with an over 2-year history of persistent nasal obstruction, sneezing, nasal itching, partial hyposmia, thick rhinorrhea and night-time cough, presented to our clinic, complaining of mild frontal headache and facial pain for the past 2 days. He had experienced recurrent similar headache episodes during the past 6 months coinciding with worsening of nasal congestion that improved with ibuprofen. He has been taking oral desloratadine occasionally (2.5 mg once a day) for 2–3 week periods with partial improvement of sneezing and rhinorrhea. Skin prick test (SPT) had revealed allergen hypersensitivity against house dust mites (*Dermatophagoides pteronyssinus*) and simple office spirometry showed a normal pattern.

F. Mariño-Sánchez (✉)
Unidad de Rinología y Cirugía de Base de Cráneo, Servicio de Otorrinolaringología, Hospital Universitario Ramón y Cajal, Madrid, Spain

INGENIO, Immunoal.lèrgia Respiratòria Clínica i Experimental (IRCE), Institut d'Investigacions Biomèdiques August Pi i Sunyer (IDIBAPS), Barcelona, Catalunya, Spain

CIBER de Enfermedades Respiratorias (CIBERES), Barcelona, Catalunya, Spain

Á. Carrillo
Unidad de Rinología y Cirugía de Base de Cráneo, Servicio de Otorrinolaringología, Hospital Universitario Ramón y Cajal, Madrid, Spain

M. Valls-Mateus
Unitat de Rinologia i Clinica de l'Olfacte, Servei d'Otorinolaringologia, Hospital Clínic i Universitari, Barcelona, Catalunya, Spain

J. Mullol
INGENIO, Immunoal.lèrgia Respiratòria Clínica i Experimental (IRCE), Institut d'Investigacions Biomèdiques August Pi i Sunyer (IDIBAPS), Barcelona, Catalunya, Spain

CIBER de Enfermedades Respiratorias (CIBERES), Barcelona, Catalunya, Spain

Unitat de Rinologia i Clinica de l'Olfacte, Servei d'Otorinolaringologia, Hospital Clínic i Universitari, Barcelona, Catalunya, Spain

N. Rezaei (ed.), *Pediatric Allergy*, https://doi.org/10.1007/978-3-030-18282-3_9

Q1. What is the most likely diagnosis?

A. Persistent allergic rhinitis
B. Recurrent acute rhinosinusitis
C. Migraine
D. Chronic rhinosinusitis with acute exacerbation
E. Answers A and D are correct

Answer*: The correct answer is* ***E****.*

The patient fulfills clinical diagnostic criteria for persistent allergic rhinitis (PER). Nevertheless, some of his symptoms are likely of sinonasal origin. PER is an IgE-mediated inflammatory response of the nasal mucous membranes after exposure to inhaled allergens. Persistent symptoms (more than 4 days/week and more than 4 weeks/year) might include rhinorrhea (anterior or posterior nasal drainage), nasal congestion, nasal itching, and/or sneezing [1]. In addition, partial improvement of symptoms with an antihistaminic drug (desloratadine) and positive SPT (*Dermatophagoides pteronyssinus*) support the diagnosis [1].

Chronic rhinosinusitis (CRS) in children is defined as an inflammation of the mucosa of the nose and the paranasal sinuses, characterized by at least 12 weeks of at least two symptoms, one of them being nasal blockage/obstruction/congestion or nasal discharge (anterior/posterior nasal drip), with facial pain/pressure or reduction/loss of smell with or without cough, accompanied by endoscopic signs of disease or relevant CT scan changes [2]. Cough is a more common symptom in children compared to adults, and headache in children is often a manifestation of rhinosinusitis rather than rhinitis [3]. With only four of the above symptoms, the probability of having CRS is over 93% [4]. Our patient can therefore be considered as having CRS, presenting with all of the above five symptoms. Confirmation of sinus disease using an objective measure is required because the symptoms could be non-specific and mimicked by several other entities [5]. As in this case, CRS may also be subject to acute exacerbations. To be considered a recurrent acute rhinosinusitis (ARS) there should be complete resolution of symptoms between episodes [2], which was not true for our patient.

Allergic rhinitis seems to be an important contributing factor and a comorbid condition in pediatric CRS [6]. Markers of atopy are more frequent in pediatric patients with CRS [7–9]. Due to the marked heterogeneity in definition of allergic rhinitis and CRS, the role of allergy in CRS remains, controversial [10].

Finally, the diagnosis of migraine is highly unlikely because of the patient's symptoms. Headache is mild, not clearly unilateral, and it appears simultaneously with nasal symptoms.

Q2. Which one of the following is the best initial procedure for the differential diagnosis?

A. Plain X radiograph (Waters's projection) of paranasal sinuses
B. Nasal endoscopy
C. CT scan of paranasal sinuses
D. Cranial MRI
E. Electroencephalography

***Answer**: The correct answer is **B**.*

The first step, when having a clinical suspicion of allergic rhinitis or CRS, is to perform a comprehensive anamnesis and physical examination including a nasal endoscopy. The latter is an excellent diagnostic tool (the "gold standard") since it allows the visualization of the middle and superior meatus as well as the nasopharynx and mucociliary drainage pathways. Nasal endoscopy may help to detect typical mucosal changes, such as purulent rhinorrhea, adenoid hyperplasia, mucosal edema and/or nasal polyps at the middle meatus [11].

Plain sinus X-rays are insensitive and of limited use for the diagnosis of rhinosinusitis due to the high rates of false positive and negative results and underestimation of bony and soft tissue pathology compared to CT scan and MRI [2].

The CT scan is the imaging "gold standard" and provides useful information about the bony structures and air cavities of the paranasal sinuses. However, it has no place in the routine initial evaluation and diagnosis of rhinosinusitis, except where there are unilateral signs and symptoms, unclear diagnosis, severe or difficult-to-treat disease, signs of extra-sinusal complications [2], or when planning a functional endoscopic sinus surgery.

MRI is currently used for evaluation of sinus disease only as a complementary study in cases where the soft tissues is involved, such as aggressive sinus infection with ocular/intracranial involvement, invasive fungal sinusitis in immunocompromised patients or in the evaluation of sinonasal tumors [12].

In our case, nasal endoscopy revealed enlarged and pale inferior turbinates, mild adenoidal hyperplasia and bilateral mucopurulent discharge in superior and middle meatus.

Q3. Best medical practice that should take place before initial treatment is:

A. Evaluation of disease severity by visual analogue score
B. Nasal swab culture
C. Dilated-pupil fundus examination
D. Serum-specific IgE (Phadiatop) testing for inhalant allergens
E. Observation and therapeutic abstention for 5–7 days

***Answer**: The correct answer is **A**.*

The importance of measuring the quality of life in children with medical problems is gaining momentum in pediatric practice. The visual analogue scale (VAS) is a sensitive and widely used and validated tool in studies evaluating disease severity and the effects of medical or surgical interventions in patients with CRS [2]. VAS is additionally useful in allergic rhinitis as it can be used in all age groups, including preschool children [13, 14]. Recently, the MACVIA (Contre les MAladies Chroniques pour un VIeillissement Actif) guidelines proposed a new algorithm to optimize disease monitoring, defining well-controlled allergic rhinitis as a VAS of 2 cm or less out of 10 cm, and proposing a VAS cut-off value of 5 cm or more out of 10 cm to refer patients to specialist, step-up or step-down treatment and for defining controlled and uncontrolled patients [15].

Microbiological investigations are not required for the diagnosis of CRS in routine practice [2]. Recently, some studies have established the relationship between superantigens of staphylococcus aureus and the severity and persistence of CRS with nasal polyps [16]. Nevertheless, the differences found in bacterial populations between patients with CRS and healthy population are not significant [17].

The dilated-pupil fundus examination, would be indicated only in the case of suspected intracranial or orbital complication of CRS. In those situations, a CT scan and/or MRI should be performed [12].

Serum specific IgE is helpful when the diagnosis of allergy is uncertain. Serum-specific IgE results correlate closely to those of SPT and nasal allergen challenges. Some methods use a mixture of several allergens in a single assay as screening tests for the diagnosis of allergic diseases in children [18]. Based on these tests, one can say whether the patient is allergic or nonallergic and additional investigations are needed of the cause of rhinitis is to be identified [1]. In this case a positive SPT for house dust mites was enough to confirm the diagnosis of PER.

Observation and therapeutic abstention are hard to admit for a patient with clear clinical signs and symptoms of a CRS exacerbation. The total symptom VAS score for allergic rhinitis was 4 cm out of 10 cm.

Q4. Most appropriate initial treatment is:

A. Intranasal budesonide
B. Intranasal fluticasone and nasal saline irrigations
C. Oral amoxicillin clavulanate
D. Long-term oral clarithromycin
E. Intranasal irrigation with surfactant and ceftazidime

***Answer**: The correct answer is **B**.*

According to the MACVIA guidelines [15] well controlled allergic rhinitis is defined as a VAS of 2 cm or less out of 10 cm. Consequently, in this patient we should step up the medical treatment.

Use of INCs, such as fluticasone or mometasone, in patients with CRS with and without polyps, as well as in patients with allergic rhinitis has been shown to be effective by multiple studies and as such, they are recommended as first choice treatment of these conditions [3]. INCs improve all the symptoms by downregulating cytokines and eosinophils infiltration [1].

Intranasal budesonide is not recommended in children due to its high bioavailability (>30%). New INCs (mometasone and fluticasone) have favorable pharmacokinetic characteristics that further minimize systemic bioavailability (<1%), thereby limiting the risk for systemic adverse events [19].

Exacerbations of CRS should be treated like ARS [2]. ARS usually resolves without antibiotic treatment [2, 6]. Use of oral amoxicillin-clavulanate does not change the clinical course of ARS nor the incidence of complications compared with placebo [20]. Antibiotic therapy in ARS should be initially reserved for patients with high fever or severe (unilateral) facial pain [2, 21].

Benefit of saline irrigation is symptomatic treatment has also been shown by meta-analyses [22]. Additionally, long term use of nasal saline irrigation reduces the need for functional endoscopic sinus surgery and CT imaging in pediatric CRS [6]. Finally, use of macrolides at low doses and over a prolonged period [2], intranasal antibiotics or nasal irrigation with surfactant have not shown any clinical benefit [23].

After 14 days of MP-AzeFlu (intranasal formulation of azelastine hydrochloride and fluticasone propionate in a single spray) the patient's headache, sneezing and nasal itching improved, and continued with MP-AzeFlu alone for three additional months. However, he still complained of persistent nasal congestion and thick rhinorrhea.

Q5. Which one of the following is the most appropriate next step in the management of this patient's condition?

A. Empiric therapy for gastro-esophageal reflux
B. Long-term oral doxycycline
C. Short course (8–10 days) of oral prednisone
D. Short course of amoxicillin-clavulanate and CT scan
E. Answers C and D are correct

Answer*: The correct answer is* ***E****.*

Although INCs and saline irrigation are first line treatments for CRS, some patients with refractory disease may benefit from short course of antibiotics [24]. The initial selection of the antimicrobial therapy is generally empiric and is based on the expected microbiology of the sinus infection. Amoxicillin-clavulanate (45 mg/kg per day divided every 12 h for at least 3 weeks) is the first-line oral agent for most patients [25]. Systemic corticosteroids have been proved to be effective on CRS [2] and may add additional benefits to the treatment with oral antibiotics [26]. Treatment with oral macrolides over a prolonged period has not shown great utility in CRS without polyps, specially if IgE is elevated.

CT scan is useful to detect anatomic disorders that can hamper the drainage of the sinuses. In addition, CT is indicated in order to plan an endoscopic sinus surgery [2].

To date, there is no solid evidence to support the role of gastroesophageal reflux as a factor in pediatric CRS treatment failure [2, 27]. Furthermore, the use of proton pump inhibitors has been implicated with increased risk of respiratory infections in children [28].

After a 5-day course of oral prednisone and 3 weeks of amoxicillin-clavulanate, CT scan revealed bilateral maxillary and sphenoid sinuses opacification (Fig. 9.1). The patient still complained of nasal congestion and cough.

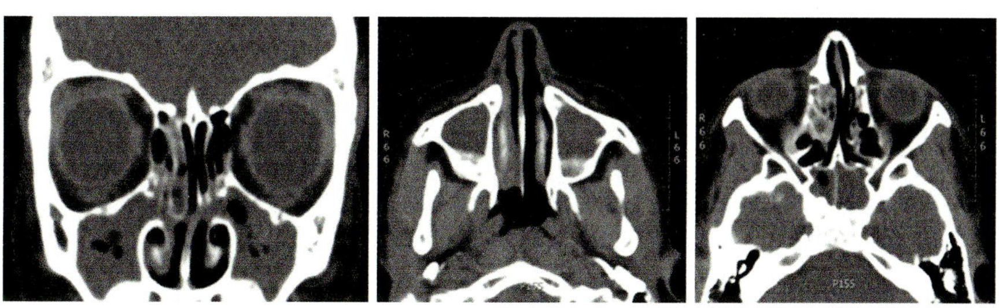

Fig. 9.1 Computed tomography scan of paranasal sinuses showing right inferior turbinate enlargement, an almost complete bilateral sphenoid and maxillary sinuses opacification, and a right anterior ethmoid sinus partial opacification

Q6. Which one of the following is the most appropriate next step in the diagnosis and management of this patient's condition?

A. Sweat test for cystic fibrosis
B. Spirometry and bronchodilator test
C. Consider referral to an otorhinolaryngologist for functional endoscopic sinus surgery +/− adenoidectomy.
D. Nasal decongestants
E. Options A, B and C

Answer: *The correct answer is* ***E***.

A significant proportion of patients with allergic rhinitis and CRS continue to experience bothersome symptoms despite adequate treatment. This group, with so-called severe chronic upper airway disease (SCUAD), pose a therapeutic challenge [29].

Additional testing to complete the differential diagnosis workup for refractory CRS in children may include: testing for a primary immunodeficiency, i.e. quantitative immunoglobulins, immune profile, vaccine titers, sweat chloride test and genetic testing for cystic fibrosis, and nasal or bronchial biopsy and genetic testing for primary ciliary dyskinesia [6]. Rhinosinusitis may often be the presenting form of milder cystic fibrosis phenotypes with borderline abnormal concentration of sweat electrolytes [30].

The potential comorbidity of CRS and allergic rhinitis with asthma should also be assessed by spirometry with the bronchodilator test [2]. Patients with CRS and asthma, depict a more severe inflammatory response in the upper airway mucosa compared to patients with CRS alone [5].

Finally, when no improvement is seen with medical treatment, referral to an otorhinolaryngologist is warranted, as functional endoscopic sinus surgery (FESS) with or without adenoidectomy might be considered [31]. FESS will not only correct the anatomical factors that exacerbate sinonasal obstruction, but also the delivery of topical medications to the sinusal mucosa [2]. Finally, nasal decongestants are not recommended in children for the treatment of PER [1] or CRS [2], due to their potential adverse effects.

Practical Points

- Uncontrolled persistent allergic rhinitis and rhinosinusitis are often found together in pediatric patients
- State-of-the-art guidelines like ARIA and EPOS provide clinicians with evidence-based treatment algorithms for allergic rhinitis and rhinosinusitis, respectively
- The primary treatment of pediatric rhinosinusitis and persistent allergic rhinitis includes intranasal corticosteroids and saline irrigations
- Concomitant anatomic nasal deformities, global airway dysfunction, and systemic diseases should be excluded, in patients with persistent symptoms despite standard therapy

References

1. Bousquet J, Khaltaev N, Cruz AA, Denburg J, Fokkens WJ, Togias A, Zuberbier T, Baena-Cagnani CE, Canonica GW, van Weel C, Agache I, Ait-Khaled N, Bachert C, Blaiss MS, Bonini S, Boulet LP, Bousquet PJ, Camargos P, Carlsen KH, Chen Y, Custovic A, Dahl R, Demoly P, Douagui H, Durham SR, van Wijk RG, Kalayci O, Kaliner MA, Kim YY, Kowalski ML, Kuna P, Le LT, Lemiere C, Li J, Lockey RF, Mavale-Manuel S, Meltzer EO, Mohammad Y, Mullol J, Naclerio R, O'Hehir RE, Ohta K, Ouedraogo S, Palkonen S, Papadopoulos N, Passalacqua G, Pawankar R, Popov TA, Rabe KF, Rosado-Pinto J, Scadding GK, Simons FE, Toskala E, Valovirta E, van Cauwenberge P, Wang DY, Wickman M, Yawn BP, Yorgancioglu A, Yusuf OM, Zar H, Annesi-Maesano I, Bateman ED, Ben Kheder A, Boakye DA, Bouchard J, Burney P, Busse WW, Chan-Yeung M, Chavannes NH, Chuchalin A, Dolen WK, Emuzyte R, Grouse L, Humbert M, Jackson C, Johnston SL, Keith PK, Kemp JP, Klossek JM, Larenas-Linnemann D, Lipworth B, Malo JL, Marshall GD, Naspitz C, Nekam K, Niggemann B, Nizankowska-Mogilnicka E, Okamoto Y, Orru MP, Potter P, Price D, Stoloff SW, Vandenplas O, Viegi G, Williams D. Allergic Rhinitis and its Impact on Asthma (ARIA) 2008 update (in collaboration with the World Health Organization, GA(2)LEN and AllerGen). Allergy 2008;63 Suppl 86:8–160.
2. Fokkens WJ, Lund VJ, Mullol J, Bachert C, Alobid I, Baroody F, Cohen N, Cervin A, Douglas R, Gevaert P, Georgalas C, Goossens H, Harvey R, Hellings P, Hopkins C, Jones N, Joos G, Kalogjera L, Kern B, Kowalski M, Price D, Riechelmann H, Schlosser R, Senior B, Thomas M, Toskala E, Voegels R, Wang de Y, Wormald PJ. European position paper on rhinosinusitis and nasal polyps 2012. Rhinology Suppl. 2012(23):p. 3. Preceding table of contents, 1–298.
3. Roberts G, Xatzipsalti M, Borrego LM, Custovic A, Halken S, Hellings PW, Papadopoulos NG, Rotiroti G, Scadding G, Timmermans F, Valovirta E. Paediatric rhinitis: position paper of the European Academy of Allergy and Clinical Immunology. Allergy. 2013;68(9):1102–16.
4. Leo G, Incorvaia C, Cazzavillan A, Consonni D. May chronic rhinosinusitis in children be diagnosed by clinical symptoms? Int J Pediatr Otorhinolaryngol. 2015;79(6):825–8.
5. Bachert C, Pawankar R, Zhang L, Bunnag C, Fokkens WJ, Hamilos DL, Jirapongsananuruk O, Kern R, Meltzer EO, Mullol J, Naclerio R, Pilan R, Rhee CS, Suzaki H, Voegels R, Blaiss M. ICON: chronic rhinosinusitis. World Allergy Organ J. 2014;7(1):25.
6. Badr DT, Gaffin JM, Phipatanakul W. Pediatric rhinosinusitis. Curr Treat Options Allergy. 2016;3(3):268–81.
7. Veling MC. The role of allergy in pediatric rhinosinusitis. Curr Opin Otolaryngol Head Neck Surg. 2013;21(3):271–6.
8. Gutman M, Torres A, Keen KJ, Houser SM. Prevalence of allergy in patients with chronic rhinosinusitis. Otolaryngol Head Neck Surg. 2004;130(5):545–52.
9. Gelincik A, Buyukozturk S, Aslan I, Aydin S, Ozseker F, Colakoglu B, Dal M. Allergic vs non-allergic rhinitis: which is more predisposing to chronic rhinosinusitis? Ann Allergy Asthma Immunol. 2008;101(1):18–22.
10. Halderman AA, Tully LJ. The role of allergy in chronic rhinosinusitis. Otolaryngol Clin N Am. 2017;50(6):1077–90.
11. Seidman MD, Gurgel RK, Lin SY, Schwartz SR, Baroody FM, Bonner JR, Dawson DE, Dykewicz MS, Hackell JM, Han JK, Ishman SL, Krouse HJ, Malekzadeh S, Mims JW, Omole FS, Reddy WD, Wallace DV, Walsh SA, Warren BE, Wilson MN, Nnacheta LC. Clinical practice guideline: allergic rhinitis. Otolaryngol Head Neck Surg. 2015;152(1 Suppl):S1–43.
12. Cornelius RS, Martin J, Wippold FJ 2nd, Aiken AH, Angtuaco EJ, Berger KL, Brown DC, Davis PC, CT MC Jr, Mechtler LL, Nussenbaum B, Roth CJ, Seidenwurm DJ. ACR appropriateness criteria sinonasal disease. J Am Coll Radiol. 2013;10(4):241–6.
13. Morais-Almeida M, Santos N, Pereira AM, Branco-Ferreira M, Nunes C, Bousquet J, Fonseca JA. Prevalence and classification of rhinitis in preschool children in Portugal: a nationwide study. Allergy. 2013;68(10):1278–88.
14. Klimek L, Bergmann KC, Biedermann T, Bousquet J, Hellings P, Jung K, Merk H, Olze H, Schlenter W, Stock P, Ring J, Wagenmann M, Wehrmann W, Mosges R, Pfaar O. Visual analogue scales (VAS): measuring instruments for the documentation of symptoms and therapy monitoring in cases of allergic rhinitis in everyday health care: position paper of the German

Society of Allergology (AeDA) and the German Society of Allergy and Clinical Immunology (DGAKI), ENT Section, in collaboration with the working group on Clinical Immunology, Allergology and Environmental Medicine of the German Society of Otorhinolaryngology, Head and Neck Surgery (DGHNOKHC). Allergo J Int. 2017;26(1):16–24.
15. Bousquet J, Schunemann HJ, Hellings PW, Arnavielhe S, Bachert C, Bedbrook A, Bergmann KC, Bosnic-Anticevich S, Brozek J, Calderon M, Canonica GW, Casale TB, Chavannes NH, Cox L, Chrystyn H, Cruz AA, Dahl R, De Carlo G, Demoly P, Devillier P, Dray G, Fletcher M, Fokkens WJ, Fonseca J, Gonzalez-Diaz SN, Grouse L, Keil T, Kuna P, Larenas-Linnemann D, Lodrup Carlsen KC, Meltzer EO, Mullol J, Muraro A, Naclerio RN, Palkonen S, Papadopoulos NG, Passalacqua G, Price D, Ryan D, Samolinski B, Scadding GK, Sheikh A, Spertini F, Valiulis A, Valovirta E, Walker S, Wickman M, Yorgancioglu A, Haahtela T, Zuberbier T. MACVIA clinical decision algorithm in adolescents and adults with allergic rhinitis. J Allergy Clin Immunol. 2016;138(2):367–74.e2.
16. Ou J, Wang J, Xu Y, Tao ZZ, Kong YG, Chen SM, Shi WD. Staphylococcus aureus superantigens are associated with chronic rhinosinusitis with nasal polyps: a meta-analysis. Eur Arch Otorhinolaryngol. 2014;271(10):2729–36.
17. Mahdavinia M, Keshavarzian A, Tobin MC, Landay AL, Schleimer RP. A comprehensive review of the nasal microbiome in chronic rhinosinusitis (CRS). Clin Exp Allergy. 2016;46(1):21–41.
18. van Toorenenbergen AW, Oranje AP, Vermeulen AM, Aarsen RS. IgE antibody screening in children. Evaluation of the phadiatop paediatric. Allergy. 1991;46(3):180–5.
19. Sastre J, Mosges R. Local and systemic safety of intranasal corticosteroids. J Investig Allergol Clin Immunol. 2012;22(1):1–12.
20. Sabino HA, Valera FC, Aragon DC, Fantucci MZ, Titoneli CC, Martinez R, Anselmo-Lima WT, Tamashiro E. Amoxicillin-clavulanate for patients with acute exacerbation of chronic rhinosinusitis: a prospective, double-blinded, placebo-controlled trial. Int Forum Allergy Rhinol. 2017;7(2):135–42.
21. Fokkens WJ, Hoffmans R, Thomas M. Avoid prescribing antibiotics in acute rhinosinusitis. BMJ. 2014;349:g5703.
22. Wang YH, Ku MS, Sun HL, Lue KH. Efficacy of nasal irrigation in the treatment of acute sinusitis in atopic children. J Microbiol Immunol Infect. 2014;47(1):63–9.
23. Snidvongs K, Thanaviratananich S. Update on intranasal medications in rhinosinusitis. Curr Allergy Asthma Rep. 2017;17(7):47.
24. Brietzke SE, Shin JJ, Choi S, Lee JT, Parikh SR, Pena M, Prager JD, Ramadan H, Veling M, Corrigan M, Rosenfeld RM. Clinical consensus statement: pediatric chronic rhinosinusitis. Otolaryngol Head Neck Surg. 2014;151(4):542–53.
25. Brook I. The role of antibiotics in pediatric chronic rhinosinusitis. Laryngoscope Investig Otolaryngol. 2017;3:104–8.
26. Ozturk F, Bakirtas A, Ileri F, Turktas I. Efficacy and tolerability of systemic methylprednisolone in children and adolescents with chronic rhinosinusitis: a double-blind, placebo-controlled randomized trial. J Allergy Clin Immunol. 2011;128(2):348–52.
27. Leason SR, Barham HP, Oakley G, Rimmer J, DelGaudio JM, Christensen JM, Sacks R, Harvey RJ. Association of gastro-oesophageal reflux and chronic rhinosinusitis: systematic review and meta-analysis. Rhinology. 2017;55(1):3–16.
28. Chung EY, Yardley J. Are there risks associated with empiric acid suppression treatment of infants and children suspected of having gastroesophageal reflux disease? Hosp Pediatr. 2013;3(1):16–23.
29. Hellings PW, Fokkens WJ, Akdis C, Bachert C, Cingi C, Dietz de Loos D, Gevaert P, Hox V, Kalogjera L, Lund V, Mullol J, Papadopoulos NG, Passalacqua G, Rondon C, Scadding G, Timmermans M, Toskala E, Zhang N, Bousquet J. Uncontrolled allergic rhinitis and chronic rhinosinusitis: where do we stand today? Allergy. 2013;68(1):1–7.
30. Mishra A, Greaves R, Massie J. The relevance of sweat testing for the diagnosis of cystic fibrosis in the genomic era. Clin Biochem Rev. 2005;4:135–53.
31. Vlastarakos PV, Fetta M, Segas JV, Maragoudakis P, Nikolopoulos TP. Functional endoscopic sinus surgery improves sinus-related symptoms and quality of life in children with chronic rhinosinusitis: a systematic analysis and meta-analysis of published interventional studies. Clin Pediatr (Phila). 2013;52(12):1091–7.

Chapter 10
Annoying Nasal Itching and Rhinorrhea

Franklin Mariño-Sánchez, Meritxell Valls-Mateus, and Joaquim Mullol

An 8-year-old girl with more than a 12-month history of rhinitis with daily nasal obstruction, sneezing, nasal itching, and rhinorrhea, presented to our clinic. Her nasal symptoms affected her sleep, daily activities and school performance. She had been using intranasal fluticasone (100 μg once a day) for the past 3 months with no improvement. Her parents assured they had administered the treatment every day.

She had been diagnosed with extrinsic asthma 4 years ago, but she only requires rescue β-agonists occasionally. Skin prick tests had revealed hypersensitivity against house dust mites (*Dermatophagoides pteronyssinus*, *Dermatophagoides farinae*) and *Parietaria judaica*. Additionally, during the past 2 months, her parents had noticed snoring while sleeping, but no daytime hypersomnia was present.

F. Mariño-Sánchez (✉)
Unidad de Rinología y Cirugía de Base de Cráneo, Servicio de Otorrinolaringología, Hospital Universitario Ramón y Cajal, Madrid, Spain

INGENIO, Immunoal.lèrgia Respiratòria Clínica i Experimental (IRCE), Institut d'Investigacions Biomèdiques August Pi i Sunyer (IDIBAPS), Barcelona, Catalunya, Spain

CIBER de Enfermedades Respiratorias (CIBERES), Barcelona, Catalunya, Spain
e-mail: jmullol@clinic.cat

M. Valls-Mateus
Unitat de Rinologia i Clinica de l'Olfacte, Servei d'Otorinolaringologia, Hospital Clínic i Universitari, Barcelona, Catalunya, Spain

J. Mullol
INGENIO, Immunoal.lèrgia Respiratòria Clínica i Experimental (IRCE), Institut d'Investigacions Biomèdiques August Pi i Sunyer (IDIBAPS), Barcelona, Catalunya, Spain

CIBER de Enfermedades Respiratorias (CIBERES), Barcelona, Catalunya, Spain

Unitat de Rinologia i Clinica de l'Olfacte, Servei d'Otorinolaringologia, Hospital Clínic i Universitari, Barcelona, Catalunya, Spain

N. Rezaei (ed.), *Pediatric Allergy*, https://doi.org/10.1007/978-3-030-18282-3_10

Q1. Which one of the following examinations is the best that should take precedence over other steps for the differential diagnosis?

A. Paranasal sinus plain X radiograph (Waters's projection)
B. Lateral nasopharynx plain X radiograph
C. Spirometry with bronchial provocation test
D. Nasal endoscopy
E. Polysomnography

Answer*: The correct answer is* ***D****.*

In the initial evaluation of an allergic rhinitis patient the physician should include a comprehensive medical history and physical examination. In this examination, nasal endoscopy will provide valuable information regarding nasal anatomy such as the presence of a deviated septum, turbinate enlargement, nasal polyps or adenoid hyperplasia. These obstructive disorders can cause nasal congestion or obstruction and prevent full efficacy of intranasal medical therapy. With the evolution of CT, conventional radiology has lost relevance in recent decades in the diagnosis of inflammatory sinonasal disorders, where there are multiple structures superimposed with different radiological densities, making it hard to differentiate the contours. Today, a lateral nasopharynx radiograph might only be useful in establishing the degree of obstruction of the pharyngeal tonsil, the presence of turbinate's tail enlargement and palatal tonsil hyperplasia [1], although nasal endoscopy and oral examination will already provide this information. The plain radiograph of sinuses in the Waters projection gives only limited information in the diagnosis of acute sinusitis of the maxillary sinuses, while providing very poor view of the remaining sinuses [2].

Current asthma guidelines endorse tailoring of asthma management according to the degree of disease control, which is defined by symptoms management and to a lesser extent by lung function and markers of airway inflammation [3]. In this clinical case spirometry could be useful for asthma follow up, since bronchial obstruction may be present in asymptomatic asthmatic children [4]. Other lung function tests such as assessment of bronchial hyperresponsiveness by provocation tests may be reserved for selected children with exercise limitations, poor symptom perception, atypical asthma symptoms, difficult or uncontrolled asthma [5]. Polysomnography may be indicated, according the snoring history and despite the absence of daytime hypersomnia that does not exclude obstructive sleep apnea syndrome [6], but before requesting any diagnostic studies, nasal endoscopy must be performed in order to exclude obstructive anatomic factors or subacute/chronic sinonasal disease [7–9].

In our case, nasal endoscopy revealed a septal deformity obstructing the right nasal fossa, including the valve area (Fig. 10.1a), an enlarged left inferior turbinate (Fig. 10.1b), and hyperplasic adenoids partially obstructing choanas (Fig. 10.1c).

Q2. What is the best treatment option for this patient?

A. Oral H_1 antihistamines
B. Intranasal formulation of fluticasone/azelastine (MP-AzeFlu)
C. Intranasal corticosteroid (INC)

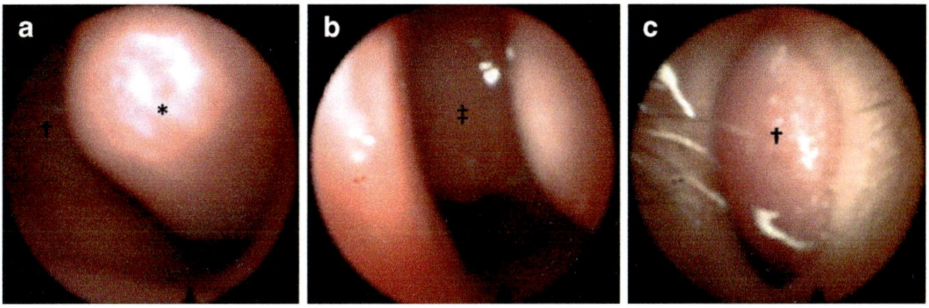

Fig. 10.1 Pediatric nasal fiberscope. (**a**) Left nasal cavity showing an enlarged obstructive inferior turbinate (*) contacting nasal septum (†); (**b**) left choanae showing a partially obstructive hyperplasic adenoid tissue (‡); (**c**) right nostril showing an anterior nasal deformity (†) with subluxation of caudal border of quadrangular cartilage which contacts lateral nasal wall, precluding further introduction of fiberscope

D. Leukotriene receptor antagonist
E. Oral corticosteroids

***Answer**: The correct answer is **B**.*

According to m-ARIA guidelines [10], this patient has a severe persistent rhinitis. The MACVIA guidelines recommends use of a combination of intranasal fluticasone propionate and azelastine hydrochloride in a single device (MP-AzeFlu), when monotherapy with either an intranasal H_1-antihistamine or an INC is ineffective to control symptoms [11]. LTs receptor antagonists are considered less effective than INCs [12]. If control is not achieved with MP-AzeFlu, it is possible that an additional short course of oral steroids (10–15 mg prednisolone for 3–7 days for school age children) might help [11]. Patients whose symptoms are uncontrolled with this treatment should be considered as having severe chronic upper airway disease (SCUAD) and might benefit from specialist referral.

Q3. Other features of the condition that should be properly addressed are?

A. Treatment adherence
B. Environmental measures to avoid allergen exposure
C. Asthma control
D. Tonsils size
E. All of the above

***Answer**: The correct answer is **E**.*

In addition to the nonadherence or lack of adherence, poor intranasal device technique should be evaluated as a potential reason for treatment failure [13]. Allergen avoidance should also be explained and encouraged. Regarding allergic comorbidities, better asthma control increases the probability of improvement with medical treatment [7]. In this case tonsils size should also be addressed regarding patients history of snoring. After 6 weeks of intranasal formulation of fluticasone/azelastine, and treatment adherence corroborated, the girl did not show any symptoms improvement.

Q4. Which one of the following is correct in relation to next step in the management of the patient's condition?

A. Sublingual immunotherapy should be initiated, re-evaluating the possibility of referral to an ENT surgeon one year later
B. Nasal surgery should be avoided until the girl is 16–18 years old to avoid adverse effects on maxillofacial development
C. Adenoid surgery alone would probably relief symptoms substantially with no adverse effects on facial growing
D. The patient should be referred to an ENT surgeon in order to propose a minor septoplasty, turbinoplasty, and adenoidectomy

Answer: *The correct answer is* ***D***.

Nasal endoscopy in this patient revealed an obstructive septal deviation, a severe turbinate enlargement in the contralateral nasal cavity and partially obstructive adenoids. To adequately address her symptoms, all three items should be surgically corrected using conservative techniques with the goal of providing a patent nasal airway and allow the entrance of intranasal therapy. Regarding face growth, the largest follow-up study in pediatric septoplasty concluded that this technique may be indicated in selected cases of obstructing nasal septum deformities [14]. Importantly, when performed via endonasal approach, avoiding a large resection of cartilage helps not to interfere with the normal growing nasal process.

Sublingual immunotherapy (SLIT) could be an initial approach for treating respiratory allergic disease, yet the lack of perceived efficacy in the first year of treatment would probably result in patient's discontinuation of therapy [15]. This patient has a low chance to see significant improvement in her quality of life if her nasal anatomical problems are not surgically addressed [9].

Q5. After surgery, which of the following options is the most appropriate long-term management?

A. Specific allergen immunotherapy
B. Intranasal corticosteroid
C. Oral H1 antihistamines on demand
D. If she is asymptomatic, she would not need long-term follow-up
E. Options A and B

Answer: *The correct answer is* ***E***.

After surgery, her nasal obstruction will probably improve. Nevertheless, she will still be allergic and will need INC. Although inferior turbinoplasty is very effective in the treatment of nasal obstruction in children, preexisting allergy might increase the risk for recurrence at long-term follow-up [16]. A high probability of relapse has been reported 36–60 months after surgery if no additional treatment is prescribed postoperatively [17]. Despite single allergen vaccines being more effective than vaccines containing allergen mixtures [18], specific allergen immunotherapy (AIT) is the only therapy which has the capacity to alter the natural course of the disease.

Practical Points

- Nasal examination, mainly nasal endoscopy, is necessary in patients with severe rhinitis, specially in those showing resistance to medical treatment
- Nasal examination would help to differentially diagnose nasal obstructive disorders and other sinonasal inflammatory conditions, and to potentially propose surgical procedures in order to improve nasal symptoms, disease severity, and patient's quality of life
- The intranasal formulation of fluticasone propionate and azelastine hydrochloride in a single device is indicated when an intranasal corticosteroid in monotherapy does not provide an adequate control of symptoms
- In children with a severe obstructive septal deformity, a conservative endonasal septoplasty may effectively improve nasal obstruction, not interfering with the normal maxillofacial development
- In allergic patients, a proper long-term follow-up and treatment is essential to avoid relapse of nasal obstruction after inferior turbinate surgery

References

1. Acar M, Kankilic ES, Koksal AO, Yilmaz AA, Kocaoz D. Method of the diagnosis of adenoid hypertrophy for physicians: adenoid-nasopharynx ratio. J Craniofac Surg. 2014;25(5):e438–40.
2. Konen E, Faibel M, Kleinbaum Y, Wolf M, Lusky A, Hoffman C, Eyal A, Tadmor R. The value of the occipitomental (Waters') view in diagnosis of sinusitis: a comparative study with computed tomography. Clin Radiol. 2000;55(11):856–60.
3. Pijnenburg MW, Baraldi E, Brand PLP, Carlsen K-H, Eber E, Frischer T, Hedlin G, Kulkarni N, Lex C, Mäkelä MJ, Mantzouranis E, Moeller A, Pavord I, Piacentini G, Price D, Rottier BL, Saglani S, Sly PD, Szefler SJ, Tonia T, Turner S, Wooler E, Carlsen KCL. Monitoring asthma in children. Eur Respir J. 2015;45(4):906–25.
4. Rietveld S, Everaerd W. Perceptions of asthma by adolescents at home. Chest. 2000;117(2):434–9.
5. Moeller A, Carlsen K-H, Sly PD, Baraldi E, Piacentini G, Pavord I, Lex C, Saglani S. Monitoring asthma in childhood: lung function, bronchial responsiveness and inflammation. Eur Respir Rev. 2015;24(136):204–15.
6. Beck SE, Marcus CL. Pediatric polysomnography. Sleep Med Clin. 2009;4(3):393–406.
7. Marino-Sanchez FS, Valls-Mateus M, Ruiz-Echevarria K, Alobid I, Cardenas-Escalante P, Jimenez-Feijoo R, Lozano-Blasco J, Giner-Munoz MT, Rodriguez-Jorge J, Haag O, Plaza-Martin AM, Mullol J. Nasal OBSTRUCTIVE Disorders induce medical treatment failure in Pediatric Persistent Allergic Rhinitis (The NODPAR Study). Pediatr Allergy Immunol. 2017;28(2):176–84.
8. Marino-Sanchez F, Valls-Mateus M, Cardenas-Escalante P, Haag O, Ruiz-Echevarria K, Jimenez-Feijoo R, Lozano-Blasco J, Giner-Munoz MT, Plaza-Martin AM, Mullol J. Influence of nasal septum deformity on nasal obstruction, disease severity, and medical treatment response among children and adolescents with persistent allergic rhinitis. Int J Pediatr Otorhinolaryngol. 2017;95:145–54.
9. Valls-Mateus M, Marino-Sanchez F, Ruiz-Echevarria K, Cardenas-Escalante P, Jimenez-Feijoo R, Blasco-Lozano J, Giner-Munoz MT, Haag O, Alobid I, Plaza Martin AM, Mullol

J. Nasal obstructive disorders impair health-related quality of life in adolescents with persistent allergic rhinitis: a real-life study. Pediatr Allergy Immunol. 2017;28(5):438–45.

10. Montoro J, Del Cuvillo A, Mullol J, Molina X, Bartra J, Davila I, Ferrer M, Jauregui I, Sastre J, Valero A. Validation of the modified allergic rhinitis and its impact on asthma (ARIA) severity classification in allergic rhinitis children: the PEDRIAL study. Allergy. 2012;67(11):1437–42.
11. Bousquet J, Schunemann HJ, Hellings PW, Arnavielhe S, Bachert C, Bedbrook A, Bergmann KC, Bosnic-Anticevich S, Brozek J, Calderon M, Canonica GW, Casale TB, Chavannes NH, Cox L, Chrystyn H, Cruz AA, Dahl R, De Carlo G, Demoly P, Devillier P, Dray G, Fletcher M, Fokkens WJ, Fonseca J, Gonzalez-Diaz SN, Grouse L, Keil T, Kuna P, Larenas-Linnemann D, Lodrup Carlsen KC, Meltzer EO, Mullol J, Muraro A, Naclerio RN, Palkonen S, Papadopoulos NG, Passalacqua G, Price D, Ryan D, Samolinski B, Scadding GK, Sheikh A, Spertini F, Valiulis A, Valovirta E, Walker S, Wickman M, Yorgancioglu A, Haahtela T, Zuberbier T. MACVIA clinical decision algorithm in adolescents and adults with allergic rhinitis. J Allergy Clin Immunol. 2016;138(2):367–74.e2.
12. Tamada T, Ichinose M. Leukotriene receptor antagonists and antiallergy drugs. Handb Exp Pharmacol. 2017;237:153–69.
13. Ocak E, Kocaoz D, Acar B. How can we improve medical adherence to intranasal corticosteroids in children? Int J Pediatr Otorhinolaryngol. 2017;100:194–7.
14. Tasca I, Compadretti GC. Nasal growth after pediatric septoplasty at long-term follow-up. Am J Rhinol Allergy. 2011;25(1):e7–12.
15. Wang T, Li Y, Wang F, Zhou C. Nonadherence to sublingual immunotherapy in allergic rhinitis: a real-life analysis. Int Forum Allergy Rhinol. 2017;7(4):389–92.
16. Arganbright JM, Jensen EL, Mattingly J, Gao D, Chan KH. Utility of inferior turbinoplasty for the treatment of nasal obstruction in children: a 10-year review. JAMA Otolaryngol Head Neck Surg. 2015;141(10):901–4.
17. De Corso E, Bastanza G, Di Donfrancesco V, Guidi ML, Morelli Sbarra G, Passali GC, Poscia A, de Waure C, Paludetti G, Galli J. Radiofrequency volumetric inferior turbinate reduction: long-term clinical results. Acta Otorhinolaryngol Ital. 2016;36(3):199–205.
18. Halken S, Larenas-Linnemann D, Roberts G, Calderon MA, Angier E, Pfaar O, Ryan DD, Agache I, Ansotegui I, Arasi S, Du Toit G, Fernandez-Rivas M, Geerth van Wijk R, Jutel M, Kleine-Tebbe J, Lau S, Matricardi PM, Pajno GB, Papadopoulos NG, Penagos M, Santos AF, Sturm GJ, Timmermans F, Van Ree R, Varga EM, Wahn U, Kristiansen M, Dhami S, Sheikh A, Antonella M. EAACI guidelines on allergen immunotherapy: prevention of allergy. Pediatr Allergy Immunol. 2017;28(8):728–45.

Chapter 11
Progressive Headaches and Right Eye Proptosis

Gordon Myers, Michael E. Dunham, and Luke A. Wall

An 18-year-old male presented to the emergency department with right eye proptosis and complaint of "blurry vision". Frontal headaches and tenderness around his right eye had been present over the last month with progressive visual changes since last week. He has otherwise felt well and has been afebrile. He has a history of cystic acne, allergic rhinitis, and chronic sinusitis. He was treated with antibiotics for a sinus infection several weeks ago but did not experience any benefit. His personal or family history is negative for atopy or recurrent infections. He denies recent travel and has lived in the Southeastern United States (Gulf of Mexico coastal region) for his entire life. Physical examination revealed significant proptosis of the right eye with intact extraocular motion. Nasal polyps were visible bilaterally. CT scan demonstrated an extremely heterogeneous opacification with multifocal high-density areas within the frontal, ethmoid and sphenoid sinuses. Multiple sinuses demonstrated expansion, with bowing of the sinus wall causing distortion of the nasal cavity, as well as optic nerve displacement causing the right eye proptosis. Some bone erosion was evident in the walls of the sinuses, but no invasion to the surrounding tissue (Fig. 11.1a–c).

Q1. Which diagnosis is most likely?

A. Invasive fungal sinusitis
B. Orbital cellulitis
C. Allergic fungal rhinosinusitis
D. Chronic rhinitis with nasal polyposis

Answer*: The correct answer is* ***C****.*

G. Myers · L. A. Wall (✉)
Section of Allergy Immunology, Department of Pediatrics, Children's Hospital, Louisiana State University School of Medicine, New Orleans, LA, USA
e-mail: lwall@lsuhsc.edu

M. E. Dunham
Pediatric Otolaryngology, Children's Hospital, Louisiana State University School of Medicine, New Orleans, LA, USA

N. Rezaei (ed.), *Pediatric Allergy*, https://doi.org/10.1007/978-3-030-18282-3_11

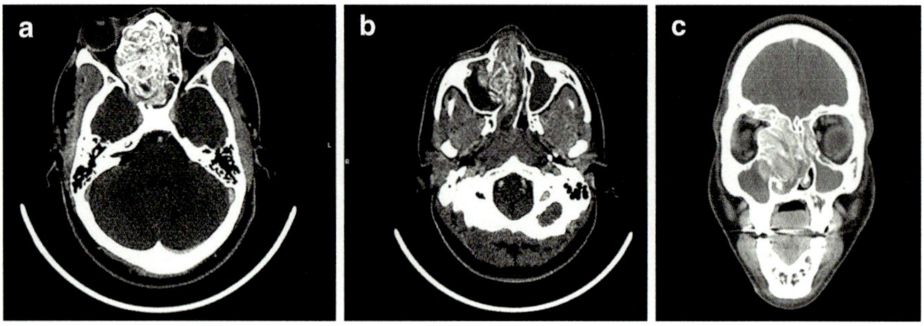

Fig. 11.1 Para nasal sinus computed tomography scan of a patient with progressive headaches and right eye proptosis. An extremely heterogeneous opacification with multifocal high-density areas is seen within the frontal, ethmoid and sphenoid sinuses (**a**, **b**). Multiple sinuses demonstrated expansion causing distortion of the nasal cavity and optic nerve displacement (**c**)

The patient's clinical presentation and CT findings are most consistent with allergic fungal rhinosinusitis (AFRS). The classic CT findings demonstrate heterogeneous material with hyper-dense signals in opacified sinuses. The evidence of bulging and boney erosion of sinus wall on CT scan (without invasion) is also consistent with AFRS [1]. The patient's surgical procedure produced specimens of thick allergic mucin with eosinophils, fungal hyphae and Charcot-Leyden crystals. The allergic mucus is characteristic, and is often described as having "peanut butter" consistency [2].

The past history of cystic acne and chronic sinus infections in the setting of proptosis could suggest a bacterial cause for the pathology. However, an orbital cellulitis causing proptosis of this degree would typically have more impressive physical exam findings. In addition, the patient would often be febrile and ill-appearing. Also, the symptoms in the case above had a chronic and indolent onset, unlike the acute or subacute onset of orbital cellulitis.

The patient is immunocompetent and non-diabetic so invasive fungal sinusitis is not likely. Meanwhile it is important to rule out this disease as a potentially fatal condition [3].

Chronic rhinitis with nasal polyposis is associated with aspirin exacerbated respiratory disease (AERD). In AERD, patients with nasal polyposis have asthma and experience severe exacerbation when taking aspirin (the classic Samter's triad). However, the condition does not involve fungal sinusitis [3].

Q2. Which of the following is considered necessary for diagnosis?

A. Type I hypersensitivity to fungal allergens
B. Peripheral blood eosinophilia
C. Elevated total IgE in serum
D. All of the above
E. None of the above

Answer: *The correct answer is* ***A***.

By definition, patients with AFRS have to be allergic to one or more fungi. Typically, they develop an allergy to the fungus that colonizes the mucin in their sinuses. Either via skin prick test (SPT) or serum specific-IgE, testing for potential allergic sensitization is critical to confirm the diagnosis and start therapy [3]. While it is common to have an elevated total serum IgE in the setting of AFRS it is not one of the diagnostic criteria [2]. Likewise, eosinophilia in peripheral blood is a minor criterion but is not required for diagnosis [3].

Q3. Which of the following is not required for diagnosis?

A. Nasal polyposis
B. Characteristic CT findings
C. Fungal cultures
D. Positive fungal stain
E. Eosinophilic mucin without invasion

***Answer**: The correct answer is **C**.*

Diagnosis of AFRS has five major requirements (Table 11.1): (1) type I hypersensitivity, (2) eosinophilic mucin in one or more sinus cavities *without* invasion, (3) characteristic CT findings, (4) nasal polyposis, and (5) positive fungal stain [3]. Patients must meet all of these major criteria to qualify for this diagnosis. While it would seem logical for the patient with AFRS to be required to have a documented fungal culture, specification of fungi from biopsy samples remains to be inaccurate and difficult [1]. The yield of fungal cultures varies between research reports but ranges from 64–100% [2]. As a positive fungal culture is hard to attain, it is not a required aspect of diagnosis. When successful, the most common isolated culprits are *Bipolaris, Curvularia, Exserohilum*, and *Alternaria* spp. The ethmoid sinuses are most commonly affected [2].

Q4. In view of these findings, which of the following would be an appropriate treatment regimen for the patient?

A. Allergen immunotherapy/AIT
B. Intranasal steroid sprays and antihistamines
C. Oral corticosteroid medication
D. Sinus surgery
E. All of the above

***Answer**: The correct answer is **E**.*

Table 11.1 Diagnostic criteria for allergic fungal rhinosinusitis

Major	Minor
Type I hypersensitivity to fungi	Asthma
Nasal polyposis	Unilateral disease
Characteristic CT findings	Bone erosion
Eosinophilic mucin without invasion	Fungal cultures
Positive fungal stain	Charcot-Leyden crystals
	Eosinophilia in blood

Some studies support the use of AIT for AFRS. In an effort to reduce the allergic burden, the patient receives immunotherapy to both fungal and non-fungal allergens diagnosed by SPT or in vitro serum specific-IgE [2]. Surgical evacuation of the allergic mucin, is considered necessary and the best time to start immunotherapy is shortly after surgery [2]. The use of intranasal corticosteroids (INCs) and antihistamines is well documented and continues to alleviate some of the more bothersome symptoms [3]. Although oral corticosteroids have been found effective for symptomatic management of AFRS, prolonged courses are usually required for full alleviation of symptoms. It is important to find the minimal therapeutic dose to prevent development of steroid-induced side effects [3].

Q5. Which of the following scenarios is most consistent with the natural course of the disease despite aggressive medical therapy?

A. The disease typically remains in remission with no recurrence or further symptoms
B. Occasional symptoms might occur but to recurrence of the polyps or fungus ball
C. Recurrence of polyps despite strict therapeutic adherence, requiring surgical intervention
D. The disease tends to progressively worsen after the age 40

Answer: *The correct answer is* ***C***.

Despite immunotherapy, INCs, antihistamines and oral corticosteroids, patients often redevelop nasal polyps which might require repeated surgical intervention. The disease tends to become more medically manageable once patients reach their 30s and 40s [3]. There are future therapies on the horizon, including biologic agents such as the monoclonal antibody omalizumab which has shown to be an effective therapy to reduce polyposis, and even alleviate asthma and allergic rhinitis [4, 5]. However, more studies need to be done to further elucidate efficacy of Omalizumab and other biologic drugs as potential adjuvant therapies. Research is also conducted on the use of systemic and intranasal antifungal therapies [3].

Practical Points

- Allergic fungal rhinosinusitis is a distinct subtype of chronic rhinosinusitis with nasal polyposis
- The diagnosis of allergic fungal rhinosinusitis has five major criteria: (1) type I hypersensitivity to fungus, (2) eosinophilic mucin in one or more sinus cavities without invasion, (3) characteristic CT scan findings, (4) nasal polyposis, and (5) positive fungal stain
- Epidemiologically, the majority of patients with allergic fungal rhinosinusitis reside in the southeastern United States
- Treatment options include a combination of endoscopic sinus surgery, systemic and topical glucocorticoids, and immunotherapy to fungal and non-fungal allergens. Preliminary studies support the use of omalizumab

References

1. Hamilos DL. Allergic fungal rhinitis and rhinosinusitis. Proc Am Thorac Soc. 2010;7(3):245–52.
2. Glass D, Amedee RG. Allergic fungal rhinosinusitis: a review. Ochsner J. 2011;11(3):271–5.
3. Peters AT, Spector S, Hsu J, Hamilos DL, Baroody FM, Chandra RK, Grammer LC, Kennedy DW, Cohen NA, Kaliner MA, Wald ER, Karagianis A, Slavin RG. Diagnosis and management of rhinosinusitis: a practice parameter update. Allergy Rhinol (Providence). 2014;113(4):347–85.
4. Evans MO 2nd, Coop CA. Novel treatment of allergic fungal sinusitis using omalizumab. Allergy Rhinol (Providence). 2014;5(3):172–4.
5. Gan EC, Habib AR, Rajwani A, Javer AR. Omalizumab therapy for refractory allergic fungal rhinosinusitis patients with moderate or severe asthma. Am J Otolaryngol. 2015;36(5):672–7.

Chapter 12
Persistence of Rhinorrhea After Use of Nasal Spray

Farzaneh Rahmani and Maryam Rahmani

An 11-year-old girl presents to the allergy clinic after 4 weeks of using intranasal corticosteroids (INCs) for her allergic rhinitis. She reported nasal congestion along with conjunctival congestion and rhinorrhoea, through the year (perennial) with seasonal exacerbations. She had also tried allergen avoidance as she believed Oat tree perpetuated her symptoms, with no success. She didn't have nasal polyps and her examination only showed nasal mucosal congestion and cobblestoning. She was prescribed with oral antihistamines twice daily and INC as beclomethasone dipropionate (BDP) (Beclex® 100 μg) twice daily. She reports no improvement in her symptoms as her rhinorrhoea persists along with nasal congestion and a recently emerged headache. She says she feels slightly better after taking antihistamines and is able to do well at the school, although feeling a bit drowsy. You ask her to use her nasal spray in your office to see if she is doing it right:

Q1. Which of the following is <u>not</u> true about the correct use of INCs:

A. Both nostrils should be gently cleared before administration by blowing out or use of normal saline
B. Tilt head forwards so that the tip of the applicator points toward nasopharynx
C. Breath in with mouth and one nostril closed while pressing the spray applicator in the other nostril

F. Rahmani
Student's Scientific Research Center (SSRC), Tehran University of Medical Sciences, Tehran, Iran

NeuroImaging Network (NIN), Universal Scientific Education and Research Network (USERN), Tehran, Iran
e-mail: f-rahmani@alumnus.tums.ac.ir

M. Rahmani (✉)
Shahid Beheshti University of Medical Sciences (SBMU), Tehran, Iran

N. Rezaei (ed.), *Pediatric Allergy*, https://doi.org/10.1007/978-3-030-18282-3_12

D. Avoid sneezing right after using the spray
E. All options are correct

Answer: *The correct answer is* ***B.***

INCs are the first choice medical therapy for uncomplicated allergic rhinitis. With increasing number of children being diagnosed with allergic rhinitis, patient education on the correct use and potential side effects of INCs is mandatory. Patients or their caregiver should be advised to gently shake the canister several times before use and prime the applicator in first use by squirting the spray into the air until a fine mist comes out. Gentle blowing out of both nostrils guarantees drug efficacy and parents should be made aware of this fact, if the patient is unable to do so based on his/her age. Bioavailability of most INCs are relatively low so that systemic/local side effects are exquisitely rare if the drug is properly absorbed through nasal turbinate mucosa, rather than being ingested [1]. The tip of the applicator should point toward the lateral wall of the nose but not the nasal septum or the nasopharynx. Perforation of the nasal septum is one rare outcome of wrong direction of INCs application. Proper technique of use also helps avoiding common side effects like nasal mucosal drying, sneezing, and irritation of throat.

Q2. The patient's mother too suffers from seasonal allergic rhinitis and takes budesonide aqueous nasal spray (BANS) (Rhinocort Acqua®). She is concerned whether a different corticosteroid might help relieve her daughter's symptoms. Which statement is correct?

A. Different brands of the same drug have the same rate of side effects
B. Different INCs have not shown any difference in efficacy controlling symptoms of allergic rhinitis in adults
C. Mometasone is superior to beclomethasone for prevention of patient's perennial symptoms
D. Different INCs are comparable in efficacy in children
E. Answers B and D are correct

Answer: *The correct answer is* ***E.***

Beclomethasone, budesonide, ciclesonide, flunisolide, fluticasone furoate, fluticasone propionate, mometasone, and triamcinolone are among the common corticosteroids used in INC preparations with no proven superiority in treatment of allergic rhinitis. Studies also support no additional comparative efficacy/safety for mometasone furoate nasal spray (MFNS) over beclomethasone or for beclomethasone over fluticasone [2, 3]. There is no overall difference is safety and efficacy of BANS, fluticasone propionate nasal spray (FPNS), MFNS, or triamcinolone aqueous nasal spray (TANS) in treatment of allergic rhinitis in children or adults [4]. There is also no difference in efficacy of oral betamethasone tablet over MFNS in reducing seasonal allergy symptoms, nasal and conjunctival congestion, itching, or rhinorrhea [5].

There is no doubt that different brands might face different tolerability by the patients and it is probable that this girl does not experience headache as a side effect using another INC preparation. Headaches, particularly if associated with epistaxis, might suggest systemic side effects like rise in blood pressure and headaches with blurred vision can suggest a rise in intraocular pressure in patients previously diagnosed with glaucoma [1].

Q3. The patient's mother is concerned about the potential effect of INC on hormonal status and growth of her daughter. Which statement is correct?

A. There are a few reports suggesting significant growth retardation with aqueous BDP
B. INCs are generally safe in management of childhood AR
C. Intranasal fluticasone furoate has no effect on adrenal suppression
D. All of the above

***Answer**: The correct answer is **D**.*

In one study published in the Paediatrics in 2000, a group reported a significant growth suppression (as much as 0.9 cm) in children receiving twice daily aqueous BDP. They showed a suppression of growth rate as early as one month after initiation of therapy and the effect being solely dependent on corticosteroid use but not age, gender, or baseline height. This effect was irrespective of alterations in hypothalamic-pituitary-adrenocortical axis [6]. Indeed this was the only study to suggest suppression of growth with INCs. Subsequent studies with BANS, MFANS, triamcinolone acetonide, or fluticasone furoate (FF) have failed to prove similar results. Clinicians can reassure patients about this side effect with new corticosteroids [1], at least for short-term courses.

A report by FDA states "when the results of the hypothalamic-pituitary-adrenal axis assessments described above are taken as a whole, an effect of intranasal FF on adrenal function cannot be ruled out, especially in pediatric patients" [7]. Following these explanations, both patient and her mother requested to be prescribed with another steroid other than BDP.

Finally, although oral corticosteroids are known to be risk factors for development of cataracts, no such side effect is demonstrated for intranasal corticosteroids. An increase in intraocular pressure is a side effect of inhaled corticosteroids and INCs, and patients with a history of glaucoma or cataracts should be warned about emergence of sudden changes in their vision, vomiting, or ciliary injection [1]. There was no such history in our patient or her mother. We assured both the patient and her mother about her medication changed to mometasone furoate (Nasonex®) and she was recommended to return for follow-up in 4 weeks.

Practical Points

- With the increasing number of children being diagnosed with allergic rhinitis, patient education on the correct use and potential side effects of intranasal corticosteroids (INCs) is mandatory
- Gentle blowing out of both nostrils before application of the drug guarantees efficacy of INCs
- Proper technique of use also helps avoiding of common side effects like nasal mucosal drying, sneezing, or irritation of throat
- Topical side effects are not an indication for discontinuation of INCs
- Clinicians can reassure patients on the absence of potential for growth suppression in chronic use of INCs with new corticosteroids

References

1. Sheth K. Evaluating the safety of intranasal steroids in the treatment of allergic rhinitis. Allergy Asthma Clin Immunol. 2008;4(3):125–9.
2. Drouin M, Yang WH, Bertrand B, Van Cauwenberge P, Clement P, Dalby K, Darnell R, Ernst TM, Hebert J, Karlsson G, Luciuk G, Mazza J, Roovers M, Ruoppi P, Seppey M, Stern M, Suonpaa J, Sussman G, Tan KY, Tse K, Widjaja P, Jensen P, Nolop K, Lutsky BN. Once daily mometasone furoate aqueous nasal spray is as effective as twice daily beclomethasone dipropionate for treating perennial allergic rhinitis patients. Allergy Asthma Clin Immunol. 1996;77(2):153–60.
3. Mandl M, Nolop K, Lutsky BN. Comparison of once daily mometasone furoate (Nasonex) and fluticasone propionate aqueous nasal sprays for the treatment of perennial rhinitis. 194-079 Study Group. Allergy Asthma Clin Immunol. 1997;79(4):370–8.
4. Herman H. Once-daily administration of intranasal corticosteroids for allergic rhinitis: a comparative review of efficacy, safety, patient preference, and cost. Am J Rhinol. 2007;21(1):70–9.
5. Karaki M, Akiyama K, Mori N. Efficacy of intranasal steroid spray (mometasone furoate) on treatment of patients with seasonal allergic rhinitis: comparison with oral corticosteroids. Auris Nasus Larynx. 2013;40(3):277–81.
6. Skoner DP, Rachelefsky GS, Meltzer EO, Chervinsky P, Morris RM, Seltzer JM, Storms WW, Wood RA. Detection of growth suppression in children during treatment with intranasal beclomethasone dipropionate. Pediatrics. 2000;105(2):E23.
7. FDA. 2007. https://www.gsksource.com/pharma/content/dam/GlaxoSmithKline/US/en/Prescribing_Information/Veramyst/pdf/VERAMYST-PI-PIL.PDF.

Chapter 13
Bloody Streaks in Stool

Samin Sharafian

A male infant, was first seen at the age of 5 months due to recurrent loose stools since 2 months ago. Stools were non-mucoid and there was a history of occasional bloody streaks in the stools. There was no associated vomiting or fever. He was exclusively breastfed since birth without any maternal dietary restriction.

Q1. Based on patient's history, which diagnosis best fits his condition?

A. Food protein-induced enterocolitis syndrome
B. Cow's milk protein-induced proctocolitis
C. Protein induced enteropathy
D. IgE-mediated food allergy

Answer: *The correct answer is* ***B***.

Food-protein induced enterocolitis syndrome (FPIES) is most commonly seen in infants between 1 week to 3 months of age who present with protracted vomiting and diarrhea, occasionally resulting in dehydration [1, 2]. Similar to FPIES, cow's milk protein-induced proctocolitis is a non-IgE-mediated gastrointestinal food allergy, presenting in the first few months of life. Although such reactions often are caused by cow's milk or soy protein hypersensitivity, most occur in exclusively breastfed infants and are related to cow's milk protein in maternal diet. Typically, infants do not appear ill, often have normally formed stools and are discovered due to the presence of blood (gross or occult) in their stool. Blood loss is usually minor but occasionally can produce anemia. Bloody stool should typically resolve within a few days of allergen avoidance. Following 6 months to 2 years of allergen avoidance, symptoms disappear in most children with cow's milk and soy protein-induced proctocolitis, but occasional refractory cases are seen too [1, 2].

S. Sharafian (✉)
Department of Allergy and Clinical Immunology, Bushehr University of Medical Sciences, School of Medicine, Bushehr, Iran

N. Rezaei (ed.), *Pediatric Allergy*, https://doi.org/10.1007/978-3-030-18282-3_13

In most infants, vomiting is the primary sign of FPIES, occurring 1–4 h after feeding. Continued exposure may result in bloody diarrhea, anemia, abdominal distention, and failure to thrive.

Diagnosis is established when elimination of the suspected allergen leads to resolution of all symptoms within 72 hours and oral food challenge with the suspected allergen reproduces the symptoms. Secondary disaccharidase deficiency due to FPEIS might uncommonly persist longer and may result in ongoing diarrhea for up to 2 weeks, even after allergen avoidance.

Dietary protein-induced enteropathy (excluding celiac disease) usually manifests in the first several months of life with diarrhea, poor weight gain, and mild to moderate steatorrhea in about 80% of patients. Symptoms include protracted diarrhea, vomiting in up to two thirds of patients, failure to thrive, and malabsorption. Relevant lab findings include: presence of reducing substances in the stools, increased fecal fat, and abnormal d-xylose absorption. Cow's milk hypersensitivity is the most frequent cause of this syndrome, but FPIES is also associated with sensitivity to soy, egg, wheat, rice, chicken, and fish.

Q2. Which of the following tests will most probably give you the underlying diagnosis in this patient?

A. Skin prick test
B. Specific IgE for foods in question
C. Skin patch test
D. Positive histamine release test to the food in question
E. Elimination and controlled food challenge

Answer: *The correct answer is* ***E***.

The diagnosis can be established when elimination of the responsible allergen leads to resolution of hematochezia, usually with dramatic improvement within 72 h of appropriate food allergen elimination. Yet, complete clearance and resolution of mucosal lesions may take up to 1 month. Reintroduction of the allergen leads to recurrence of symptoms within several hours to days. Sigmoidoscopy findings vary, ranging from areas of patchy mucosal injection to severe friability with small, aphthoid ulcerations and bleeding. Lesions are usually confined to the distal large bowel. Colonic biopsy reveals a prominent eosinophilic infiltrate in the colonic villi, crypt epithelia and the lamina propria. In severe lesions crypt destruction and neutrophils are prominent.

Q3. It was impossible to convince the mother to continue breastfeeding. Which formula would you recommend?

A. Standard first infant formula
B. Extensively hydrolyzed cow's milk based formula
C. Partially hydrolyzed cow's milk based formula
D. Soy based formula
E. Answers B, C and D

Answer: *The correct answer is* ***E***.

Elimination diets are frequently used in the diagnosis and management of adverse food reactions. Foods suspected of provoking allergic disorders are completely omitted from the diet. The success of these diets depend on the identification of the correct allergen(s), the ability of the patient to maintain a diet completely free of all forms of the offending allergen(s), and the assumption that other factors do not provoke similar symptoms during the period of study. Unfortunately, these conditions are rarely met altogether. In a young infant reacting to cow's milk formula, resolution of symptoms after substitution with a casein hydrolysate (e.g., Alimentum®, Nutramigen®) or with an elemental amino acid-based formula (e.g., Neocate®, EleCare®) are highly suggestive of cow's milk or other food allergies, respectively. This might also suggest lactose intolerance.

Q4. Which of the following dietetic measures reduces the risk for development of food allergy and atopic eczema in "high-risk" infants?

A. Exclusive breastfeeding during at least 6 months
B. Avoidance of cow's milk products during at least the first year of life
C. Exclusive breastfeeding and/or a documented hypoallergenic formula during the first 4 months of life
D. Exclusive breastfeeding and/or a documented hypoallergenic formula during the first 2 months of life
E. Avoidance of hyperallergenic food such as cow's milk, hens' egg, peanut, tree nuts and fish the first year of life

Answer*: The correct answer is* ***C****.*

According to the recommendations for prevention follow the 2008 American Academy of Pediatrics clinical report, breastfeeding is encouraged for all infants [3]. Hydrolyzed infant formulas are suggested for infants at risk, while complementary food including potential allergens are not restricted after 4–6 months (of course not for infants experiencing allergic reactions to those food). Maternal diet during pregnancy should be healthy and balanced as evidence to support avoidance of potential food allergens, during pregnancy are lacking. Early dietary intervention in high risk infants can reduce the risk for developing food allergy and eczema, but does not appear to modify the natural course of the allergic march in the long run.

Practical Points

- Food-protein induced enterocolitis syndrome (FPIES) is a disorder most commonly seen in infants between 1–3 weeks of age, with gross or microscopic hematochezia
- The reaction is most common in exclusively breast fed infants as a result of cow's milk or soy protein in mothers diet
- Elimination of the responsible allergen leads to resolution of hematochezia within 72 h

References

1. Cherian S, Varshney P. Food protein-induced enterocolitis syndrome (FPIES): review of recent guidelines. Curr Allergy Asthma Rep. 2018;18(4):28.
2. Leonard SA, Pecora V, Fiocchi AG, Nowak-Wegrzyn A. Food protein-induced enterocolitis syndrome: a review of the new guidelines. World Allergy Organ J. 2018;11(1):4.
3. Greer FR, Sicherer SH, Burks AW, American Academy of Pediatrics Committee on Nutrition; American Academy of Pediatrics Section on Allergy and Immunology. Effects of early nutritional interventions on the development of atopic disease in infants and children: the role of maternal dietary restriction, breastfeeding, timing of introduction of complementary foods, and hydrolyzed formulas. Pediatrics. 2008;121(1):183–91.

Chapter 14
Vomiting and Angioedema After Eating Chocolate

Farzaneh Rahmani

A 2-year-old girl was brought up to the emergency room by her parents, due to protracted vomiting, breathlessness, and emergence of severe swelling on her lips and face, minutes after ingestion of a chocolate cream in a party. Her parents had known about their daughter probable allergy to nuts, as she frequently experienced itching, urticaria and mild angioedema after having tree nut, soy beans or processed nut-containing mixed bars. The chocolate cream of suspicion contained peanut cream, and almond particles, to which they were not sure if she had ever been exposed. Anaphylaxis management protocol was started for her with epinephrine and methylprednisolone.

Q1. All the following statements are correct about peanut allergy, <u>except</u>:

A. It is one of the most common causes of food allergy worldwide
B. Severe multisystem reactions are uncommon with this type of allergy
C. Development of tolerance is common in peanut allergy
D. Co-allergy to other nuts, such as tree nut is common
E. First exposure commonly occurs in early childhood

Answer: *The correct answer is* ***B***.

Allergy to nuts and seeds is amongst the most common food allergies worldwide. Prevalence of peanut allergy reaches to up to 1–2% in United States, while the condition is considered to be rare in most Asian countries. Besides a personal or family history of atopy, early exposure to peanut oil in skin care products and

F. Rahmani (✉)
Students Scientific Research Center (SSRC), Tehran University of Medical Sciences, Tehran, Iran

NeuroImaging Network (NIN), Universal Scientific Education and Research Network (USERN), Tehran, Iran
e-mail: f-rahmani@alumnus.tums.ac.ir

N. Rezaei (ed.), *Pediatric Allergy*, https://doi.org/10.1007/978-3-030-18282-3_14

household exposures are considered risk factors for childhood peanut allergy. Sensitization to peanut occurs early after birth and most children (approx. 75%) show symptoms during first direct exposure to the suspected nut/seed [1]. Age at onset is between 1–2 years old in many western studies, but it is suspected to be higher in Asian countries. Tolerance is uncommon in peanut allergy with only 10–20% of young children being desensitized in a 10-year follow up. Up to one half of children with peanut allergy are also allergic to tree nuts, and co-allergy to other nuts occurs in up to one half of patients with tree nut allergy. Systemic reaction is common and is seen in at least half of all IgE-mediated acute reactions to peanut. Peanut and tree nut allergy account for the majority of food-induced anaphylactic reactions [1].

Being aware of their child's allergy to nuts, her parents had tried to prevent exposure to nuts whenever possible. As their daughter was recovering, they wanted to make sure of the culprit food to be able to exert avoidance measures.

Q2. Which of the following statements is true about the diagnosis of peanut allergy?

A. A history of food-induced reaction with typical allergic symptoms, after ingestion of peanut is enough to establish the diagnosis
B. Diagnosis requires a history of allergic reaction with "oral" exposure/ingestion of peanut rather than topical or inhaled exposure
C. Skin prick test should be avoided when peanut allergy is suspected due to a high risk of anaphylaxis
D. Placebo-controlled oral food challenge test is gold-standard and first step in diagnosis of food allergy
E. A skin prick test survey with a number of suspected food items should be first step in workup of this patient

Answer: *The correct answer is* ***E***.

A reliable history of allergic reactions with exposure to a common/likely food item, along with involvement of two or more organ systems established the diagnosis of anaphylaxis in this girl and hence her allergy to peanut. Anaphylactic reaction can interfere with the results of skin prick test and less probably to specific IgE (sIgE) radioallergosorbent test (RAST) [2]. It is therefore plausible to maintain comprehensive avoidance from all suspected nuts and also provide the parents with epinephrine autoinjector, until the follow-up visit. When the suspected nut is identified, RAST can strongly predict clinical reactivity to peanut. Positive IgE and clinical history together disclose the diagnosis in most patients [3]. When clinical history is vague or sIgE levels are equivocal, a double-blind placebo-controlled oral food challenge (OFC) with items of suspect from prick test can be performed to establish a consensus over the culprit item [3].

Skin prick test was negative for almond (3 mm), tree nut (4 mm) and marginally positive for peanut (7 mm) (histamine control = 3 mm). Peanut sIgE by ImmunoCAP was 13 IU/mL (levels between 13 to 15 IU/mL have a 95–99% positive predictive value). OFC with peanut in allergy clinic reproduced wheezing and urticaria in the girl, confirming her diagnosis.

Q3. All of the following are true regarding allergen avoidance in patients with peanut allergy, except:

A. It is reasonable to measure tree-nut-sIgE, before filling it free for use
B. The girl should be advised to abstain from eating any kind of nut by the age she is able to identify different nuts
C. Accidental exposure to peanut is uncommon, provided that the parents watchfully control their daughter's diet
D. Concomitant use of NSAIDS or exercise may provoke anaphylaxis with items previously proven to be safe or providing only mild reaction
E. Contamination of food items with peanut and hidden peanut ingredients of food items are common causes of accidental exposure to peanut

Answer: *The correct answer is* ***C***.

Co-allergy to other nuts is quite common in patients with peanut allergy (33–50% for tree nut allergy) and the girl should abstain from all nuts, unless they are cleared by skin prick test with or without sIgE levels. Cross contamination of other food products with peanut is common, especially with bakery or pastry products, where shared food containers and handling objects are used for different products [2]. Parents are strongly recommended to read all food labels and beware of hidden food items in products, especially if ingredients labels are missing or incomplete. Children often misidentify peanuts with other nuts and vice versa and this poses a challenge to the parents to be able to control accidental ingestion of peanuts in young children.

Practical Points

- Allergy to nuts is amongst the most common food allergies worldwide
- Co-allergy to peanut and three nut is common
- Radioallergosorbent test (RAST) can strongly predict clinical reactivity to peanut
- Double-blind placebo-controlled oral food challenge is gold-standard in diagnosis of food allergy

References

1. Liu M, Burks AW, Green TD. Tree nut allergy: risk factors for development, mitigation of reaction risk and current efforts in desensitization. Expert Rev Clin Immunol. 2015;11(5):673–9.
2. Smeekens JM, Bagley K, Kulis M. Tree nut allergies: allergen homology, cross-reactivity, and implications for therapy. Clin Exp Allergy. 2018;48(7):762–72.
3. Stiefel G, Anagnostou K, Boyle RJ, Brathwaite N, Ewan P, Fox AT, Huber P, Luyt D, Till SJ, Venter C, Clark AT. BSACI guideline for the diagnosis and management of peanut and tree nut allergy. Clin Exp Allergy. 2017;47(6):719–39.

Chapter 15
Facial Angioedema Following Smoothie Ingestion

Alexandra Langlois and Moshe Ben Shoshan

An 18-month-old girl was referred to the emergency department with diffuse urticaria and facial angioedema. A few minutes after ingestion of a smoothie containing whey protein powder, the patient developed cough and 45 min later, a rash and facial angioedema. The parents treated her with 10 mg diphenhydramine. On arrival to the emergency room, 2 h after ingestion of the smoothie, she presented angioedema, generalized urticaria, persistent cough and wheezing on auscultation. The reaction occurred 2 h after waking up in the morning and the parents indicated that they had not given her any medication that morning.

The smoothie contained fruits, juice, ice, and whey protein. There were notably no nuts or peanuts. She had no known allergies and her diet was varied. However, her parents had been recommended to put her on a milk avoidance diet since a few months ago because of abdominal discomfort. She also had an upper respiratory tract infection for the last few days. Parents reported that patient had no prior symptoms consistent with asthma or eczema. Her parents were both previously diagnosed with hay fever.

At the emergency room, she was treated with intramuscular epinephrine with rapid resolution of symptoms. She was discharged from the emergency room after 6 h of observation. Six hours later they returned to the emergency room due to recurrence of hives and angioedema. A tryptase level, drawn 2.5 h after her initial presentation to the emergency room, was elevated (22.7 μg/L (reference range: 0–11.4 μg/L)). A level drawn 2 days later was normal (5.4 μg/L). Specific IgE (sIgE) levels of for milk protein was 1.3 AU/mL. Her skin prick testing for milk was positive at 6 mm/20 mm (wheal/flare).

A. Langlois (✉) · M. B. Shoshan
Division of Pediatric Allergy, Dermatology and Clinical Immunology, Department of Pediatrics, Montreal Children's Hospital, McGill University Health Centre, Montreal, QC, Canada
e-mail: alexandra.langlois@mail.mcgill.ca

N. Rezaei (ed.), *Pediatric Allergy*, https://doi.org/10.1007/978-3-030-18282-3_15

Q1. Which statement best lists the differential diagnoses is order of likelihood?

A. Asthma exacerbation, anaphylaxis, viral urticaria
B. Anaphylaxis, viral upper respiratory tract infection with urticaria, asthma exacerbation
C. Anaphylaxis, mastocytosis, viral urticaria
D. Chronic spontaneous urticaria, viral urticaria, mastocytosis

Answer: *The correct answer is **B**.*

The most important diagnosis to consider is anaphylaxis. Anaphylaxis is a clinical diagnosis and should be diagnosed and treated promptly to prevent morbidity and potential fatality.

According to the most commonly cited criteria, anaphylaxis is likely when any one of the three below scenarios are fulfilled [1]:

1. Acute onset of an illness (minutes to several hours) with involvement of the skin, mucosal tissue or both and at least one of the following:
   (a) Respiratory compromise
   (b) Reduced blood pressure or associated symptoms of end-organ dysfunction
2. Two or more of the following that occur rapidly after exposure to a likely allergen in a patient with
   (a) Involvement of the skin-mucosal tissue
   (b) Respiratory compromise
   (c) Reduced blood pressure or associated symptoms
   (d) Persistent gastrointestinal symptoms
3. Reduced blood pressure after exposure to known allergen in a patient with
   (a) Low blood pressure (less than 90 mmHg for adult or age-specific for children) or greater than 30%.

In this particular case, asthma cannot explain the urticaria and angioedema. Mastocytosis, a disorder characterized by increased number of mast cells [2], is unlikely given that there had been only one episode consistent with mast cell activation and that baseline tryptase was within the normal range [3]. A viral illness could present with similar symptoms, but is less likely given the clear association with a potential trigger (the smoothie), the rapid resolution of symptoms with epinephrine administration and elevated level of tryptase during reaction. The symptoms are also not consistent with chronic spontaneous urticaria (CSU). CSU is defined as the presence of hives, angioedema or both, occurring for at least 6 consecutive weeks with no associated trigger [4].

Q2. What is the first-line treatment?

A. Epinephrine 1:1000, 0.01 mg/kg IV
B. Diphenhydramine 1 mg/kg PO/IV/IM

C. Epinephrine 1:1000, 0.1 mg/kg IM
D. Epinephrine 1:1000, 0.01 mg/kg IM

Answer*: The correct answer is* ***D****.*

For optimal management of anaphylaxis, a dose of 0.01 mg/kg of 1:1000 epinephrine solution or 1 mg/mL (maximum dose 0.5 mg) should be administered promptly in the anterolateral aspect of the quadriceps. This mode of administration has shown higher and faster plasma peak [5]. The epinephrine dose can be repeated every 5–15 min based on the clinical status of the patient. Anti-histamines and steroids play only a secondary role and should not delay administration of epinephrine when indicated [6].

Q3. What was the reason for the girls return to the emergency department?

A. Biphasic anaphylactic reaction
B. Bipolar anaphylactic reaction
C. Protracted anaphylactic reaction
D. Delayed anaphylactic reaction

Answer*: The correct answer is* ***A****.*

The patient demonstrated a biphasic reaction. The most widely cited definition of biphasic anaphylaxis is recurrence of symptoms after initial resolution, despite no further exposure. Secondary phase of reaction can occur following an asymptomatic interval of at least 1 h to up to 72 h. The reported incidence varies from 3% to 23% [7] and the risk significantly increases when epinephrine is not administered promptly and in patients with severe reactions [8]. Protracted reactions are defined as anaphylactic reactions that last for hours, days and sometimes weeks after exposure. Delayed reactions are rare cases of anaphylaxis with onset hours after the exposure to the allergen [9].

Q4. The major cause of anaphylaxis in children is:

A. Venom
B. Drug
C. Food
D. Unknown

Answer*: The correct answer is* ***C****.*

Foods are major cause of anaphylaxis world-wide [10]. While in North America and Europe peanut and tree nut are reported to be the major culprits [11–13], shellfish is reportedly the major anaphylaxis trigger in Asia children [14, 15].

Q5. Which statement does not apply to milk allergy?

A. Whey protein contains alpha-lactalbumin, β-lactoglobulin, and lactoferrin.
B. A high proportion of patient will tolerate milk in baked goods
C. All IgE-mediated milk allergic patient should avoid beef
D. Milk-allergic patient are susceptible to failure to thrive, calcium and vitamin D deficiency

Answer*: The correct answer is* ***C****.*

The main allergens are caseins and whey protein. Caseins are heat-stable proteins whereas heat-labile whey proteins are alpha-lactalbumin (Bos d 4), beta-lactoglobulin (Bos d 5) and lactoferrin (Bos d lactoferrin). Most patients are sensitized to various proteins in the milk [16], not just one component. About 75% of milk-allergic patients tolerate milk in baked goods [17, 18]. Beef is tolerated in the vast majority of patients diagnosed with milk allergy [19, 20]. Once a diagnosis of milk allergy is confirmed, elimination of milk is paramount but bears the risk of developing failure to thrive, calcium and vitamin D deficiency.

Q6. Which statement is <u>not</u> true about serum tryptase level?

A. The optimal timing to draw a tryptase level is 15 min to 3 h after initial symptoms develop
B. Tryptase levels are lower in neonates compared to teenagers
C. An elevated tryptase value is suggestive of anaphylaxis
D. High baseline levels of tryptase are consistent with mastocytosis

Answer: *The correct answer is* ***B***.

Tryptase levels are highest during the first 3 months of life and decrease progressively until 9–12 months of age [21]. The elevated tryptase is also a useful marker in confirming atypical presentations of anaphylaxis. An elevated tryptase level is suggestive of anaphylaxis but a normal value does not rule it out [3]. If tryptase level stays elevated when measured at baseline, the clinician should consider systemic mastocytosis [2].

Practical Points

- IgE-mediated milk allergy is a frequent food allergy that presents with various symptoms usually within 2 h after exposure
- Prompt diagnosis and management with intramuscular epinephrine is paramount
- Biphasic anaphylactic reactions can be seen especially when there is a delay in epinephrine administration and more severe presentations
- Comparing tryptase levels during reaction with baseline levels can confirm the diagnosis of anaphylaxis

References

1. Sampson HA, Munoz-Furlong A, Campbell RL, Adkinson NF Jr, Bock SA, Branum A, Brown SG, Camargo CA Jr, Cydulka R, Galli SJ, Gidudu J, Gruchalla RS, Harlor AD Jr, Hepner DL, Lewis LM, Lieberman PL, Metcalfe DD, O'Connor R, Muraro A, Rudman A, Schmitt C, Scherrer D, Simons FE, Thomas S, Wood JP, Decker WW. Second symposium on the definition and management of anaphylaxis: summary report—second National Institute of Allergy and Infectious Disease/Food Allergy and Anaphylaxis Network symposium. Ann Emerg Med. 2006;47(4):373–80.
2. Le M, Miedzybrodzki B, Olynych T, Chapdelaine H, Ben-Shoshan M. Natural history and treatment of cutaneous and systemic mastocytosis. Postgrad Med. 2017;129(8):896–901.

3. De Schryver S, Halbrich M, Clarke A, La Vieille S, Eisman H, Alizadehfar R, Joseph L, Morris J, Ben-Shoshan M. Tryptase levels in children presenting with anaphylaxis: temporal trends and associated factors. J Allergy Clin Immunol. 2016;137(4):1138–42.
4. Netchiporouk E, Sasseville D, Moreau L, Habel Y, Rahme E, Ben-Shoshan M. Evaluating comorbidities, natural history, and predictors of early resolution in a cohort of children with chronic urticaria. JAMA Dermatol. 2017;153(12):1236–42.
5. Simons FE, Roberts JR, Gu X, Simons KJ. Epinephrine absorption in children with a history of anaphylaxis. J Allergy Clin Immunol. 1998;101(1 Pt 1):33–7.
6. Simons FE, Ebisawa M, Sanchez-Borges M, Thong BY, Worm M, Tanno LK, Lockey RF, El-Gamal YM, Brown SG, Park HS, Sheikh A. 2015 update of the evidence base: World Allergy Organization anaphylaxis guidelines. World Allergy Organ J. 2015;8(1):32.
7. Alqurashi W, Ellis AK. Do corticosteroids prevent biphasic anaphylaxis? J Allergy Clin Immunol Pract. 2017;5(5):1194–205.
8. Alqurashi W, Stiell I, Chan K, Neto G, Alsadoon A, Wells G. Epidemiology and clinical predictors of biphasic reactions in children with anaphylaxis. Ann Allergy Asthma Immunol. 2015;115(3):217–23 e2.
9. Bircher AJ, Hofmeier KS, Link S, Heijnen I. Food allergy to the carbohydrate galactose-alpha-1,3-galactose (alpha-gal): four case reports and a review. Eur J Dermatol. 2017;27(1):3–9.
10. Ben Shoshan M, Clarke AE. Anaphylaxis: past, present and future. Allergy. 2011;66(1):1–14.
11. Hochstadter E, Clarke A, De SS, LaVieille S, Alizadehfar R, Joseph L, Eisman H, Ben-Shoshan M. Increasing visits for anaphylaxis and the benefits of early epinephrine administration: a 4-year study at a pediatric emergency department in Montreal, Canada. J Allergy Clin Immunol. 2016;137(6):1888–1890.e4.
12. Decker WW, Campbell RL, Manivannan V, Luke A, St Sauver JL, Weaver A, Bellolio MF, Bergstralh EJ, Stead LG, Li JT. The etiology and incidence of anaphylaxis in Rochester, Minnesota: a report from the Rochester Epidemiology Project. J Allergy Clin Immunol. 2008;122(6):1161–5.
13. Vetander M, Helander D, Flodstrom C, Ostblom E, Alfven T, Ly DH, Hedlin G, Lilja G, Nilsson C, Wickman M. Anaphylaxis and reactions to foods in children—a population-based case study of emergency department visits. Clin Exp Allergy. 2012;42(4):568–77.
14. Lee AJ, Gerez I, Shek LP, Lee BW. Shellfish allergy—an Asia-Pacific perspective. Asian Pac J Allergy Immunol. 2012;30(1):3–10.
15. Piromrat K, Chinratanapisit S, Trathong S. Anaphylaxis in an emergency department: a 2-year study in a tertiary-care hospital. Asian Pac J Allergy Immunol. 2008;26(2–3):121–8.
16. Fiocchi A, Brozek J, Schunemann H, Bahna SL, von Berg A, Beyer K, Bozzola M, Bradsher J, Compalati E, Ebisawa M, Guzman MA, Li H, Heine RG, Keith P, Lack G, Landi M, Martelli A, Rance F, Sampson H, Stein A, Terracciano L, Vieths S, World Allergy Organization Special Committee on Food A. World Allergy Organization (WAO) Diagnosis and Rationale for Action against Cow's Milk Allergy (DRACMA) guidelines. Pediatr Allergy Immunol 2010;21 Suppl 21:1–125.
17. Gupta RS, Springston EE, Warrier MR, Smith B, Kumar R, Pongracic J, Holl JL. The prevalence, severity, and distribution of childhood food allergy in the United States. Pediatrics. 2011;128(1):e9–17.
18. Kim JS, Nowak-Wegrzyn A, Sicherer SH, Noone S, Moshier EL, Sampson HA. Dietary baked milk accelerates the resolution of cow's milk allergy in children. J Allergy Clin Immunol. 2011;128(1):125–31 e2.
19. Martelli A, De Chiara A, Corvo M, Restani P, Fiocchi A. Beef allergy in children with cow's milk allergy; cow's milk allergy in children with beef allergy. Ann Allergy Asthma Immunol. 2002;89(6 Suppl 1):38–43.
20. Werfel SJ, Cooke SK, Sampson HA. Clinical reactivity to beef in children allergic to cow's milk. J Allergy Clin Immunol. 1997;99(3):293–300.
21. Belhocine W, Ibrahim Z, Grandne V, Buffat C, Robert P, Gras D, Cleach I, Bongrand P, Carayon P, Vitte J. Total serum tryptase levels are higher in young infants. Pediatric Allerg Immunol. 2011;22(6):600–7.

Chapter 16
Itchy Eyes and Rhinorrhea When Playing with Her Dog

Eva Macías, Milagros Lázaro, and Ignacio Dávila

A 12-year-old girl diagnosed with rhino-conjunctivitis and asthma with sensitization to pollen and fungal spores has been followed-up on an outpatient basis in our service. She has owned a dog for more than 10 years. Five years ago, she started to complain of itchy eyes, rhinorrhea and sneezing when playing with the dog. In the last 2 years she has developed episodes of dry nonproductive cough, dyspnea and shortness of breath after contacting the dog, causing the dog to be kept outside the house. Soon after, she began presenting the same symptoms every time she contacted a cat in a relative's home.

During her last routine visit, the patient reports that in the last 4 months she has had several episodes of itching of the oral cavity and lip edema, which appeared 5 min after the ingestion of pork. They have also appeared after ingesting pork ham, bacon, pork loin and pork sausages. She has tolerated chicken and veal sausages as well as the meats of other mammals.

Skin prick test (SPT) was performed with a locally adapted battery of aeroallergens that includes both domestic and storage dust mite, fungal spores, grass pollen, weeds and trees, as well as battery of animals that include horse, rabbit, cat, hamster and dog. Her results were positive for grass pollen, *Alternaria* spp., dog dander and cat dander and negative for the rest of allergens. SPT with a pork meat extract was also positive.

Her serum total IgE was elevated and specific IgE (sIgE) against cat albumin, pork albumin (nSus s), pork meat and bovine albumin were positive. sIgE against uteroglobin (rFel d 1) and sIgE to alpha-gal were negative. The sIgE against nCan f 1, rCan f 2, rCan f 3 and rCan f 5 came back positive.

E. Macías · M. Lázaro (✉) · I. Dávila
Allergy Department, University Hospital of Salamanca, Salamanca, Spain

N. Rezaei (ed.), *Pediatric Allergy*, https://doi.org/10.1007/978-3-030-18282-3_16

Q1. Which of the following is the most likely true?

A. Pork albumin are the primary sensitizing antigen
B. Dog and cat serum albumins are the primary sensitizing antigens
C. Cross-reactivity between the albumins of the different animals is not responsible for the symptoms of the patient
D. Allergy to pork meat has no relationship with her previous cat allergy

Answer*: The correct answer is* ***B****.*

This atopic patient initially presented symptoms of rhino-conjunctivitis and asthma due to contact with her dog. Later she developed symptoms when contacting with a cat and finally symptoms after the consumption of pork meat. In fact, a clinically relevant reactivity to meats has been demonstrated, which points to a cross-reactivity and not to a sensitization with meat-specific epitopes. Keeping with this, cross-reactive IgE antibodies that bind to various mammalian albumins have been described, notably in the so-called pork-cat syndrome. Her symptoms induced by cat and dog exposure are presumably due to cross-reactivity of cat and dog albumin. The subsequent symptoms induced by the consumption of pork meat are mediated by sensitization to pork albumin. This sequence of events, which begins with the sensitization to an aeroallergen and leads to allergic symptoms in response to food, is due to cross-reactivity and has also been described as "pollen-fruit-vegetable" and "feather-egg" syndrome. This cross-reactivity is most common among young atopic patients [1–7].

Q2. Which of following is the most likely diagnosis?

A. Allergy caused by alpha-gal
B. Allergy to albumins of meat origin
C. Allergy to mammalian meat
D. Pork-cat syndrome

Answer*: The correct answer is* ***D****.*

The timing of the reaction is very helpful in differentiating the pork-cat syndrome from a delayed anaphylaxis caused by IgE to alpha-gal. Both food allergies are IgE mediated, and mammalian meat is involved. However, symptoms of pork-cat syndrome can occur rapidly and may present initially with oral pruritus during the meal. In general, reactions to pork begin within 20–30 min of consumption, often with mild gastrointestinal symptoms, such as abdominal cramping, yet fatal reactions of anaphylaxis with pork have also been described. The patient does not have allergies to all mammalian meats, since she tolerates beef meat without problems [1–7].

Q3. Based on the clinical diagnosis, which of the following recommendations would be most appropriate for the patient?

A. Remove all types of meats from the diet of the patient, given the risk of developing allergies to all types of meats
B. The patient can continue to eat all kinds of meat, including pork and beef
C. The patient will only withdraw pork from the diet
D. The patient will withdraw both pork and beef meat from the diet, since sIgE to bovine albumin is positive

Answer*: The correct answer is* ***C****.*

While patients with sIgE to alpha-gal have positive immunoassay results for bovine and porcine meat, patients with a pork-cat syndrome show a variable degree of cross-reactivity with bovine albumin. Thus certain patients with pork-cat syndrome can tolerate beef, whereas other cannot. We should not recommend avoidance of beef unless patients report symptoms associated with eating beef, which was not the case of our patient [1–7].

Practical Points

- The pork-cat syndrome is an uncommon allergic reaction
- The IgE-mediated response in the patient is a result of cross-reactivity between albumins of the different species of mammalians
- We present a patient sensitized to cat and dog albumins, with symptoms after the consumption of pork due to cross-reactivity with pork albumin

References

1. Drouet M, Sabbah A. The pork/cat syndrome or crossed reactivity between cat epithelia and pork meat. Monogr Allergy. 1996;32:164–73.
2. Konradsen JR, Fujisawa T, van Hage M, Hedlin G, Hilger C, Kleine-Tebbe J, Matsui EC, Roberts G, Ronmark E, Platts-Mills TA. Allergy to furry animals: new insights, diagnostic approaches, and challenges. J Allergy Clin Immunol. 2015;135(3):616–25.
3. Posthumus J, James HR, Lane CJ, Matos LA, Platts-Mills TA, Commins SP. Initial description of pork-cat syndrome in the United States. J Allergy Clin Immunol. 2013;131(3):923–5.
4. Hilger C, Kohnen M, Grigioni F, Lehners C, Hentges F. Allergic cross-reactions between cat and pig serum albumin. Study at the protein and DNA levels. Allergy. 1997;52(2):179–87.
5. Commins SP, Satinover SM, Hosen J, Mozena J, Borish L, Lewis BD, Woodfolk JA, Platts-Mills TA. Delayed anaphylaxis, angioedema, or urticaria after consumption of red meat in patients with IgE antibodies specific for galactose-alpha-1,3-galactose. J Allergy Clin Immunol. 2009;123(2):426–33.
6. Drouet M, Sabbah A, Le Sellin J, Bonneau JC, Gay G, Dubois-Gosnet C. Fatal anaphylaxis after eating wild boar meat in a patient with pork-cat syndrome. Allerg Immunol. 2001;33(4):163–5.
7. Savi E, Rossi A, Incorvaia C. Cat-pork syndrome: a case report with a three years follow-up. Eur Ann Allergy Clin Immunol. 2006;38(10):366–8.

Chapter 17
Acute Reaction After Drinking Formula Milk

Kok Wee Chong, Wenyin Loh, and Jan Hau Lee

A 4-year old boy with no previous known food allergies developed an acute reaction after drinking formula milk. He was well prior to presentation and had been drinking cow's milk formula since birth. On the day of presentation, he drank a new milk formula from a newly opened tin (different product from the same brand) for the first time. Twenty minutes later, he developed itch in both eyes, incessant coughing with rhinorrhea, followed by severe eye swelling. There was no vomiting, shortness of breath, or drowsiness.

In past medical history he had a history of recurrent viral-induced wheeze but no eczema or allergic rhinitis. A previous skin prick test (SPT) was positive to house dust mite. Upon arrival at the emergency department, he was alert and his vital signs were normal. He was noted to have generalized urticaria with bilateral eye angioedema. There was no wheeze and physical examination was unremarkable.

Q1. Which of the following is the most likely diagnosis?

A. Cow's milk protein allergy
B. House dust mite allergy
C. Lactose intolerance
D. Allergy to supplement in the cow's milk formula

Answer: *The correct answer is* ***D***.

The acute symptoms are in keeping with an IgE-mediated allergic reaction. This patient has been tolerating cow's milk since birth. Thus, it is highly unlikely that he has developed a new onset cow's milk protein allergy at the age of 4 years. House dust

K. W. Chong · W. Loh
Allergy Service, Department of Paediatric Medicine, KK Women's and Children's Hospital, Singapore, Singapore

J. H. Lee (✉)
Children's Intensive Care Unit, KK Women's and Children's Hospital, Singapore, Singapore
e-mail: lee.jan.hau@singhealth.com.sg

N. Rezaei (ed.), *Pediatric Allergy*, https://doi.org/10.1007/978-3-030-18282-3_17

mite allergy causing an acute flare of allergic rhinitis may result in a similar clinical presentation. However, this patient had no known history of allergic rhinitis, and the acute reaction appears to be temporally related to the milk feed, hence making Answer B less favorable. Oral mite anaphylaxis (also known as Pancake syndrome) is a well-described entity characterized by the occurrence of severe allergic symptoms beginning immediately after eating foods contaminated with domestic mites [1]. It has been suggested that high temperatures and humidity in tropical and subtropical regions may promote dust mite propagation in contaminated flour. This is less likely in this case, since the milk was from a newly opened tin and this is a syndrome most commonly associated with flour and has not been reported with milk powder. Lactose intolerance is often confused with cow's milk protein allergy. Lactose intolerance is an inability to digest lactose, the main sugar in milk, which gives rise to gastrointestinal symptoms such as diarrhea, flatulence and abdominal pain. It is caused by a deficiency of the intestinal enzyme, lactase. The symptoms presented in this case are not in keeping with a diagnosis of lactose intolerance. An allergic reaction to a supplement that had been added to the formula is hence most plausible. A comparison of the new milk powder and the one which he had been tolerating, revealed that addition of prebiotics was the main difference between both formulas. In particular, supplementation of commercially available milk formulations with the prebiotic, galacto-oligosaccharide (GOS), has been a growing trend in recent years and GOS allergy and anaphylaxis has been reported in the Asian region in the past few years [2, 3]. Till date, all GOS-allergic patients reported in literature have shown reaction following their first known exposure. GOS allergy is the most likely cause in this case.

Q2. All of the following statements are true about food allergens, except:

A. The part of the food allergen that is responsible for IgE binding can be a sequential or conformational epitope
B. Food allergens are always proteins
C. The glycan portion of glycoproteins (carbohydrates bound to proteins) is generally not immunogenic
D. Allergic reactions to class II food allergens result from primary sensitization to homologous allergens from a different source

Answer*: The correct answer is* ***B****.*

The part of the food allergen that is responsible for IgE binding, also known as B-cell epitopes, can be a sequential or conformational epitope. Sequential epitopes refer to stretches of consecutive amino acids that bind to variable part of the IgE molecule, while in conformational epitopes the folded protein in its 3-dimensional shape binds to the IgE, although the amino acids involved in the binding site are located discontinuously. The majority of B-cell epitopes of food allergens are conformational. Allergens are traditionally thought to be proteins or substances bound to proteins and carbohydrates on their own are generally deemed to be poorly immunogenic. This is due to the small molecular size of most mammalian carbohydrates, making it unlikely to cross-link IgE on mast cells. Glycans are naturally occurring chains of simple sugars that when attached to a protein carrier, are able to bind to IgE and induce an allergic response. An example would be the oligosaccharide galactose-α-1,3-galactose (α-Gal), a sugar chain commonly found as part of glycoproteins and glycolipids in mammals, which is involved in red meat allergy. GOS, which is a pure carbohydrate, has been shown to be immunogenic when coupled with carrier proteins in animal models [4], and it is suggested that in patients with GOS allergy it is a ubiquitous cell-surface protein [2].

Q3. What would be the acute management of this child?

A. Intramuscular adrenaline at 0.01 mg/Kg of 1:1000 with intramuscular diphenhydramine
B. Oral prednisolone with oral second generation anti-histamine (e.g., cetirizine)
C. Oral second generation antihistamine (e.g., cetirizine) with nebulized salbutamol
D. Oral second generation antihistamine (e.g., cetirizine)

***Answer**: The correct answer is **D**.*

The patient presented with cutaneous symptoms of urticaria with angioedema, as well as mild respiratory symptoms of cough and rhinorrhea. These symptoms alone are not consistent with a diagnosis of anaphylaxis. Hence only an oral second generation anti-histamine such as cetirizine would be indicated in immediate management of this patient. However, the patient should be monitored for progression of symptoms and intramuscular adrenaline would be indicated if anaphylaxis develops.

Q4. Which one of the following is the most appropriate next step in the evaluation of this patient's condition?

A. Cow's milk specific serum IgE
B. Skin prick test to cow's milk, implicated milk powder, GOS
C. Serum tryptase levels
D. Basophil activation test to GOS

***Answer**: The correct answer is **B**.*

The most appropriate next step in the evaluation would be to perform a SPT to cow's milk, the implicated milk powder and GOS. This would exclude a cow's milk protein allergy and confirm the trigger to be a supplement in the new formula, which in this case would be GOS. Measurement of cow's milk specific IgE (sIgE) is unlikely to be useful in a child who is well-tolerating cow's milk. Serum tryptase levels may be raised in anaphylaxis but do not help recognizing the trigger. Basophil activation test may be useful in the evaluation of GOS allergy, but it is not routinely available in clinical practice.

The patient's SPT results were: histamine = 5.0 mm, diluent = 0 mm, cow's milk = 0 mm, implicated milk powder = 5.5 mm and GOS = 7.0 mm.

Q5. What option below gives the appropriate management plans for this patient?

A. Avoid GOS and all formula milk, prescribe an adrenaline autoinjector
B. Avoid GOS, all cow's milk and dairy products, prescribe an anaphylaxis action plan
C. Avoid GOS, prescribe an anaphylaxis action plan and an adrenaline-auto injector
D. Avoid GOS, probiotics, prescribe an anaphylaxis action plan and an adrenaline autoinjector

Answer*: The correct answer is* ***C****.*

The most important step in management of this patient would be strict avoidance of all food products containing GOS. There is a risk of anaphylaxis with future exposure to GOS. Milk products not containing GOS are safe and allowed. Probiotics are defined as live bacteria that provide a beneficial effect when administered in adequate amounts and should not be confused with prebiotics which are indigestible carbohydrates serving as substrates for bacteria in the colon. Provision of an individualized anaphylaxis action plan written clearly in simple, nonmedical language will aid in recognition and treatment of further reactions. Prescription of an adrenaline autoinjector can be considered, especially if there is a risk of inadvertent exposure. The absolute indications for prescription of an adrenaline autoinjector include [5]:

- Previous anaphylaxis triggered by food, latex, or aeroallergens
- Previous exercise-induced anaphylaxis
- Previous idiopathic anaphylaxis
- Co-existing unstable or moderate to severe, persistent asthma and a food allergy
- Venom allergy in children with more than cutaneous/mucosal systemic reactions
- Underlying mast cell disorders or elevated baseline serum tryptase concentrations together with any previous systemic allergic reactions to insect stings.

The prescription of an adrenaline autoinjector should be considered if any of the following additional factors is present:

- Previous mild-to-moderate allergic reaction to peanut and/or tree nut
- Teenager or young adult with a food allergy
- Remoteness from medical help and previous mild-to-moderate allergic reaction to a food, venom, latex, or aeroallergens
- Previous mild-to-moderate allergic reaction to traces of food

Practical Points

- Cow's milk and egg allergy are the most common causes of food allergy in children
- Most patients develop natural tolerance by first year of age
- Acute onset of symptoms such as urticaria, angioedema, nausea, vomiting, wheezing following food ingestion, should prompt a diagnosis of food allergy
- Allergy to galacto-oligosaccharides, a prebiotic carbohydrate, has been recently described in atopic patients in South-East Asia
- Galacto-oligosaccharides allergy is contrary to conventional understanding that allergens are proteins or glycoproteins

References

1. Sánchez-Borges M, Suárez-Chacon R, Capriles-Hulett A, Caballero-Fonseca F, Iraola V, Fernández-Caldas E. Pancake syndrome (oral mite anaphylaxis). World Allergy Organ J. 2009;2(5):91–6.
2. Chiang WC, Huang CH, Llanora GV, Gerez I, Goh SH, Shek LP, Nauta AJ, Van Doorn WA, Bindels J, Ulfman LH, Knipping K, Delsing DJ, Knol EF, Lee BW. Anaphylaxis to cow's milk formula containing short-chain galacto-oligosaccharide. J Allergy Clin Immunol. 2012;130(6):1361–7.
3. Soh JY, Huang CH, Chiang WC, Llanora GV, Lee AJ, Loh W, Chin YL, Tay VY, Chan YH, Dianne D, Lee BW. Anaphylaxis to galacto-oligosaccharides--an evaluation in an atopic population in Singapore. Allergy. 2015;70(8):1020–3.
4. Kaneko K, Watanabe Y, Kimura K, Matsumoto K, Mizobuchi T, Onoue M. Development of hypoallergenic galacto-oligosaccharides on the basis of allergen analysis. Biosci Biotechnol Biochem. 2014;78(1):100–8.
5. Muraro A, Roberts G, Worm M, Bilo MB, Brockow K, Fernandez Rivas M, Santos AF, Zolkipli ZQ, Bellou A, Beyer K, Bindslev-Jensen C, Cardona V, Clark AT, Demoly P, Dubois AE, DunnGalvin A, Eigenmann P, Halken S, Harada L, Lack G, Jutel M, Niggemann B, Rueff F, Timmermans F, Vlieg-Boerstra BJ, Werfel T, Dhami S, Panesar S, Akdis CA, Sheikh A. Anaphylaxis: guidelines from the European Academy of Allergy and Clinical Immunology. Allergy. 2014;69(8):1026–45.

Chapter 18
Recurrent Itchy Mouth

Charmi Patel and Punita Ponda

A 14-year-old girl presents with a complaint of an itchy mouth when eating fresh pitted fruits such as cherries, plums, peaches, apricots, nectarines and apples since many years ago. She can tolerate these fruits if they are cooked or dried. She also reports itchy mouth after eating almonds and itchy throat after eating raw hazelnut, but can tolerate roasted almond paste and almond flavoring. She is unsure if she has had roasted hazelnut.

She also complains of nasal congestion and sneezing during the springtime since 10 years of age. Her symptoms are now well-controlled on "as need" antihistamines and an intranasal corticosteroids (INC) spray during February to August. Family history was remarkable for a mother with allergic rhinitis and childhood asthma and her personal history was positive for anemia. Physical examination is remarkable for allergic shiners and pale, bluish edematous inferior nasal turbinates. Skin prick test (SPT) for aeroallergens is positive for dust mites, cockroach, cat, dog, trees including birch, elm, alder, oak, mulberry, red top grass and ragweed. SPT was positive for hazelnut (10.5 mm) and negative for almond. Her laboratory studies included a specific IgE (sIgE) measurement with ImmunoCAP which was 2.24 AU/mL for hazelnut.

Q1. Which one of the following is most likely the diagnosis?

A. Pollen food syndrome (PFS)
B. Food allergy

C. Patel
Division of Allergy and Immunology, Department of Medicine, Albany Medical Center, Albany Medical College, Albany, NY, USA

P. Ponda (✉)
Division of Allergy and Immunology, Cohen Children's Hospital of New York, Donald and Barbara Zucker School of Medicine at Hofstra/Northwell, Great Neck, NY, USA
e-mail: pponda@northwell.edu

N. Rezaei (ed.), *Pediatric Allergy*, https://doi.org/10.1007/978-3-030-18282-3_18

C. Irritant contact dermatitis
D. Chronic urticaria

Answer: *The correct answer is* ***A***.

Pollen food allergy syndrome is a common form of food allergy manifested by itching and or localized mild swelling of the mouth or throat immediately after ingestion of raw fruits, vegetables or nuts. This is due to pollen-related molecular mimicry in the food item, producing a contact urticaria in the mouth and oropharynx [1]. As the protein is denatured by heating, patients usually tolerate the cooked form of the food. Pollen-food syndrome (PFS) occurs in patients with concomitant pollen allergy. Although pollen food allergy syndrome is a type of food allergy, "food allergy" alone is not the most accurate diagnosis.

Irritant contact dermatitis due to certain foods being chemical irritants, is seen in chefs and food handlers. These patients present without itching, but with burning sensation, erythema, edema, vesicles, bullae, and oozing at the site of repetitive contact [2]. In most cases, the affected sites are exposed areas such as the dorsum of hands, face, and neck. Chronic urticaria simply implies the presence of recurrent urticaria for at least 6 weeks [3] and does not comply with our patient's history.

Q2. All of the following statement are correct about the evaluation of the patient, except:

A. Prick to prick is the best modality of testing
B. Skin prick testing using traditional food extracts is the most sensitive and specific method of testing
C. Specific component testing to hazelnut and peanut is helpful in risk stratifying for graded oral challenge in these patients
D. Skin prick testing to various pollen extracts are necessary for diagnosis

Answer: *The correct answer is* ***B***.

Diagnosis of PFS comprises of: 1) typical clinical symptoms evoked by the culprit plant/food with 2) evidence of sensitization to the corresponding pollen and 3) a known correlation between the food and pollen to which the patient is sensitized [4]. The preferred method of prick test for PFS is prick-by-prick skin testing with fresh foods. Component testing is helpful in risk stratification of systemic reactions with peanut and hazelnut. Commercial food extracts lack sensitivity for PFS as the culprit allergens tend to get destroyed during the extract production process [5].

Q3. Which component for hazelnut is expected to be elevated in this patient?

A. Ara h 8
B. Ara h 2
C. Cor a 1
D. Cor a 14

Answer: *The correct answer is* ***C***.

Cor a 1 is homologous with birch pollen allergen for hazelnut and is typically associated with oropharyngeal symptoms and often with tolerance to most forms of hazelnut [6, 7]. Ara h 8 is a birch allergen homologue for peanut associated with milder symptoms in the oropharyngeal region and low likelihood of systemic reactions especially when there is an isolated elevation in Ara h 8 IgE levels in the absence of IgE to Ara h 1, Ara h 2, or Ara h 3 [8]. Those sensitized to Cor a 9 or 14 are more likely to have systemic reactions [9]. Anti-COR a 1 component in our patient was 2.20 UA/mL, while her COR a 8, COR a 14 and COR a 9 are <0.10 AU/mL.

Q4. Which of the proteins cross-react with the culprit fruits?

A. Profilin
B. Bet v 1
C. Hev b 6.02
D. Lipid transfer proteins

Answer*: The correct answer is* ***B****.*

Bet v 1 is part of the PR10 protein family and is the major birch pollen allergen which accounts for cross-reactivity with apple, cherry, apricot, pear, carrot, celery, parsley, hazelnut and peanut [1]. Profilins are small actin binding proteins in all eukaryotic cells that can be "panallergens" found in several fruits and vegetables [10]. Bet v 2 was the first profilin identified [1, 10]. Profilins are culprits for celery-mugwort-spice syndrome [1]. Hev b 6.02 is the major latex allergen and contributes to latex fruit syndrome with banana, avocado, chestnut, and more commonly to kiwi [11]. Additionally, Hev b 2 (endo-β1, 3-glucanase), Hev b7 (patatin-like protein), Hev b 8 (profilin) and Hev b 12 (non-specific lipid transfer protein) are other members of this family, also implicated in latex fruit syndrome [11]. Lipid transfer proteins have low molecular mass and compact structure that are resistant to heating and proteases [1], thereby, bearing serious potential to induce systemic allergic reactions [1]. Gly m 1 is a lipid transfer protein, and a major allergen in soybean [1].

Q5. Which of the pollen-food associations are correct?

A. Ragweed: celery, carrot, bell pepper, fennel and black pepper
B. Orchard grass: cantaloupe, honeydew, watermelon, and zucchini
C. Birch: cantaloupe, celery, peanut, tomato and white potato
D. Mugwort: mustard, garlic, fennel and coriander

Answer*: The correct answer is* ***D****.*

Mugwort-associated PFS is typically with celery, carrot, parsley, caraway, fennel, black pepper, coriander, aniseed, mustard, cauliflower, cabbage, broccoli, bell pepper, garlic, onion and peach.

Ragweed association PFS occurs with melons (cantaloupe, honeydew, watermelon), banana, zucchini and cucumber. Orchard-grass-association includes; melon (cantaloupe, honeydew, watermelon), white potato, tomato and peanut.

Table 18.1 Most common food-pollen syndrome associations

Birch	Rosaceae: apple, peach, plum, pear, cherry, apricot, almond
	Apiaceae: carrot, celery, parsley, caraway, fennel, coriander, aniseed
	Fabaceae: soybean, peanut
	Betulaceae: hazelnut
Ragweed	Cucurbitaceae: cantaloupe, honeydew, watermelon, zucchini, cucumber
	Musaceae: banana
Mugwort	Apiaceae: celery, carrot, parsley, caraway, fennel, coriander, aniseed
	Brassicaceae: mustard, cauliflower, cabbage, broccoli
	Liliaceae: garlic, onion
	Rosaceae: peach
	Solanaceae: bell pepper
	Piperaceae: black pepper
Orchard	Cucurbitaceae: cantaloupe, honeydew, watermelon
	Solanaceae: white potato, tomato
	Fabaceae: peanut
Timothy	Amaranthaceae: Swiss chard
	Rutaceae: orange
Plane (sycamore) [12–14]	Hazelnut, peach, apple, kiwi, peanut, corn, chickpea, lettuce, and green beans

Birch-association includes; apple, peach, plum, pear, cherry, apricot, almond, carrot, celery, parsley, caraway, fennel, coriander, aniseed, soybean, peanut and hazelnut. Table 18.1 shows some of the most common correct PFS associations [12–14].

Practical Points

- Pollen-food allergy syndrome is caused by cross reactivity of pollen-related protein with raw fruits, vegetables and nuts
- Symptoms are a result of contact urticaria in the oral and oropharyngeal mucosa
- Prick to prick is the best diagnostic method for pollen food syndrome in combination with typical history
- For certain nuts such as peanut and hazelnut, component testing can be helpful for diagnosis
- Patients can continue to have cooked or heated foods as tolerated

References

1. Nowak-Węgrzyn A, Burks AW, Sampson HA. Reactions to foods. In: Middleton's allergy: principles and practice. 8th ed. Philadelphia, PA: Saunders; 2014. p. 1310–39.
2. Smith HR, Basketter DA, McFadden JP. Irritant dermatitis, irritancy and its role in allergic contact dermatitis. Clin Exp Dermatol. 2002;27(2):138–46.
3. Zuberbier T, Aberer W, Asero R, Bindslev-Jensen C, Brzoza Z, Canonica GW, Church MK, Ensina LF, Gimenez-Arnau A, Godse K, Goncalo M, Grattan C, Hebert J, Hide M, Kaplan A, Kapp A, Abdul Latiff AH, Mathelier-Fusade P, Metz M, Nast A, Saini SS, Sanchez-Borges M, Schmid-Grendelmeier P, Simons FE, Staubach P, Sussman G, Toubi E, Vena GA, Wedi B, Zhu XJ, Maurer M. European Academy of A, Clinical I, Global A, Asthma European N, European Dermatology F, World Allergy O. The EAACI/GA(2) LEN/EDF/WAO Guideline for the definition, classification, diagnosis, and management of urticaria: the 2013 revision and update. Allergy. 2014;69(7):868–87.
4. Price A, Ramachandran S, Smith GP, Stevenson ML, Pomeranz MK, Cohen DE. Oral allergy syndrome (pollen-food allergy syndrome). Dermatitis. 2015;26(2):78–88.
5. Vieths S, Hoffmann A, Holzhauser T, Muller U, Reindl J, Haustein D. Factors influencing the quality of food extracts for in vitro and in vivo diagnosis. Allergy. 1998;53(46 Suppl):65–71.
6. De Knop KJ, Verweij MM, Grimmelikhuijsen M, Philipse E, Hagendorens MM, Bridts CH, De Clerck LS, Stevens WJ, Ebo DG. Age-related sensitization profiles for hazelnut (Corylus avellana) in a birch-endemic region. Pediatr Allergy Immunol. 2011;22(1 Pt 2):e139–49.
7. Hansen KS, Ballmer-Weber BK, Sastre J, Lidholm J, Andersson K, Oberhofer H, Lluch-Bernal M, Ostling J, Mattsson L, Schocker F, Vieths S, Poulsen LK. Component-resolved in vitro diagnosis of hazelnut allergy in Europe. J Allergy Clin Immunol. 2009;123(5):1134–41. 41.e1-3.
8. Asarnoj A, Nilsson C, Lidholm J, Glaumann S, Ostblom E, Hedlin G, van Hage M, Lilja G, Wickman M. Peanut component Ara h 8 sensitization and tolerance to peanut. J Allergy Clin Immunol. 2012;130(2):468–72.
9. Masthoff LJN, Mattsson L, Zuidmeer-Jongejan L, Lidholm J, Andersson K, Akkerdaas JH, Versteeg SA, Garino C, Meijer Y, Kentie P, Versluis A, den Hartog Jager CF, Bruijnzeel-Koomen CAFM, Knulst AC, van Ree R, van Hoffen E, Pasmans SGMA. Sensitization to Cor a 9 and Cor a 14 is highly specific for a hazelnut allergy with objective symptoms in Dutch children and adults. J Allergy Clin Immunol. 2013;132(2):393–9.
10. Hoffmann-Sommergruber K, Mills ENC. Food allergen protein families and their structural characteristics and application in component-resolved diagnosis: new data from the EuroPrevall project. Anal Bioanal Chem. 2009;395(1):25–35.
11. Radauer C, Adhami F, Fürtler I, Wagner S, Allwardt D, Scala E, Ebner C, Hafner C, Hemmer W, Mari A, Breiteneder H. Latex-allergic patients sensitized to the major allergen hevein and hevein-like domains of class I chitinases show no increased frequency of latex-associated plant food allergy. Mol Immunol. 2011;48(4):600–9.
12. Fernández-Rivas M, van Ree R, Cuevas M. Allergy to Rosaceae fruits without related pollinosis. J Allergy Clin Immunol. 1997;100(6):728–33.
13. Pascal M, Munoz-Cano R, Reina Z, Palacin A, Vilella R, Picado C, Juan M, Sanchez-Lopez J, Rueda M, Salcedo G, Valero A, Yague J, Bartra J. Lipid transfer protein syndrome: clinical pattern, cofactor effect and profile of molecular sensitization to plant-foods and pollens. Clin Exp Allergy. 2012;42(10):1529–39.
14. Gao Z-S, Yang Z-W, Wu S-D, Wang H-Y, Liu M-L, Mao W-L, Wang J, Gadermaier G, Ferreira F, Zheng M, Van Ree R. Peach allergy in China: a dominant role for mugwort pollen lipid transfer protein as a primary sensitizer. J Allergy Clin Immunol. 2013;131(1):224–6.e3.

Chapter 19
Recurrent Wheals When He Exercised

Makiko Hiragun, Shunsuke Takahagi, and Michihiro Hide

A 16-year-old Japanese boy presented with a 6-year history of recurrent wheals when he exercised. The wheals tended to appear after he had shrimp. The attacks had never been accompanied by systemic symptoms, such as dyspnea and loss of consciousness. No wheals were induced either when he had shrimp without subsequent exercise or when he exercised without eating shrimp. He had a history of atopic dermatitis and allergic rhinitis since childhood. Laboratory data showed that total serum IgE was 462 IU/mL (reference range: 170–232 IU/mL), while specific IgE (sIgE) titers to shrimp, wheat, gluten and omega-5 gliadin were under detection limit (i.e. <0.34 U_A/mL) (ImmunoCAP™, Thermo Scientific, Tokyo, Japan). No significant skin reactions were induced in skin prick test (SPT) by using commercially available extracts from wheat, bread and shrimp (Torii, Tokyo, Japan).

Q1. Which one of the following is the most likely diagnosis?

A. Chronic spontaneous urticaria
B. Cholinergic urticaria
C. Solar urticaria
D. Food-dependent exercise-induced anaphylaxis

Answer*: The correct answer is* ***D****.*

Classic food allergy is an IgE-mediated hypersensitivity to a certain food, producing a series of allergic symptoms approximately 15–30 min post-ingestion of the causative agent. Food-dependent exercise-induced anaphylaxis (FDEIA) is a unique type of food allergy characterized by allergic reactions evoked by exercise mostly within 2 h after the ingestion of the culprit food [1, 2]. Importantly, neither the food

M. Hiragun · S. Takahagi · M. Hide (✉)
Department of Dermatology, Institute of Biomedical and Health Sciences, Hiroshima University, Hiroshima, Japan

N. Rezaei (ed.), *Pediatric Allergy*, https://doi.org/10.1007/978-3-030-18282-3_19

ingestion nor the exercise alone can induce the allergic symptoms in a patient with FDEIA. A variety of foods have been identified as allergens for FDEIA, in various geographical regions. In Japan, wheat is the most frequent causative food, followed by shrimp. Clinically history of our patients implies a shrimp-associated FDEIA. Surprisingly, no evidence of the hypersensitivity to shrimp was noted in SPT with commercially available shrimp extract.

As for the mechanism of the induction of allergic reactions in FDEIA, it is important to note that sIgE to wheat antigens such as omega-5 gliadin can be found in sera of most patients with wheat-associated FDEIA (WDEIA) [1]. One theory suggests that physical exercise disrupts normal physical barrier of the gastrointestinal tract mucosa, resulting in the absorption of undigested food antigens. Critically, gliadin levels increase in sera of patients with WDEIA, acutely after exercise post-wheat intake [1]. Thus, FDEIA is speculated to arise from both the absorption of undigested causative antigen by the exercise and the IgE-mediated hypersensitivity to the absorbed antigen [1, 3].

Q2. Which one of the following is the most appropriate next step evaluation of this patient's condition?

A. Check for specific IgE to common food items
B. Skin prick test by using whole shrimp antigen
C. Intradermal skin test using commercially available shrimp extracts
D. Oral provocation test for shrimp

Answer: *The correct answer is* ***B***.

In our case, wheal and flare were induced by SPT utilizing fresh meat of white pacific shrimp (*Litopenaeus vannamei*), but not against those of black tiger shrimp (*Penaeus monodon*) and northern shrimp (*Pandalus borealis*) (Fig. 19.1). We finally made a diagnosis of FDEIA due to white pacific shrimp.

A challenge test of exercise with the oral provocation of a putative causal food is necessary for more reliable diagnosis of FDEIA. However, skin test, either by prick or intradermal injection with food extracts, is performed in necessary, as provocation test may result in the induction of a life-threatening attack.

SPT is readily performed using extracts of suspected foods, with identified allergens in shrimps, tropomyosin, arginine kinase, sarcoplasmic calcium-binding protein, myosin light chain, troponin C and triosephosphate isomerase, or using whole shrimp for prick to prick test [4]. However, the causative shrimp antigen associated with FDEIA has not yet been elucidated. Commercially available shrimp extracts usually consist of 2 or 3 kinds of shrimp extracts, but may not represent all shrimp antigens. Therefore, SPT using causative shrimp meat is important, especially when SPT using commercially available antigens are negative. Generally, intradermal skin test is more sensitive than SPT, but yields high false negative results. Moreover, the potential risk of anaphylaxis by intradermal skin test should be considered if the patient is extremely sensitive to the antigen.

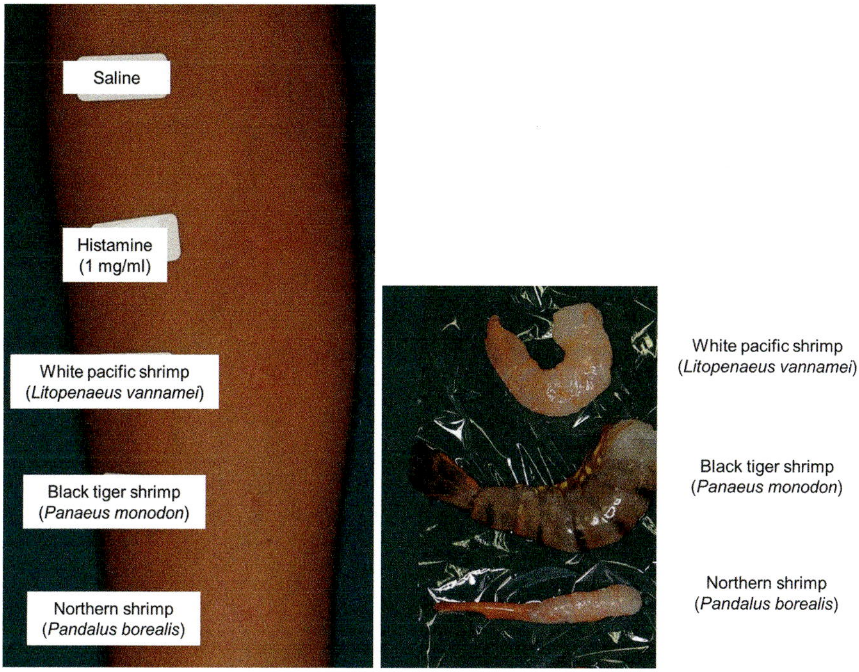

Fig. 19.1 Skin prick tests utilizing fresh meat of white pacific shrimp (*Litopenaeus vannamei*), black tiger shrimp (*Penaeus monodon*) and northern shrimp (*Pandalus borealis*)

Q3. Which one of the following is the most appropriate medical aid in case his allergic reaction progresses to systemic symptoms, such as dyspnea and loss of consciousness?

A. Topical antihistamine ointment
B. Oral non-sedative antihistamine
C. Systemic corticosteroid
D. Oral cyclosporine
E. Intramuscular injection of epinephrine

Answer: *The correct answer is* ***E***.

Attacks of FDEIA frequently progress to anaphylaxis accompanied with wheezing, dyspnea and loss of consciousness, in which prompt intervention is critical. International guidelines concur on the importance of the intramuscular administration of epinephrine, 0.3 mg/body for adults and 0.01 mg/kg for children, as the first choice in anaphylaxis. Epinephrine is the only medication that reduces the rate of hospitalization and death [5]. The prescription of the epinephrine autoinjectors and education on avoidance and management of anaphylaxis are also recommended because anaphylaxis usually occurs in the absence of healthcare professionals with the rapid progression to the life-threatening emergency.

Q4. Which one of the following is the most adequate instruction for this patient?

A. To avoid both shrimp and exercise
B. To avoid exercise 4 h after eating shrimp
C. To avoid only shrimp
D. To avoid only exercise
E. No restriction on eating shrimp and exercising

Answer: *The correct answer is **B**.*

Patients diagnosed with FDEIA should avoid exercise at least for 2 h, or safely for 4 h, after eating the causative food. While the physician should refrain from the excessive removal of the food and exercise, patients who develop symptoms occasionally without the apparent triggering exercise, should be advised to avoid having the causal food in any context.

Q5. Which one of the following is <u>least</u> likely to provoke an attack after this patient eating the causative shrimp?

A. Taking bath
B. Cleaning
C. Taking oral aspirin
D. Sleeping

Answer: *The correct answer is **D**.*

Since the threshold of the attack was affected by various factors such as patients' general conditions and intake of medicines, the attack of FDEIA was not necessarily induced by the heavy exercise. Even non-heavy daily activities, such as taking a bath, singing and/or cleaning after eating a causative food can be sometimes relevant to the attack of FDEIA. Importantly, intake of aspirin or NSAIDs in combination with the culprit food item can trigger the attack by enhancing antigen uptake across the intestinal epithelium and/or by perpetuating direct activation of mast cells through IgE-mediated cross-linking of antigen binding [1].

Practical Points

- This patient with shrimp-associated Food-dependent exercise-induced anaphylaxis (FDEIA) showed hypersensitivity to only the white pacific shrimp
- Both serum shrimp-sIgE and skin prick test by the commercially available kit and shrimp extract were negative in this patient
- The hypersensitivity to white pacific shrimp was proved only by the skin prick test utilizing fresh white pacific shrimp meat, leading to the diagnosis of shrimp-associated FDEIA
- Avoidance of exercise for at least 2 h after having the causative food is essential for patients with FDEIA
- Once life-threatening anaphylaxis occurs, intramuscular epinephrine must be promptly administered regardless of the trigger

References

1. Morita E, Matsuo H, Chinuki Y, Takahashi H, Dahlström J, Tanaka A. Food-dependent exercise-induced anaphylaxis -importance of omega-5 gliadin and HMW-glutenin as causative antigens for wheat-dependent exercise-induced anaphylaxis. Allergol Int. 2009;58(4):493–8.
2. Harada S, Horikawa T, Ashida M, Kamo T, Nishioka E, Ichihashi M. Aspirin enhances the induction of type I allergic symptoms when combined with food and exercise in patients with food-dependent exercise-induced anaphylaxis. Br J Dermatol. 2001;145(2):336–9.
3. Matsuo H, Morimoto K, Akaki T, Kaneko S, Kusatake K, Kuroda T, Niihara H, Hide M, Morita E. Exercise and aspirin increase levels of circulating gliadin peptides in patients with wheat-dependent exercise-induced anaphylaxis. Clin Exp Allergy. 2005;35(4):461–6.
4. Matsuo H, Yokooji T, Taogoshi T. Common food allergens and their IgE-binding epitopes. Allergol Int. 2015;64(4):332–43.
5. Simons FE, Ebisawa M, Sanchez-Borges M, Thong BY, Worm M, Tanno LK, Lockey RF, El-Gamal YM, Brown SG, Park HS, Sheikh A. 2015 update of the evidence base: World Allergy Organization anaphylaxis guidelines. World Allergy Organ J. 2015;8(1):32.

Chapter 20
Reflux and Failure to Thrive

David A. Hill

A 2-year-old patient was seen at Children's Hospital of Philadelphia for symptoms of vomiting, regurgitation, and poor growth and development. Regurgitation and vomiting started at 14 months of age, and she subsequently dropped from the 15th to the 5th percentile for weight. Developmentally, she was unsteady ambulating independently and had a mild speech delay. She had not experienced hives, respiratory distress, or associated diarrhea. The patient was exclusively breast fed until 6 months of age when her parents introduced complementary foods. At the time of presentation, her diet comprised of milk, egg, wheat, soy, oat, rice, pork, fish, turkey, peanut and other legumes, tree nuts, banana, pear, and avocado. Her personal medical history was otherwise uneventful, though her family history was notable for IgE-mediated food allergy in her mother and brother, and allergic rhinitis in her father. Other than a cat at home, her social history was unremarkable.

A thorough physical examination was notable for an alert, but small child with a benign abdominal exam. Skin-prick allergy testing was performed for common allergenic foods and was negative. Due to her predominantly gastrointestinal symptoms, the patient was placed on an optimal gastric acid suppression regimen with a proton pump inhibitor (PPI) and scheduled for an esophagogastroduodenal endoscopy (EGD). Six weeks after initiation of PPI therapy. EGD revealed 75 eosinophils per high-power microscopy field in the mucosa of the distal esophagus (Fig. 20.1a). The patient was instructed to eliminate milk, egg, and soy. Six weeks after initiating food elimination, her symptoms improved and a repeat EGD revealed normal esophageal mucosa without eosinophilic infiltration (Fig. 20.1b). The patient's growth and developmental delay improved over the course of the following months. Six and 12 months later, milk and soy were re-introduced into the patient's diet,

D. A. Hill (✉)
Division of Allergy and Immunology, Department of Pediatrics,
Children's Hospital of Philadelphia, Philadelphia, PA, USA
e-mail: hilld3@email.chop.edu

N. Rezaei (ed.), *Pediatric Allergy*, https://doi.org/10.1007/978-3-030-18282-3_20

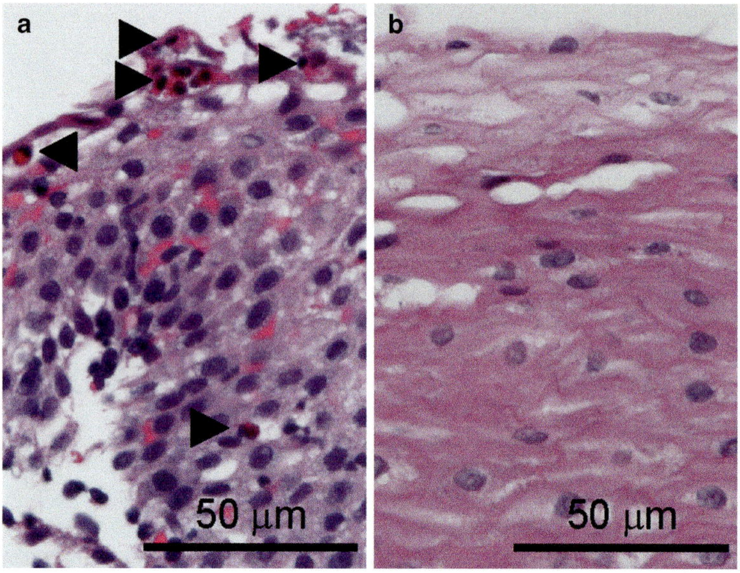

Fig. 20.1 Hematoxylin and eosin staining of esophageal tissue sections from a patient with eosinophilic esophagitis before (**a**), and after 6 weeks of food avoidance resulting in remission (**b**). Eosinophils are marked with arrows

without re-accumulation of mucosal eosinophils on repeat EGD. Accidental egg consumption at the age of 3.5 years resulted in return of gastrointestinal symptoms, and subsequent EGD revealed eosinophil infiltration.

Q1. Which of the one following is the most likely diagnosis?

A. IgE-mediated food allergy
B. Eosinophilic gastritis
C. Food Protein-Induced Enterocolitis Syndrome
D. Eosinophilic esophagitis
E. Gastroesophageal reflux disease

Answer: *The correct answer is* ***D***.

The patient's presentation and EGD results are consistent with a diagnosis of eosinophilic esophagitis (EoE). EoE is a chronic allergic inflammatory disease that, if left untreated, can result in significant impairment in the quality of life secondary to odynophagia, food impaction, esophageal stricture formation, and in rare and extreme cases esophageal rupture [1, 2]. When a diagnosis of EoE is made, it is imperative that measures be taken to eliminate or control inflammation, via either food avoidance or use of swallowed topical steroid preparations, for both symptomatic relief and prevention of complications [3].

Q2. Which one of the following is the most common laboratory or histologic finding in this condition?

A. Neutropenia
B. Eosinophil infiltrates and epithelial barrier defects
C. Elevated allergen-specific serum IgE level
D. Peripheral eosinophilia
E. Th17 cell-mediated esophageal fibrosis

Answer: *The correct answer is **B**.*

From a histopathological point of view, EoE is characterized by esophageal eosinophil infiltrates and epithelial barrier defects [4]. A clinical diagnosis is made by the presence of 15 or more eosinophils per high-power field in one or more of at least four esophageal biopsy specimens obtained via EGD [5].

Q3. Which of the following foods are the most common causes of the patient's disease process?

A. Peanut, meats, wheat, and soy
B. Milk, egg, wheat, and soy
C. Egg, milk, peanut, and tree nuts
D. Legumes, wheat, beef, and soy
E. Oat, egg, peanut, and soy

Answer: *The correct answer is **B**.*

The most common foods that cause EoE are milk, egg, wheat, soy, corn, and meats (Table 20.1) [6, 7]. Consistent with EoE falling on the allergic spectrum, the inflammation observed in EoE responds to allergen avoidance and/or topical steroid applications [8–10]. Elemental diets are highly effective in inducing histologic and clinical remission in children with EoE, though adherence to these diets is frequently

Table 20.1 Most common cause of Eosinophilic Esophagitis (EOE)

Food	Percentage in all EOE
Milk	35%
Egg	13%
Wheat	12%
Soy	9%
Corn	6%
Beef	5%
Chicken	5%
Peanut	3%
Potato	3%
Pork	3%
Rice	2%
Other	2%

poor [11, 12]. Alternative diets have been examined such as empiric elimination diets, based on the most commonly identified etiologic foods, and allergy testing-directed diets [13].

Q4. One would consider EGD endoscopy in all of the following conditions, except:

A. A 3-year-old girl with atopic history, regurgitation, and halitosis
B. A 10-year-old girl with odynophagia, who ingests soy
C. A 5-year-old boy with abdominal pain and distention after ingestion of milk
D. A 12-month infant with coffee ground vomiting
E. A 4-year old boy with gel-like, dark feces and a history of intermittent colicky abdominal pain for the last 12 h

***Answer**: The correct answer is **E**.*

Practical Points

- Eosinophilic esophagitis (EoE) is a chronic allergic inflammatory disease that can cause significant impairment in quality of life
- It is imperative to take measures to eliminate or control inflammation in EoE for both symptomatic relief and the prevention of esophageal strictures
- Patient history, and not cutaneous allergy testing, is the most useful source of information to determine if a patient requires endoscopic evaluation for EoE

References

1. DeBrosse CW, Franciosi JP, King EC, Butz BK, Greenberg AB, Collins MH, Abonia JP, Assa'ad A, Putnam PE, Rothenberg ME. Long-term outcomes in pediatric-onset esophageal eosinophilia. J Allergy Clin Immunol. 2011;128(1):132–8.
2. Hill DA, Spergel JM. The immunologic mechanisms of eosinophilic esophagitis. Curr Allergy Asthma Rep. 2016;16(2):9.
3. Schoepfer AM, Safroneeva E, Bussmann C, Kuchen T, Portmann S, Simon HU, Straumann A. Delay in diagnosis of eosinophilic esophagitis increases risk for stricture formation in a time-dependent manner. Gastroenterology. 2013;145(6):1230–6.e1-2.
4. Simon D, Radonjic-Hosli S, Straumann A, Yousefi S, Simon HU. Active eosinophilic esophagitis is characterized by epithelial barrier defects and eosinophil extracellular trap formation. Allergy. 2015;70(4):443–52.
5. Dellon ES, Liacouras CA, Molina-Infante J, Furuta GT, Spergel JM, Zevit N, Spechler SJ, Attwood SE, Straumann A, Aceves SS, Alexander JA, Atkins D, Arva NC, Blanchard C, Bonis PA, Book WM, Capocelli KE, Chehade M, Cheng E, Collins MH, Davis CM, Dias JA, Di Lorenzo C, Dohil R, Dupont C, Falk GW, Ferreira CT, Fox A, Gonsalves NP, Gupta SK, Katzka DA, Kinoshita Y, Menard-Katcher C, Kodroff E, Metz DC, Miehlke S, Muir AB, Mukkada VA, Murch S, Nurko S, Ohtsuka Y, Orel R, Papadopoulou A, Peterson KA, Philpott H, Putnam PE,

Richter JE, Rosen R, Rothenberg ME, Schoepfer A, Scott MM, Shah N, Sheikh J, Souza RF, Strobel MJ, Talley NJ, Vaezi MF, Vandenplas Y, Vieira MC, Walker MM, Wechsler JB, Wershil BK, Wen T, Yang G-Y, Hirano I, Bredenoord AJ. Updated international consensus diagnostic criteria for eosinophilic esophagitis: proceedings of the AGREE conference. Gastroenterology. 2018;155(4):1022–1033.e10.

6. Hill DA, Dudley JW, Spergel JM. The prevalence of eosinophilic esophagitis in pediatric patients with IgE-mediated food allergy. J Allergy Clin Immunol Pract. 2017;5(2):369–75.
7. Spergel JM, Brown-Whitehorn TF, Cianferoni A, Shuker M, Wang ML, Verma R, Liacouras CA. Identification of causative foods in children with eosinophilic esophagitis treated with an elimination diet. J Allergy Clin Immunol. 2012;130(2):461–7.e5.
8. Aceves SS, Bastian JF, Newbury RO, Dohil R. Oral viscous budesonide: a potential new therapy for eosinophilic esophagitis in children. Am J Gastroenterol. 2007;102(10):2271–9. quiz 80.
9. Konikoff MR, Noel RJ, Blanchard C, Kirby C, Jameson SC, Buckmeier BK, Akers R, Cohen MB, Collins MH, Assa'ad AH, Aceves SS, Putnam PE, Rothenberg ME. A randomized, double-blind, placebo-controlled trial of fluticasone propionate for pediatric eosinophilic esophagitis. Gastroenterology. 2006;131(5):1381–91.
10. Dohil R, Newbury R, Fox L, Bastian J, Aceves S. Oral viscous budesonide is effective in children with eosinophilic esophagitis in a randomized, placebo-controlled trial. Gastroenterology. 2010;139(2):418–29.
11. Markowitz JE, Spergel JM, Ruchelli E, Liacouras CA. Elemental diet is an effective treatment for eosinophilic esophagitis in children and adolescents. Am J Gastroenterol. 2003;98(4):777–82.
12. Peterson KA, Byrne KR, Vinson LA, Ying J, Boynton KK, Fang JC, Gleich GJ, Adler DG, Clayton F. Elemental diet induces histologic response in adult eosinophilic esophagitis. Am J Gastroenterol. 2013;108(5):759–66.
13. Lucendo AJ. Meta-analysis-based guidance for dietary management in eosinophilic esophagitis. Curr Gastroenterol Rep. 2015;17(10):464.

Chapter 21
Abdominal Rash and a History of Hirschsprung

Mahboubeh Mansouri

Our patients was a 10-year-old boy, who was consulted due to an eczematous rash in the abdominal region. He had a history of severe constipation since 10 days old. A colostomy had been performed after confirming the diagnosis of Hirschsprung at 6 years old. However soiling and constipation continued after re-anastomosis and pull through surgery. The boy also had multiple episodes of diarrhea and fever, leading to repetitive hospitalizations. As the constipation did not respond to any treatment, an appendicostomy was performed, yet rectorrhagia and bleeding from the site of surgery, nausea and vomiting had persisted then after.

In his past medical history, the boy was diagnosed with asthma. He also had refractory seizures from 3 years old which were irresponsive to a number of anticonvulsive drugs. The boy had developed several episodes of drug allergy reactions as a consequence of antiepileptic drugs as well. All other laboratory findings including autoantibody screening, immunoglobulin levels, stool exams for parasites, as well as all radiological evaluations were normal.

In one colonic mucosal biopsy, ulcerative surfaces and severe infiltration of acute inflammatory cells with eosinophil dominance was reported. His CBC was normal apart from eosinophilia (700/μL) and anemia (Hb: 9 mg/dL). Skin prick test was highly positive for weed and tree pollens and foods like egg yolk, peanut, and soy.

Q1. What is the most probable diagnosis?

A. HIV disease
B. Inflammatory bowel disease
C. Primary immunodeficiency diseases
D. Eosinophilic associated gastrointestinal disorders

M. Mansouri (✉)
Department of Immunology and Allergy, Mofid Children's Hospital, Shahid Beheshti University of Medical Sciences, Tehran, Iran
e-mail: m.mansouri@sbmu.ac.ir

N. Rezaei (ed.), *Pediatric Allergy*, https://doi.org/10.1007/978-3-030-18282-3_21

Answer*: The correct answer is* ***D****.*

Eosinophilic gastrointestinal disorders (EGIDs) are defined by abnormal eosinophilic infiltration of different segments of the gastrointestinal tract in the absence of secondary causes, including collagen vascular disease, malignancy, or parasitic infections [1].

Clinical manifestations depend on the involved sites and layers and may include abdominal pain, nausea, vomiting, diarrhea, weight loss, gastrointestinal bleeding, intestinal malabsorption, even ascites or protein loosing enteropathy (PLE) [2]. Anemia with or without apparent gastrointestinal bleeding is an important clinical finding to look for [2].

Q2. All of the below findings are in favor of eosinophilic associated gastrointestinal disorders, except:

A. No response to elimination diets
B. Normal tissue pathology
C. Absence of peripheral eosinophilia
D. Negative skin prick test for food allergens

Answer*: The correct answer is* ***A****.*

EGIDs is considered an allergic condition and strongly associates with a higher prevalence of other allergic disorders [1]. Peripheral blood eosinophilia are not necessary for the diagnosis, and negative histological findings cannot exclude the possibility of eosinophilic gastroenteritis. Because eosinophilic infiltration is usually patchy in distribution, biopsy from multiple sites should be obtained.

Q3. What classification of hypersensitivity reactions is the main immunological mechanisms involved in EGID?

A. IgE-mediated reaction (type 1)
B. Antibody-mediated cell cytotoxicity (type 2)
C. Immune complex disease (type 3)
D. Cell-mediated hypersensitivity reactions (type 4)

Answer*: The correct answer is* ***D****.*

It is believed that cell-mediated hypersensitivity is the main immunological mechanism involved in EGID, as allergen-specific IgE (sIgE) is usually negative in most patients [2]. There is a strong association of EGID with food allergies, environmental allergies, asthma, and atopic dermatitis [3, 4]. Recently, an empiric diet, preferentially devoid of the six most common food-allergens, milk, soy, egg, wheat, peanuts, tree nuts, shellfish, and fish (six food elimination diet) has been suggested with significant improvement in patients with EGID and efficacy reaching equivalent to topical steroids [5, 6].

Q4. All of the followings are correct treatment, except:

A. Topical budesonide
B. Prednisolone
C. Six foods avoidance
D. Bone marrow transplantation

Answer*: The correct answer is* ***D****.*

All the mentioned treatments, except Answer D, are widely accepted in the treatment of EGID [7].

Practical Points

- In contrast to IgE-mediated clinical reaction in food allergy the clinical presentations in Eosinophilic associated gastrointestinal disorders (EGID) are not straight forward and might be misleading
- Clinical symptoms are variable according to the site and layer of infiltration of eosinophils in esophagus, stomach, duodenum or colon or location of eosinophil infiltration in submucosal, muscular or subserosal layers
- The diagnosis of EGID needs a high index of suspicion by the physician
- The diagnosis of EGID should be considered in the presence of any chronic symptoms in the GI tract, with or without atopic diathesis
- Multiple biopsies depending on site of the involvement, must be taken, in spite of normal look mucosa

References

1. Mansoor E, Saleh MA, Cooper GS. Prevalence of eosinophilic gastroenteritis and colitis in a population-based study, from 2012 to 2017. Clin Gastroenterol Hepatol. 2017;15(11):1733–41.
2. Tien FM, Wu JF, Jeng YM, Hsu HY, Ni YH, Chang MH, Lin DT, Chen HL. Clinical features and treatment responses of children with eosinophilic gastroenteritis. Pediatr Neonatol. 2011;52(5):272–8.
3. Schoepfer A. Diagnostic approach to eosinophilic oesophagitis: pearls and pitfalls. Best Pract Res Clin Gastroenterol. 2015;29(5):783–92.
4. Leung J, Beukema KR, Shen AH. Allergic mechanisms of Eosinophilic oesophagitis. Best Pract Res Clin Gastroenterol. 2015;29(5):709–20.
5. Wang F, Han J. Delayed eosinophilic gastroenteritis, a possible side effect of clopidogrel? Int J Cardiol. 2013;165(3):e53–4.
6. Yamada Y, Kato M, Isoda Y, Nishi A, Jinbo Y, Hayashi Y. Eosinophilic gastroenteritis treated with a multiple-food elimination diet. Allergol Int. 2014;63(Suppl 1):53–6.
7. Siewert E, Lammert F, Koppitz P, Schmidt T, Matern S. Eosinophilic gastroenteritis with severe protein-losing enteropathy: successful treatment with budesonide. Dig Liver Dis. 2006;38(1):55–9.

Chapter 22
Recurrent Sepsis-Like Episodes

Purificacion Gonzalez-Delgado and Javier Fernandez

A 16-month old girl born at full term by cesarean section was brought to our allergy clinic for workup of what was apparently a food allergy. She was exclusively breast-fed until 4 months of age, after which supplemental formula and solid foods were introduced without problems. At 11 months of age she had to be transferred to emergency department with acute profuse vomiting, pallor, lethargy, and loss of consciousness. Her family reported no history of toxin ingestion or head injury. Physical examination revealed a severely ill, irritable and unresponsive patient with a body temperature of 35.6 °C, heart rate of 130 bpm, hypotonia, hypotension (81/39 mmHg) and a Glasgow coma score between 9 and 10. She had no visible skin lesions at the onset of symptoms. She was admitted to the pediatric intensive care unit, where an extensive workup was performed, revealing metabolic acidosis (pH: 7.25, venous pCO_2: 50 mmHg, HCO_3^-: 21.3 mmol/L, base excess: −3.8 mmol/L), leukocytosis (WBC: 15,080/μL, with 69.4% neutrophils), a platelet count of 327,000/μL and a CRP level of 22 mg/L. A lumbar puncture and cranial CT scan gave normal results. An abdominal ultrasound was performed to exclude intestinal invagination. Blood, urine and stool cultures were taken.

The patient improved clinically within 1–2 h of IV fluid therapy, without antibiotic administration. She had an episode of watery diarrhea a few hours later and was discharged 24 h after admission with a diagnosis of suspected viral gastroenteritis, with all cultures returning negative.

One and two weeks later, the baby had two similar episodes, accompanied by metabolic acidosis. Symptoms again resolved within a few hours of fluid therapy, with diarrhea occurring in the following 12 h. An exhaustive study was performed,

P. Gonzalez-Delgado
Allergy Section, Alicante University General Hospital-ISABIAL, Alicante, Spain

J. Fernandez (✉)
Allergy Section, Alicante University General Hospital-ISABIAL, Alicante, Spain

Department of Clinical Medicine, Miguel Hernandez University, Alicante, Spain
e-mail: fj.fernandez@umh.es

N. Rezaei (ed.), *Pediatric Allergy*, https://doi.org/10.1007/978-3-030-18282-3_22

including screening for toxins in urine, cerebrospinal fluid analysis, serum amino acids and organic acids in urine, all giving results within normal limits. The study was completed with an electroencephalogram, cardiac ultrasound and sweat diagnostic tests, which did not reveal any significant abnormalities.

In our allergy unit, a careful clinical history was taken, revealing that the patient had ingested different species of fish (European hake, panga, white hake) 2–3 h before all the episodes, although she had tolerated fish on previous occasions since it was first introduced to her diet at 10 months of age. She had a positive family history of atopy and her mother suffered from allergic rhinitis.

Allergy tests, including a skin prick test for different foods and fish species, were negative. Total IgE was 10 IU/mL (reference range: 0–100 IU/mL) and specific IgE (sIgE) using ImmunoCAP, was negative to a series of foods and fish species.

At 20 months of age, the patient underwent an open oral food challenge (OFC) to sole fish in a hospital setting. Two hours later she developed vomiting, pallor, lethargy and hypotension. She recovered within a few hours of IV rehydration but had diarrhea a few hours later. A slight elevation in neutrophils was detected 6 h after the challenge.

We followed up and reassessed the patient every 2 years. She avoided all types of fish, and no new episodes occurred. Her height and weight were in the 50th percentiles. We performed sIgE measurement and skin tests (prick and patch tests) with fish during each assessment and the results were always negative.

To assess tolerance acquisition, another OFC to Hake fish was performed when the patient was 4 years old. Two hours after ingesting a serving of hake, she experienced vomiting with abdominal pain and pallor. She recovered spontaneously within 3 h, but had diarrhea a few hours later. No treatment was needed on this occasion.

Q1. What is the most probable diagnosis?

A. Anaphylactic reaction
B. Viral gastroenteritis
C. Toxic ingestion
D. Recurrent sepsis
E. Food protein-induced enterocolitis syndrome

Answer*: The correct answer is* ***E****.*

Anaphylactic reactions usually occur within 30 min of exposure to the allergen, and though they may start with repetitive vomiting and diarrhea, skin and respiratory symptoms are usually also present. These symptoms are absent in food-protein induced enterocolitis syndrome (FPIES). Skin testing is the most effective way to differentiate between the two conditions. FPIES is considered a non-IgE mediated food allergy, although occasionally some patients may develop sIgE to the implicated food [1].

Viral and bacterial gastroenteritis also manifest with the same symptoms as FPIES, but the recurrence of vomiting after ingestion of a certain food suggests food intolerance rather than infectious gastroenteritis or toxic ingestion. Sepsis and acute FPIES may share clinical and laboratory features, but the rapid recovery of the child after IV rehydration in all episodes with normal or slightly elevated inflammatory markers in FPIES attacks, rules out sepsis. Acute FPIES typically occurs in infancy and is characterized by profuse vomiting, diarrhea, pallor and lethargy that appear 1–4 h after food intake. Severe cases may progress to hypotension, acidosis or methemoglobinemia [1].

An uncommon chronic form of FPIES has been reported in infants younger than 4 months of age who ingest the offending food on a regular basis. This form of the disorder is characterized by chronic diarrhea, intermittent vomiting and failure to thrive [1]. The prevalence of FPIES is not well known [1]. Katz reported a 0.34% prevalence of cow's milk FPIES [2], and the incidence in Australian infants under 24 months of age was reported 15.4 in 100,000 per year [2].

The foods most commonly implicated in FPIES are cow's milk, soy and grains, although several others items have also been implicated, such as chicken, egg and nuts [3, 4]. In older children and adults, fish and shellfish are the most common relevant triggers [5, 6]. Importantly, about 30% of patients may have symptoms with more than one group of food items.

Many patients loose sensitivity by the age of 2 or 3 years, these stats are yet heterogeneous and patients who subsequently develop sIgE antibodies to the offending food, as well as patients with solid-food FPIES, are at risk to a protracted course [7]. The diagnostic criteria for FPIES have already been reported in previous publications and will also be discussed in next chapter [8, 9].

Q2. Which of the following is the most appropriate next step for assessing and managing this patient's condition?

A. Careful clinical history
B. Prick test to suspected foods
C. Patch test
D. Detection of specific IgE to foods
E. Oral food challenge

Answer: *The correct answer is* ***A***.

Diagnosis of FPIES is based on clinical history, exclusion of other causes and OFC. Infants often present with multiple reactions and an extensive evaluation and history taking is required to establish a FPIES diagnosis, especially in FPIES to solid foods. Fortunately, the causative food is identified through careful history taking in most patients and OFC should only be performed when the diagnosis is not well established, when a food trigger is not identified, or to determine whether the patient has grown out of FPIES, and the procedure should always take place in a medically supervised setting with access to fluid resuscitation. The usual recommended procedure consists of administration of 0.06–0.6 mg of food protein per kilogram of body weight in three equal doses over 30 min. In severe reactions the initial dose may be lower and the observation period between doses may be longer [8]. Complete blood counts obtained before and after challenge show an increase in the neutrophil count [1]. Specific IgE and skin prick test are not usually performed in the initial assessment, but these tests are recommended before assessing tolerance acquisition through an OFC. In positive cases the protocol must be adapted with gradually increasing doses [10].

Patch testing is not routinely performed in the diagnosis of FPIES, as conflicting results have been reported in the literature and its value is therefore unclear [11, 12].

Q3. Which one of the followings entities must be considered in the differential diagnoses of this patient?

A. Sepsis
B. Necrotizing enterocolitis
C. Pyloric stenosis
D. Inborn errors of metabolism
E. All of the above

Answer*: The correct answer is* ***E****.*

People with acute FPIES are often misdiagnosed with sepsis in the emergency room. Fever is a cardinal symptom of sepsis but can be absent in severe cases. Otherwise, leukocytosis, elevated neutrophil count, metabolic acidosis, and methemoglobinemia may be present in both conditions. Inflammatory markers can be used to differentiate between them [13].

In neonates, especially premature and low birth weight infants, necrotizing enterocolitis (NEC) is another entity that shares clinical features with FPIES. The pathognomonic sign of NEC is intramural gas on abdominal X-ray [14]. Pyloric stenosis also occurs in the first weeks of life and manifests with persistent vomiting, leading to dehydration and shock in some cases. An ultrasound scan can confirm the diagnosis [15]. Inborn errors of metabolism must be considered in differential diagnosis of metabolic acidosis. In such cases, blood ammonia, blood gases, liver and renal function tests, blood lactate, and serum and urinary amino acids should be sent [16].

Some patients with FPIES even undergo surgery due to suspicion of acute surgical abdomen [17].

In general, rapid resolution of symptoms after fluid therapy and the recurrence of episodes upon re-exposure to the offending food are characteristic of acute FPIES.

Q4. Which mechanisms or cells have been demonstrated after food challenge in FPIES?

A. Neutrophil activation
B. Absence of specific T cells involved in food antigen recognition
C. Innate immune system activation
D. TNF-alpha elevation
E. All of the above

Answer*: The correct answer is* ***E****.*

Classically, FPIES has been considered a T-cell-mediated disease. After exposure to food allergens, activated peripheral mononuclear cells upregulate TNF-α production, inducing local intestinal inflammation [18]. A broad activation of $CD4^+$, $CD8^+$, and $\gamma\delta$ lymphocytes has also been reported [19]. The role of humoral response appears to be limited in FPIES [20].

Recently, a broad systemic activation of innate immune cells including neutrophils, monocytes, eosinophils and natural killer cells has also been detected in FPIES attack [9].

Otherwise, the mechanism of antigen recognition remains unclear, and antigen-specific B or T cell responses have not been shown to expand in FPIES [21]. It has been also suggested that locally produced IgE in the intestinal mucosa exacerbates local intestinal inflammation, yet is not reflected in serum IgE levels.

Q5. Which one of the following is the most appropriate treatment in the acute phase of FPIES?

A. Adrenaline
B. Aggressive fluid resuscitation
C. Ondansetron
D. Supplemental oxygen
E. Antibiotic therapy

Answer*: The correct answer is* ***B****.*

The acute phase of severe FPIES must be treated with aggressive fluid resuscitation, as hypovolemic shock may develop. Supplemental oxygen and ventilation may also be required in severe cases. Although some authors have reported that ondansetron may shorten the duration of the reaction, more studies are needed to confirm its value in FPIES, and special caution should be administered in children, as ondansetron may prolong the QT interval [9].

Corticosteroids are sometimes administered to children with severe dehydration and hypotension, but there are a paucity of evidence on utility of this approach. Also, epinephrine is not routinely prescribed unless a concomitant IgE-mediated allergy is detected. Similarly, antibiotic therapy is not a useful tool in FPIES management.

In the long-term management of FPIES, avoidance of the offending food is a must, followed by nutritional advice and monitoring to assess tolerance. The timing of reintroduction varies, although most authors suggest a minimum of 12–18 months past the last reaction.

Practical Points

- Food-protein induced enterocolitis syndrome (FPIES) is a non-IgE mediated allergic disorder that typically occurs in infancy, characterized by profuse vomiting and diarrhea and even lethargy
- Symptoms appear 1–4 h after food intake
- Cow's milk, soy and grains are the most common triggers for FPIES
- Most patients recover at 2 or 3 years of age, but the development of specific IgE and solid-food FPIES report of a poor prognosis and prolonged course
- Diagnosis is based on clinical history, exclusion of other causes and oral food challenge
- Differential diagnoses include sepsis, acute gastrointestinal infection, surgical emergencies, metabolic and neurological disorders and other types of food allergy
- Although FPIES is considered to be a result of T-cell-mediated disorder, the pathophysiology is not well known
- The acute phase of severe FPIES must be treated with aggressive fluid resuscitation as a state of shock

References

1. Sicherer SH. Food protein-induced enterocolitis syndrome: case presentations and management lessons. J Allergy Clin Immunol. 2005;115(1):149–56.
2. Sicherer SH. Food protein-induced enterocolitis syndrome: clinical perspectives. J Pediatr Gastroenterol Nutr. 2000;30(Suppl):S45–9.
3. Mehr S, Frith K, Campbell DE. Epidemiology of food protein-induced enterocolitis syndrome. Curr Opin Allergy Clin Immunol. 2014;14(3):208–16.
4. Katz Y, Goldberg MR, Rajuan N, Cohen A, Leshno M. The prevalence and natural course of food protein-induced enterocolitis syndrome to cow's milk: a large-scale, prospective population-based study. J Allergy Clin Immunol. 2011;127(3):647–53.e1-3.
5. Mehr S, Kakakios A, Frith K, Kemp AS. Food protein-induced enterocolitis syndrome: 16-year experience. Pediatrics. 2009;123(3):e459–64.
6. Nowak-Wegrzyn A, Sampson HA, Wood RA, Sicherer SH. Food protein-induced enterocolitis syndrome caused by solid food proteins. Pediatrics. 2003;111(4 Pt 1):829–35.
7. Gonzalez-Delgado P, Caparros E, Moreno MV, Clemente F, Flores E, Velasquez L, Rubio G, Fernandez J. Clinical and immunological characteristics of a pediatric population with food protein-induced enterocolitis syndrome (FPIES) to fish. Pediatr Allergy Immunol. 2016;27(3):269–75.
8. Miceli Sopo S, Monaco S, Badina L, Barni S, Longo G, Novembre E, Viola S, Monti G. Food protein-induced enterocolitis syndrome caused by fish and/or shellfish in Italy. Pediatr Allergy Immunol. 2015;26(8):731–6.
9. Goswami R, Blazquez AB, Kosoy R, Rahman A, Nowak-Wegrzyn A, Berin MC. Systemic innate immune activation in food protein-induced enterocolitis syndrome. J Allergy Clin Immunol. 2017;139(6):1885–96.e9.
10. Caubet JC, Ford LS, Sickles L, Jarvinen KM, Sicherer SH, Sampson HA, Nowak-Wegrzyn A. Clinical features and resolution of food protein-induced enterocolitis syndrome: 10-year experience. J Allergy Clin Immunol. 2014;134(2):382–9.
11. Nowak-Wegrzyn A, Chehade M, Groetch ME, Spergel JM, Wood RA, Allen K, Atkins D, Bahna S, Barad AV, Berin C, Brown Whitehorn T, Burks AW, Caubet JC, Cianferoni A, Conte M, Davis C, Fiocchi A, Grimshaw K, Gupta R, Hofmeister B, Hwang JB, Katz Y, Konstantinou GN, Leonard SA, Lightdale J, McGhee S, Mehr S, Sopo SM, Monti G, Muraro A, Noel SK, Nomura I, Noone S, Sampson HA, Schultz F, Sicherer SH, Thompson CC, Turner PJ, Venter C, Westcott-Chavez AA, Greenhawt M. International consensus guidelines for the diagnosis and management of food protein-induced enterocolitis syndrome: executive summary-workgroup report of the Adverse Reactions to Foods Committee, American Academy of Allergy, Asthma & Immunology. J Allergy Clin Immunol. 2017;139(4):1111–26.e4.
12. Nowak-Wegrzyn A, Assa'ad AH, Bahna SL, Bock SA, Sicherer SH, Teuber SS. Work Group report: oral food challenge testing. J Allergy Clin Immunol. 2009;123(6 Suppl):S365–83.
13. Maloney J, Nowak-Wegrzyn A. Educational clinical case series for pediatric allergy and immunology: allergic proctocolitis, food protein-induced enterocolitis syndrome and allergic eosinophilic gastroenteritis with protein-losing gastroenteropathy as manifestations of non-IgE-mediated cow's milk allergy. Pediatr Allergy Immunol. 2007;18(4):360–7.
14. Fogg MI, Brown-Whitehorn TA, Pawlowski NA, Spergel JM. Atopy patch test for the diagnosis of food protein-induced enterocolitis syndrome. Pediatr Allergy Immunol. 2006;17(5):351–5.
15. Jarvinen KM, Caubet JC, Sickles L, Ford LS, Sampson HA, Nowak-Wegrzyn A. Poor utility of atopy patch test in predicting tolerance development in food protein-induced enterocolitis syndrome. Ann Allergy Asthma Immunol. 2012;109(3):221–2.
16. Fiocchi A, Claps A, Dahdah L, Brindisi G, Dionisi-Vici C, Martelli A. Differential diagnosis of food protein-induced enterocolitis syndrome. Curr Opin Allergy Clin Immunol. 2014;14(3):246–54.

17. Murch SH. Cow's-milk protein as a specific immunological trigger of necrotising enterocolitis--or food protein-induced enterocolitis syndrome in disguise? J Pediatr Gastroenterol Nutr. 2013;56(1):3–4.
18. Pandya S, Heiss K. Pyloric stenosis in pediatric surgery: an evidence-based review. Surg Clin North Am. 2012;92(3):527–39. vii–viii.
19. Jayasooriya S, Fox AT, Murch SH. Do not laparotomize food-protein-induced enterocolitis syndrome. Pediatr Emerg Care. 2007;23(3):173–5.
20. Caubet JC, Nowak-Wegrzyn A. Current understanding of the immune mechanisms of food protein-induced enterocolitis syndrome. Expert Rev Clin Immunol. 2011;7(3):317–27.
21. Caubet JC, Bencharitiwong R, Ross A, Sampson HA, Berin MC, Nowak-Wegrzyn A. Humoral and cellular responses to casein in patients with food protein-induced enterocolitis to cow's milk. J Allergy Clin Immunol. 2017;139(2):572–83.

Chapter 23
Vomiting, Lethargy and Pallor

Melanie A. Ruffner and Terri F. Brown-Whitehorn

A 5-month-old female presented to the allergy clinic for evaluation of recurrent projectile vomiting episodes followed by lethargy and pallor. She had been evaluated twice earlier in the emergency room for these complaints. The child was the product of an uncomplicated pregnancy and born by planned repeat caesarean section at term with no complications. She had been growing well and developing normally, while exclusively breastfed. Three weeks' prior to presentation in allergy clinic, rice cereal was introduced into the infant's diet for the first time. Approximately 2 h later, she developed multiple episodes of non-bloody, non-bilious vomiting with no evidence of hives, stridor, cough or wheeze. No viral prodrome had been noted, and there were no known infections in close contacts. Her mother brought her to the emergency room because she had not tolerated breastfeeding for several hours and then passed a loose stool. On exam in the emergency room, she was tachycardic and her capillary refill was 2 seconds. She was noted to be lethargic with pallor. She was admitted overnight for IV rehydration and the next morning, she had recovered and was tolerating oral intake. Her laboratory results demonstrated normal complete blood count with exception of slightly elevated WBC count of 12,500/μL with ANC of 8500/μL and 2% immature granulocytes. Blood culture was negative at 24 h. She was discharged with presumed gastroenteritis and continued with breastfeeding at home. One week later, rice cereal mixed in breast milk was again attempted and was initially tolerated. However, in 90 min she again developed recurrent vomiting followed by lethargy and pallor. On presentation in the emergency department she was noted to be tachycardic and normotensive but was unable to tolerate oral intake.

M. A. Ruffner (✉) · T. F. Brown-Whitehorn
Division of Allergy and Immunology, Children's Hospital of Philadelphia, Philadelphia, PA, USA

Department of Pediatrics, Perelman School of Medicine at the University of Pennsylvania, Philadelphia, PA, USA
e-mail: ruffnerm@email.chop.edu

N. Rezaei (ed.), *Pediatric Allergy*, https://doi.org/10.1007/978-3-030-18282-3_23

Electrolytes and liver enzymes were with normal limits. Blood counts were again normal except WBC count of 13,100/μL with ANC of 8600/μL and 3% immature granulocytes. Blood culture again was negative and following 1 day of IV fluids rehydration she improved and was discharged.

Q1. Which one of the following is the most likely underlying allergic diagnosis?

A. Food-protein induced proctocolitis
B. IgE mediated food allergy
C. Food-protein mediated enteropathy
D. Acute food protein-induced enterocolitis syndrome
E. Chronic food protein-induced enterocolitis syndrome

***Answer**: The correct answer is **D**.*

Food-protein induced enterocolitis syndrome (FPIES) is a non-IgE mediated food allergy which typically presents in young children under the age of 1 year [1]. Rarely, FPIES reactions can present later in childhood and there have been rare descriptions of FPIES to shellfish in adults [2, 3]. FPIES can present with either acute or chronic forms [1, 4, 5]. Acute FPIES presents when the food allergen is ingested intermittently, and presents with a pattern of recurrent vomiting and pallor which begins 1–4 h after ingestion of food allergen (Table 23.1 for diagnostic criteria). Depending on the severity, episodes may be accompanied by diarrhea, lethargy and can include tachycardia and hypotension requiring IV hydration. In most patients, a history of delayed reproducible reactions fitting this description is sufficient to make a diagnosis of acute FPIES [1, 6].

Chronic FPIES reactions are less common and have been reported in infants under 4 months of age ingesting milk or soy formula [4, 5]. Chronic FPIES presents with recurrent emesis, diarrhea, and failure to thrive which can progress to dehydration and metabolic acidosis in more severe cases. Removal of the offending food from the patient's diet should resolve all symptoms of presumptive FPIES. This

Table 23.1 Diagnostic criteria for patients presenting with possible FPIES

Major criteria	Delayed vomiting 1–4 h after ingestion of suspected food. No evidence of respiratory of skin symptoms of classic IgE mediated food allergy.
Minor criteria	• ≥2 episodes of vomiting after eating the same food
	• Repetitive vomiting 1–4 h after eating a different food
	• Lethargy with suspected reaction
	• Pallor with suspected reaction
	• Need for emergency room visit with suspected reaction
	• Diarrhea 5–10 h after food ingestion
	• Hypotension with suspected reaction
	• Hypothermia with suspected reaction

Diagnosis of FPIES requires history of ≥2 episodes of 1 major and ≥3 minor criteria [1]. If only one episode has occurred, then physician-supervised oral food challenge should be considered
FPIES = Food-protein induced enterocolitis syndrome

is a critical point in clinical diagnosis. If official confirmation of the diagnosis of chronic FPIES is necessary, oral food challenge (OFC) is the only method available (Table 23.1) [1]. However, physician supervision of OFC is necessary as symtoms of acute FPIES reaction can occur with reintroduction of the food. Food protein-induced proctocolitis is a common cause of painless rectal bleeding in an otherwise asymptomatic infant, and typically resolves by 1 year of age [7, 8]. Food protein-induced enteropathy is a syndrome of recurrent abdominal pain, chronic malabsorptive diarrhea, and weight loss resulting from villous atrophy and blunting [9]. Celiac disease is the most common form of food protein-induced enteropathy, but this has been described with other foods including milk and soy [10].

Q2. Which one of the following findings is true regarding laboratory workup of FPIES patients?

A. Abdominal radiography is diagnostic of FPIES
B. Leukopenia is a common finding during acute FPIES attacks
C. FPIES patients can present with acquired hemolytic anemia during acute attacks
D. Patients with chronic FPIES can present with anemia and hypoalbuminemia

***Answer**: The correct answer is **D**.*

There are no radiographic findings which are pathognomonic for FPIES. Laboratory workup is not required for diagnosis of FPIES, however, some typical laboratory findings have been described [1, 11]. Leukocytosis with left shift is seen during acute FPIES episodes. ANC increased ≥1500 above baseline is a supporting minor criteria for diagnosis of FPIES following oral food challenge in addition to lethargy, pallor, diarrhea, hypotension and hypothermia. Methemoglobinemia has been described during acute FPIES episodes, and in rare cases may require treatment with methylene blue and bicarbonate [11]. Anemia and hypoalbuminemia can be seen in chronic FPIES and are thought to be related to malnutrition due to chronic vomiting, diarrhea and failure to thrive [4]. Endoscopy is not recommended in the routine management of FPIES.

Q3. Which of the following foods have been demonstrated to cause FPIES reactions?

A. Milk and soy
B. Rice, Oat, Wheat
C. Legumes, Potato
D. All of the above

***Answer**: The correct answer is **D**.*

There is considerable geographic variation in which foods most commonly cause FPIES, which reflects early-life feeding practices as a potential risk factor. The most common food to cause FPIES is cow's milk, followed by soy and grains (rice, oat, wheat) in the United States [12–14]. In a series of FPIES patients, high cross-reactivity between groups of foods have been reported, e.g. up to 30–40% of patients with FPIES to cow's milk also react to soy [12–14]. If breast milk is tolerated it can be continued or hypoallergenic formula can be used. The majority of children with FPIES to milk tolerate extensively hydrolyzed cow's milk formula, but a minority may require amino-acid based formula [1, 15]. High levels of caution is required with the introduction of grains to patients who have FPIES to another grain as 50% have FPIES to one or more types of grain [12, 13]. Similarly, in the United States the coincidence of poultry FPIES is 40% and for soy and legume FPIES the coincidence is up to 80% [1]. Physicians should be aware of these possible risks and significant geographic variation, as they can assist in guiding food introduction to these patients. For example, lower coincidence of soy FPIES with milk FPIES has been reported in an Israeli birth cohort, and fish is a significant solid food FPIES trigger in Italy and Great Britain [16–18]. Tolerance to one food item from a food group (i.e. grains, poultry, meats, legumes) is a good prognostic sign that the child will tolerate other foods in this group.

Q4. All of the following interventions should be considered in FPIES patients, except:

A. Observation and administration of antiemetics and oral or IV rehydration during active reaction to food allergen exposure
B. Epinephrine autoinjector should be carried and used for FPIES reaction
C. Patients' families should be counseled on food avoidance and given a plan with care instructions in case of accidental ingestion of food allergens
D. Reintroduction of food allergens into the diet should be conducted by clinician-observed oral food challenge

***Answer**: The correct answer is **B**.*

Epinephrine autoinjectors are not routinely recommended for FPIES reactions. However, if patients have comorbid IgE-mediated food allergy an autoinjector should be prescribed and patients should educated about when to use the autoinjector [6]. Emergency planning for accidental ingestions with documented treatment plan is recommended for patient care of patients with IgE food allergy and v [1]. FPIES is a non-IgE mediated allergy and strict avoidance of the allergenic food(s) is the ultimate treatment option for both acute and chronic FPIES [1, 6]. Physician-supervised OFC is recommended for reintroduction of offending food to all children with a history of severe FPIES reaction [1, 15].

Q5. Which of the following is a poor prognostic indicator for resolution of FPIES?

A. Positive allergen skin prick testing to milk
B. Male gender
C. Female gender
D. Onset of FPIES symptoms before 1 year of age

***Answer**: The correct answer is **A**.*

Generally, reintroduction of the culprit food can be considered approximately 12–18 months after the last FPIES reaction, conducted by physician-supervised OFC [15]. Gender and race have not been demonstrated to influence prognosis, however there is significant variation based on geographic area. In a prospective Korean study, all milk FPIES resolved at 24 months and soy FPIES resolved at

14 months [19]. This is significantly different than data in the United States, for example, where retrospective studies indicate that 35% of patients tolerate milk at 24 months and 85% tolerate milk by 5 years. The average age of resolution for FPIES to solid foods is later than that of milk and soy [12–14]. Onset of FPIES under 1 year of age is not associated with poor prognosis for FPIES resolution.

The diagnosis of FPIES is based on clinical criteria and allergy testing is not recommended nor required for routine diagnosis. Serum specific IgE (sIgE) and skin prick test (SPT) are typically negative at initial diagnosis in FPIES patients [12–14]. However, in published series, 0–24% of patients with FPIES to milk develop evidence of specific IgE to milk over time. This is consistent with "atypical" FPIES. Caubet et al. have shown that development of milk-specific IgE to milk, predicted persistence of FPIES symptoms into young adulthood [12]. In contrast, patients with undetectable milk-specific IgE tolerated milk at a median age of 5.1 years. Therefore, food-specific IgE testing to milk may predict patients at risk of persistent FPIES, especially if symptoms including atopic dermatitis and IgE-mediated food allergy are present.

Practical Points

- Food-protein induced enterocolitis syndrome (FPIES) typically presents with a delayed onset of vomiting beginning 1–4 h after ingestion of the offending food(s)
- Classic IgE mediated symptoms including hives, flushing or respiratory symptoms are absent in FPIES
- Rarely, chronic forms of FPIES can present with frequent antigen exposure/ingestion and are characterized by vomiting, diarrhea, weight loss and failure to thrive
- Treatment of FPIES is by removal of the offending food(s) from the diet and supportive care as needed for dehydration and to optimize nutrition
- Diagnosis of FPIES is based on clinical features
- Skin testing and specific-IgE testing do not predict FPIES triggers and have little utility in this non-IgE-mediated disorder
- Prognosis of FPIES in children is generally good and the majority of patients will tolerate the offending food(s) after a period of avoidance

References

1. Nowak-Węgrzyn A, Chehade M, Groetch ME, Spergel JM, Wood RA, Allen K, Atkins D, Bahna S, Barad AV, Berin C, Brown Whitehorn T, Burks AW, Caubet JC, Cianferoni A, Conte M, Davis C, Fiocchi A, Grimshaw K, Gupta R, Hofmeister B, Hwang JB, Katz Y, Konstantinou GN, Leonard SA, Lightdale J, McGhee S, Mehr S, Sopo SM, Monti G, Muraro A, Noel SK, Nomura I, Noone S, Sampson HA, Schultz F, Sicherer SH, Thompson CC, Turner PJ, Venter C, Westcott-Chavez AA, Greenhawt M. International consensus guidelines for the diagnosis and management of food protein–induced enterocolitis syndrome: executive summary—workgroup report of the Adverse Reactions to Foods Committee, American Academy of Allergy, Asthma & Immunology. J Allergy Clin Immunol. 2017;139:1111–26.e4.

2. Fernandes BN, et al. Food protein-induced enterocolitis syndrome can occur in adults. J Allergy Clin Immunol. 2012;130:1199.
3. Tan JA, Smith WB. Non–IgE-mediated gastrointestinal food hypersensitivity syndrome in adults. J Allergy Clin Immunol Pract. 2014;2:355–7.e1.
4. Weinberger T, Feuille E, Thompson C, Nowak-Wegrzyn A. Chronic food protein-induced enterocolitis syndrome: characterization of clinical phenotype and literature review. Ann Allergy Asthma Immunol. 2016;117(3):227–33.
5. Powell GK. Milk- and soy-induced enterocolitis of infancy. Clinical features and standardization of challenge. J Pediatr. 1978;93(4):553–60.
6. Sampson HA, Aceves S, Bock SA, James J, Jones S, Lang D, Nadeau K, Nowak-Wegrzyn A, Oppenheimer J, Perry TT, Randolph C, Sicherer SH, Simon RA, Vickery BP, Wood R, Joint Task Force on Practice P, Bernstein D, Blessing-Moore J, Khan D, Lang D, Nicklas R, Oppenheimer J, Portnoy J, Randolph C, Schuller D, Spector S, Tilles SA, Wallace D, Practice Parameter W, Sampson HA, Aceves S, Bock SA, James J, Jones S, Lang D, Nadeau K, Nowak-Wegrzyn A, Oppenheimer J, Perry TT, Randolph C, Sicherer SH, Simon RA, Vickery BP, Wood R. Food allergy: a practice parameter update-2014. J Allergy Clin Immunol. 2014;134(5):1016–25.e43.
7. Machida HM, Catto Smith AG, Gall DG, Trevenen C, Scott RB. Allergic colitis in infancy: clinical and pathologic aspects. J Pediatr Gastroenterol Nutr. 1994;19(1):22–6.
8. Elizur A, Cohen M, Goldberg MR, Rajuan N, Cohen A, Leshno M, Katz Y. Cow's milk associated rectal bleeding: a population based prospective study. Pediatr Allergy Immunol. 2012;23(8):766–70.
9. Kuitunen P, Visakorpi JK, Savilahti E, Pelkonen P. Malabsorption syndrome with cow's milk intolerance. Clinical findings and course in 54 cases. Arch Dis Child. 1975;50(5):351–6.
10. Savilahti E. Food-induced malabsorption syndromes. J Pediatr Gastroenterol Nutr. 2000;30(Suppl):S61–6.
11. Pecora V, Dahdah L, Mazzina O, Vessicchio D, Fiocchi AG. The clinical prehistory of food-protein induced enterocolitis syndrome (FPIES) twenty-three children. J Allergy Clin Immunol. 2012;137:AB240.
12. Caubet JC, Ford LS, Sickles L, Järvinen KM, Sicherer SH, Sampson HA, Nowak-Węgrzyn A. Clinical features and resolution of food protein-induced enterocolitis syndrome: 10-year experience. J Allergy Clin Immunol. 2014;134:382–9.e4.
13. Ruffner MA, Ruymann K, Barni S, Cianferoni A, Brown-Whitehorn T, Spergel JM. Food protein-induced enterocolitis syndrome: insights from review of a large referral population. J Allergy Clin Immunol In Pract. 2013;1:343–9.
14. Sicherer SH, Eigenmann PA, Sampson HA. Clinical features of food protein-induced enterocolitis syndrome. J Pediatr. 1998;133:214–9.
15. Jarvinen KM, Nowak-Wegrzyn A. Food protein-induced enterocolitis syndrome (FPIES): current management strategies and review of the literature. J Allergy Clin Immunol Pract. 2013;1(4):317–22.
16. Infante S, Marco-Martin G, Sanchez-Dominguez M, Rodriguez-Fernandez A, Fuentes-Aparicio V, Alvarez-Perea A, Cabrera-Freitag P, Morales-Cabeza C, Zubeldia JM, Zapatero L. Food protein-induced enterocolitis syndrome by fish: not necessarily a restricted diet. Allergy. 2018;73:728.
17. Ludman S, Harmon M, Whiting D, Du Toit G. Clinical presentation and referral characteristics of food protein-induced enterocolitis syndrome in the United Kingdom. Ann Allergy Asthma Immunol. 2014;113:290–4.
18. Katz Y, Goldberg MR, Rajuan N, Cohen A, Leshno M. The prevalence and natural course of food protein-induced enterocolitis syndrome to cow's milk: a large-scale, prospective population-based study. J Allergy Clin Immunol. 2011;127:647–53.
19. Hwang JB, Sohn SM, Kim AS. Prospective follow-up oral food challenge in food protein-induced enterocolitis syndrome. Arch Dis Child. 2009;94(6):425–8.

Chapter 24
Nausea, Profuse Sweating, and Flushing After Eating Seafood

Sara Manti, Bianca Faraci, Annamaria Bagnato, and Caterina Cuppari

A young girl of 16 years old presented to the emergency unit with a 1-h history of headache, nausea, itchy, profuse sweating, tongue and face swelling with flushing and shortness of breath. The patient's past medical history was unremarkable for atopic predisposition and/or atopic diseases. She was not taking any drugs. Her illness began immediately after eating cooked tuna.

She reported a burning sensation in her tongue, followed by flushing, starting from her face and spreading through her body. She also described feelings of face, lips, and tongue swelling (Fig. 24.1a). In the emergency room, the patient was afebrile, had a

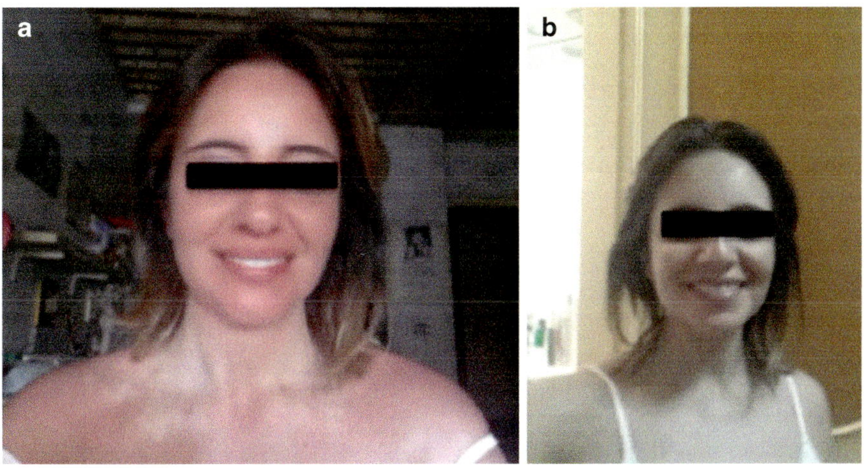

Fig. 24.1 Pictures before and after treatment in a 16-year-old girl with severe systemic reaction in a after ingestion of fish, on admission (**a**) and after 12-h in observation unit (**b**)

S. Manti (✉) · B. Faraci · A. Bagnato · C. Cuppari
Unit of Pediatric, Department of Pediatrics, University of Messina, Messina, Italy
e-mail: smanti@unime.it

N. Rezaei (ed.), *Pediatric Allergy*, https://doi.org/10.1007/978-3-030-18282-3_24

heart rate of 132 bpm, blood pressure of 126/81 mmHg, respiratory rate of 24, and intermittent arterial oxygen saturations of 91% on 3 L by nasal cannula.

She had an erythematous, itchy, papular rash over her face, neck, and torso, decreased breath sounds bilaterally with expiratory wheezes on chest auscultation, and dyspnea. During her hospital stay, she also developed diffuse abdominal pain followed by diarrhea. Her laboratory results were remarkable for a WBC count of 12,300/μL with 11,400 neutrophils/μL. Chest and abdominal radiograph findings were within normal limits.

We also describe four siblings: a 9-year old couple of female twins and two males of 10 years old and 4 years old, respectively. They all were admitted to the emergency room suffering from headache while three of them also presented a flushing. Moreover, one of the twins complained of nausea, diffuse abdominal pain and a sensation of cutaneous warmth and, she presented the most severe cutaneous reaction on her trunk and arms characterized by erythema and wheals as well as tachycardia. None of the siblings showed dyspnea or respiratory symptoms and their vital signs were normal. They all had eaten fried sardines left under the sunlight before cooking.

Q1. Presence or absence of which of the following signs or symptoms would help most in differentiation between food allergy or direct histamine toxicity/release?

A. IgE-mediated food allergy
B. Flushing disorders such as carcinoid syndrome and mast cell activation syndrome
C. Anisakiasis
D. Histamine fish poisoning or scombroid poisoning

Answer*: The correct answer is* ***D****.*

Given the unremarkable history for atopic predisposition and/or atopic diseases, the clinical presentation and its undoubted association with the ingestion of tuna, we consulted an allergologist and a diagnosis of histamine fish poisoning (HFP) was performed.

The differential diagnosis for histamine fish poisoning reactions include an IgE-mediated food allergy, flushing disorders, such as carcinoid syndrome and mast cell activation syndrome, and anisakiasis.

Although in literature the HFP is widely recognized, the cases described are very rare. In fact, given that symptoms result from excess amounts of histamine, the physical manifestations of histamine fish poisoning are similar to those of an allergic reaction, thus, HFP is often misdiagnosed as IgE-mediated fish allergy [1]. However, differently from true food allergy, HFP is mediated by mast cell- and basophil-independent mechanism of histamine toxicity [2]. Moreover, while urinary N-methylhistamine can be elevated in both histamine fish poisoning and IgE-mediated food allergy, serum tryptase and urinary prostaglandins metabolites are within normal range in HFP. This further confirms that mast cell degranulation does not occur in this pathological entity. Moreover, measurement of tryptase and urinary prostaglandins metabolites can help diagnose flushing disorders.

Similarly, in our patients, urinary N-methylhistamine was elevated and serum tryptase and urinary prostaglandins metabolite were normal.

Usually, when anisakiasis occurs, radiologic findings can reveal intestinal wall thickening, mesenteric infiltration, bowel dilatation proximal to the lesion and ascites [3]. Given the abdominal radiographs findings were unremarkable, anisakiasis diagnosis was excluded.

Q2. Which one of the following findings is least likely to be related to patients affected by HFP?

A. Cutaneous symptoms
B. Gastrointestinal symptoms
C. Systemic symptoms
D. All previous answers

Answer*: The correct answer is* ***D****.*

Clinically, HFP is characterized by cutaneous, gastrointestinal as well as systemic symptoms [4, 5], manifesting within minutes of ingesting spoiled fish [6, 7]. According to a retrospective study [8], dermatologic manifestations occur in 82.2%, gastrointestinal symptoms in 37%, neurological in 34.7%, respiratory in 17.4%, weakness and malaise in 4.3% and, finally cardiovascular symptoms in 37.8% of the patients with HFP [8].

The histamine-mediated toxicity is intrinsically benign and most symptoms resolve within 6–8 h, but feelings of malaise can last for a day or more [5]. Severe HFP cases as well as atypical presentation have been also described [5]. Particularly, severe reactions result in hypotension, bronchospasm, respiratory distress, myocardial infarction, and even refractory myocardial dysfunction requiring biventricular assist devices [5]. Vision loss and atrial tachycardia with conduction block have also been reported after eating tuna [4, 5].

Q3. Which one of the following does rule out the diagnosis of HFP in this patients?

A. Histamine levels
B. Skin prick testing
C. Prick to prick test
D. None of the above

Answer*: The correct answer is* ***D****.*

Due to the lack of specific laboratory tests and/or findings, HFP diagnosis is clinical and exclusively based on the characteristic syndrome in close proximity to fish ingestion. Attention should be given to the type of fish ingested, type and degree of cooking, a history of similar reactions in the past, and the time frame between fish ingestion and the onset of symptoms [9]. Moreover, testing the histamine levels, via high-performance liquid chromatography (HPLC), flow injection analysis (FIA) or enzyme-linked immunosorbent assay (ELISA) kit, in the incriminated fish can aid the diagnosis [10]. Generally, a dose of more than 50 mg of histamine per 100 g of fish can causes HFP [10]. If in vitro testing for tissue histamine levels in fish is not available, skin prick test (SPT) and prick to prick test can help diagnose HFP [11]. If the SPT results comes back positive only to the implicated tuna sample, diagnosis of HFP should be hypothesized. The physician should also test a control subject with fresh tuna samples, implicated sample, histamine and saline. If both the patients and the control person both develop a positive SPT to the implicated tuna, the diagnosis of HFP is confirmed.

Q4. Which one of the following treatments is most likely to benefit this patient?

A. H1 antagonists and/or H2 antagonists
B. Epinephrine
C. Intravenous fluids
D. All previous answers

Answer*: The correct answer is* ***D****.*

To date, no double-blind, placebo-controlled trials have been performed to validate treatments or the superiority of one antihistamine or combination of antihistamines over others [12]. Thus, the recommended therapeutic approach was adapted from previous case series studies. Oral H1 antagonists (e.g., diphenhydramine, cetirizine, and chlorpheniramine) are preferred for mild to moderate symptoms. H2 blockers (e.g., cimetidine, famotidine, ranitidine) can also be added.

For more severe clinical presentations, intravenous H1 and H2 blockers are the drugs of choice. Finally, intramuscular injection of epinephrine and intravenous fluids should be considered when the symptoms are particularly severe [12].

Q5. Which one of the following is the most appropriate next step in the evaluation and management of this patient's condition?

A. Avoid fish
B. Adrenaline prescription
C. Histamine antagonists
D. None of the above

Answer*: The correct answer is* ***D****.*

The pathogenesis HFP is a pseudoallergic poisoning caused by the ingestion of histamine-contaminated fish products [13]. The patient does not therefore, require abstention from causative fishes or adrenaline prescription. It is important to communicate to the patient that, in absence of a true food-allergy, future fish ingestions will be safe.

However, patients on isoniazid (INH) and monoamine oxidase inhibitors (MAOIs), which both inhibit histamine metabolism, may be at an increased risk for HFP [14]. Hence, prescribing histamine antagonists for prophylactic purposes could be considered for patients on INH or MAO inhibitors who have had a first episode [14].

Facing the clinical picture of the above described patients, we administered intravenous chlorpheniramine, hydrocortisone and fluids, nebulised salbutamol. After 12 h in an observation unit, all patients were discharged, completely asymptomatic and advice to return if any symptoms recurred (Fig. 24.1b).

Practical Points

- Histamine fish poisoning is a food-borne disease consisting of a pseudoallergic reaction caused by ingestion of histamine-contaminated fish products
- Histamine fish poisoning is often misdiagnosed as IgE-mediated fish allergy
- A well-collected clinical history allows to promptly recognize this condition and to reach a correct diagnosis
- Histamine fish poisoning can present with extremely variable and non-specific presentation
- Histamine fish poisoning should be suspected when there is a history of inadequate cooling and poor preservation of the fish

References

1. Attaran RR, Probst F. Histamine fish poisoning: a common but frequently misdiagnosed condition. Emerg Med J. 2002;19(5):474–5.
2. Brown AF. Therapeutic controversies in the management of acute anaphylaxis. J Accid Emerg Med. 1998;15(2):89–95.
3. Chung TW, et al. Radiographic findings of gastrointestinal anisakiasis: clinical and pathologic correlation. J Korean Radiol Soc. 2000;43(2):209–13.
4. M Cucunato GC, Currò A. Acute coronary syndrome and scombroid syndrome. Int J Cardiol. 2015;187:317–8.
5. Wilson BJ, Musto RJ, Ghali WA. Histamine fish poisoning in a young atopic woman. J Gen Intern Med. 2012;27(7):878–81.
6. Russell FE, Maretić Z. Scombroid poisoning: mini-review with case histories. Toxicon. 1986;24:967–73.
7. Bedry R, Gabinski C, Paty MC. Diagnosis of scombroid poisoning by measurement of plasma histamine. N Engl J Med. 2000;342:520–1.
8. Lavon O, Lurie Y, Bentur Y. Scombroid fish poisoning in Israel, 2005-2007. Isr Med Assoc J. 2008;10(11):789–92.
9. Lehane L, Olley J. Histamine fish poisoning revisited. Int J Food Microbiol. 2000;58(1-2):1–37.
10. Yesudhason P, Al-Zidjali M, Al-Zidjali A, Al-Busaidi M, Al-Waili A, Al-Mazrooei N, Al-Habsi S. Histamine levels in commercially important fresh and processed fish of Oman with reference to international standards. Food Chem. 2013;140(4):777–83.
11. Kelso JM, Lin FL. Skin testing for scombroid poisoning. Ann Allergy Asthma Immunol. 2009;103:447.
12. Feng C, Teuber S, Gershwin ME. Histamine (Scombroid) fish poisoning: a comprehensive review. Clin Rev Allergy Immunol. 2016;50(1):64–9.
13. Taylor SL, Stratton JE, Nordlee JA. Histamine poisoning (scombroid fish poisoning): an allergy-like intoxication. J Toxicol Clin Toxicol. 1989;27(4-5):225–40.
14. Uragoda CG, Kottegoda SR. Adverse reactions to isoniazid on ingestion of fish with a high histamine content. Tubercle. 1977;58(2):83–9.

Chapter 25
Acute Reaction to Influenza Vaccination

Silviya Mihaylova Novakova, Plamena Ivanova Novakova, and Maria Toncheva Staevska

A 15-year-old boy with a history of moderate asthma and previously diagnosed egg allergy, was referred to our allergy unit for consultation about safety and possibility of administration of influenza vaccination. Egg allergy was first diagnosed, when he was 10 years old, presenting with repeated angioedema and urticaria up to 20 min after drinking egg shake and after pancakes. Sensitization to egg yolk was confirmed with positive skin prick test (SPT) and elevated level of specific IgE (sIgE). The boy can consume hardboiled eggs.

Q1. Influenza vaccine is recommended for?

A. Anyone 6 months and older.
B. Children with asthma
C. Patients who are at high risk for complications from influenza
D. All of the above

Answer: *The correct answer is* ***D***.

Egg protein is present in influenza vaccines. Although rare, allergic reactions are possible in people with egg allergy. Egg-free vaccines are now available in some countries, but for adults only. Patients with egg allergy are also those at higher risk for adverse outcome from influenza infection. The annual seasonal influenza vaccine is recommended for everyone 6 months and older, especially children and adolescents at high risk for complications from influenza (e.g. children with chronic medical conditions such as pulmonary diseases like asthma) [1]. According to

S. M. Novakova (✉)
Allergy Unit, Internal Consulting Department, University Hospital "St. George", Plovdiv, Bulgaria

P. I. Novakova · M. T. Staevska
Clinic of Clinical Allergy, Medical University, Sofia, Bulgaria

N. Rezaei (ed.), *Pediatric Allergy*, https://doi.org/10.1007/978-3-030-18282-3_25

Global Initiative for Asthma (GINA) patients with moderate-severe asthma are advised to receive influenza vaccination every year [2].

Q2. What is the amount of egg protein in the available influenza vaccines?

A. ≤1 μg/0.5 ml dose for flu shots
B. 0.24 μg/0.2 ml dose for the nasal spray vaccine
C. It is a secret of the manufacturer.
D. Answers A and B are correct

***Answer**: The correct answer is **D**.*

Most vaccine manufacturers now provide the egg protein content on their influenza vaccine products. Maximum amount of ovalbumin reported by the manufacturers is ≤1 μg per 0.5 ml dose for shots and 0.24 μg/0.2 mL dose for the nasal spray vaccine [3]. Independent studies demonstrated even lower egg protein content in many vaccines than was reported by the manufacturer [3, 4]. The amounts of egg protein in influenza vaccines are low and unlikely to induce an allergic reaction. Cell-based influenza vaccines contain a significantly smaller amount of egg protein, while recombinant vaccines are completely egg free.

Q3. Do you recommend SPT before influenza vaccination?

A. Yes. In patients with a history of allergy to one of the vaccine constituents who have not received the vaccine before, a complete allergic work-up is always recommended and skin test with the vaccine itself should be performed
B. No. Skin test to the influenza vaccine before vaccination is no longer recommended
C. The decision depends on the severity of egg allergy

***Answer**: The correct answer is **B**.*

It is recommended to administer a complete allergic workup for patients presenting with a history of allergies prior to influenza vaccination [5]. However, regarding administration of influenza vaccine, numerous studies have demonstrated that it can be safely administered to even severely egg-allergic recipients, probably because of the low amount of egg protein (ovalbumin) [6, 7]

Skin test with influenza vaccine before vaccination is no longer recommended due to low sensitivity and specificity of the test in predicting serious reactions to vaccine administration [8].

Q4. Is influenza vaccine is safe for the boy in the presented case?

A. Yes, the boy can get any licensed inactivated influenza vaccine safely.
B. No, because there is a high risk of anaphylaxis.
C. Yes, the boy can be vaccinated, but only with egg-free influenza vaccine or intranasal vaccine which has low amounts of egg protein.

***Answer**: The correct answer is **A**.*

Results of studies indicate that inactivated influenza vaccine (IIV) administered in a single, age appropriate dose is well tolerated by any recipient, even those with an egg allergy [1]. Anaphylaxis is rare, even in patients with a history of severe reactions to egg. Anaphylaxis after IIV administration is equally frequent egg-allergic and non-egg-allergic recipients and no more compared to that after other universally recommended vaccines. Although the intranasal vaccine is with low amounts of egg protein, it should not be used in egg-allergic patients as there is limited data on its safety and it is also contraindicated in patients with asthma [8]. Recombinant vaccine is not approved by the FDA for children and adolescents.

Q5. What recommendations regarding influenza vaccine administration must be given to the presented case?

A. Available IIV can be given with no precaution and no serious adverse reactions are expected due to the low amounts of egg protein in the vaccine.
B. Dividing the dose of influenza vaccine is recommended in children with egg allergy.
C. Influenza vaccine can be given in an inpatient or outpatient clinical setting under the supervision of a health care provider with expertise in management of severe allergic conditions.

***Answer**: The correct answer is **C**.*

The Center for Disease Control and Prevention's Advisory Committee on Immunization Practices recommends that patients with a history of hives only after egg ingestion to receive any licensed age-appropriate influenza vaccine in a primary care physicians, office. Dividing the dose of vaccine is not recommended because enough evidence demonstrates that even the most severely egg-allergic patients can tolerate the full dose [8]. The presented case involves a 15 year-old boy previously diagnosed with asthma and a history of angioedema after eating foods containing egg. Even patients with a history of severe reactions to egg, requiring emergency medical intervention, can receive any licensed, age-appropriate vaccine. However, it is recommended that the vaccine is given in a medical setting under the supervision of a health care provider with expertise in recognizing and managing severe allergic conditions and can administer epinephrine.

Q6. Does tolerance to egg-containing foods exclude allergic reactions after influenza vaccine?

A. Yes, tolerance to egg-containing foods excludes allergic reactions after influenza vaccine
B. No, allergic reactions are not excluded in people who tolerated egg-containing foods
C. The risk of allergic reactions depends on type of egg-containing foods that are tolerated

***Answer**: The correct answer is **B**.*

Influenza vaccines contain components other than egg protein that might as well be allergenic. Allergic reactions can occur in response to components other than egg protein. People with egg allergy may tolerate foods like hard-boiled eggs and eggs in baked products. However, they experience reactions after eating lightly cooked egg (scrambled eggs, egg shake etc.), as the boy in the reported case. Tolerance to egg-containing food does not exclude egg allergy. Previous severe reaction to influenza vaccine, regardless of the component suspected, is contraindication for receiving influenza vaccine in future.

Practical Points

- The annual seasonal influenza vaccine is recommended for everyone 6 months and older
- Influenza vaccine can be safely administered to even severely egg-allergic recipient
- Tolerance to egg-containing food/vaccine does not exclude egg allergy

References

1. Committee on Infectious Diseases. Recommendations for Prevention and Control of Influenza in Children, 2017 – 2018. Pediatrics. 2017;140:e20173535.
2. Global initiative for asthma. Global strategy for asthma management and prevention. 2017. Available from: www.ginasthma.org.
3. Li JT, Rank MA, Squillace DL, Kita H. Ovalbumin content of influenza vaccines. J Allergy Clin Immunol. 2010;125(6):1412–4.
4. Yang HJ. Safety of influenza vaccination in children with allergic diseases. Clin Exp Vacc Res. 2015;4(2):137–44.
5. Caubet J-C, Terreehorst I. Adverse reactions to vaccines for infectious diseases. In: Global atlas of allergy. Zurich: European Academy of Allergy and Clinical Immunology; 2014.
6. Kelso JM, Greenhawt MJ, Li JT, Nicklas RA, Bernstein DI, Blessing-Moore J, Cox L, Khan D, Lang DM, Oppenheimer J, Portnoy JM, Randolph CR, Schuller DE, Spector SL, Tilles SA, Wallace D. Adverse reactions to vaccines practice parameter 2012 update. J Allergy Clin Immunol. 2012;130(1):25–43.
7. Wood RA. Allergic reactions to vaccines. Pediatr Allergy Immunol. 2013;24(6):521–6.
8. Kelso JM, Li JT. Adverse reactions to vaccines for infectious diseases. In: Global atlas of allergy. Zurich: European Academy of Allergy and Clinical Immunology; 2013.

Chapter 26
Extensive Rashes

Brian K. Y. Chia and Emily Y. Gan

A 3-year-old boy presented with a 6-month history of itchy rashes over the scalp, face, trunk and limbs. He had received a course of oral prednisolone from his general practitioner 2 months ago with transient improvement but has since experienced a flare of his condition. He has no family history of atopic dermatitis and no personal history of asthma or allergic rhinitis. Examination revealed widespread weepy erythematous plaques over the scalp, face, trunk and limbs with an estimated body surface area involvement of about 80% (Fig. 26.1a–e).

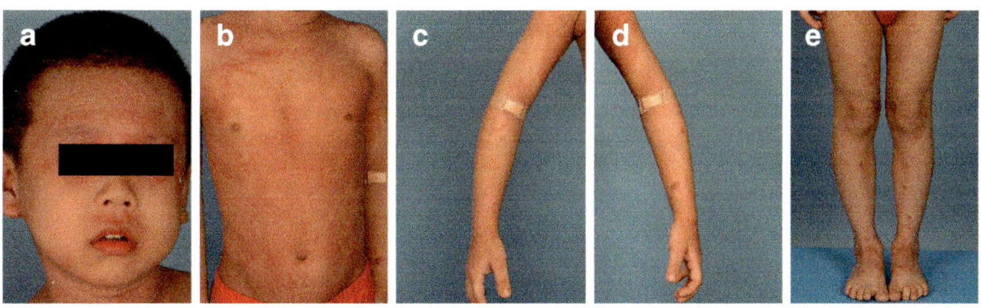

Fig. 26.1 (**a**–**e**) Erythematous plaques on face, trunk and limbs of a 3-year-old boy

B. K. Y. Chia (✉)
National Skin Centre, Singapore, Singapore
e-mail: brian.chia@mohh.com.sg

E. Y. Gan
Department of Dermatology,
KK Women's and Children's Hospital, Singapore, Singapore

N. Rezaei (ed.), *Pediatric Allergy*, https://doi.org/10.1007/978-3-030-18282-3_26

Q1. Which one of the following conditions is least likely to have cutaneous features similar to the patient's presentation?

A. Hyper IgE syndrome
B. Severe combined immunodeficiency
C. Maffucci syndrome
D. Ataxia-telangiectasia
E. Netherton syndrome

Answer*: The correct answer is* ***C****.*

The patient's clinical presentation is consistent with severe atopic dermatitis, as demonstrated by the widespread weepy erythematous plaques over the face, trunk and limbs. In addition to atopic dermatitis, multiple other conditions may also present with severe eczema-like eruptions.

Hyper IgE syndrome (HIES) is characterized by recurrent cutaneous and sinopulmonary infections, dermatitis beginning in infancy or early childhood, and extremely elevated IgE levels [1]. Patients with HIES may have a severe eczematous rash which shares many clinical features with atopic dermatitis such as pruritus, lichenification and staphylococcal superinfection [2].

Severe combined immunodeficiency (SCID) is a heterogeneous group of disorders that share clinical manifestations related to defective function of both cell-mediated and humoral immunity [3]. Patients with SCID may present with widespread seborrheic-dermatitis like eruptions. Extensive eczematous dermatitis or erythroderma may also occur in the setting of Omenn's syndrome [4].

Ataxia–telangiectasia (A-T) is characterized by oculocutaneous telangiectasias, progressive cerebellar ataxia, a variable immunodeficiency with a tendency for sinopulmonary infections, and chromosomal instability with exposure to ionizing radiation. Cutaneous findings in A-T may also include poikiloderma, an eczematous dermatitis and seborrheic dermatitis with blepharitis [4].

Netherton syndrome comprises the triad of congenital ichthyosis, trichorrhexis invaginata and atopy [5]. Patients with Netherton syndrome may present soon or after birth with generalized erythroderma and scaling or continuous peeling of the skin. In patients with severe disease, generalized ichthyosis and erythroderma may persist throughout life.

Maffucci syndrome comprises a combination of venous malformations and enchondromas, most commonly affecting the extremities. An eczematous eruption is not a usual manifestation of this condition.

Q2. Which of the following will be the most appropriate amount of topical corticosteroids to be prescribed to the patient? (Assuming twice-daily application for 1 week before next review)

A. One tube (15 g)
B. Two tubes (30 g)
C. Three tubes (45 g)
D. Four tubes (60 g)
E. Eight tubes (120 g)

***Answer**: The correct answer is **E**.*

Topical glucocorticoids are first-line anti-inflammatory treatment and have been demonstrated to have a significant effect on improving skin lesions compared to placebo [6]. Application of TCSs should follow the finger-tip unit (FTU) rule. A FTU is the amount of ointment expressed from a tube with a 5 mm diameter nozzle and measured from the distal skin crease to the tip of the index finger. This amounts to 0.5 g of the topical medication and is an adequate amount for application of two adult palm areas, which is approximately 2% of the body surface area (BSA) [7]. In general, infants require 1/5 of the adult dose, children require 2/5 of the adult dose and adolescents 2/3 of the adult dose [8].

In the patient above, an estimated 80% of the BSA is involved. Thus, the amount of corticosteroids needed per application would be $80/2 \times 0.5\ g \times 2/5 = 8\ g$.

Assuming twice a day application over a period of a week, the total required would be $8\ g \times 2 \times 7 = 112\ g$ (approximately eight tubes)

Q3. In terms of treatment of pruritus in this patient, which of the following statements is most accurate?

A. Newer non-sedating antihistamines (e.g. loratadine, cetirizine or fexofenadine) demonstrate little to no relief of pruritus
B. Topical antihistamines appear to have more significant efficacy in treatment of pruritus compared to oral antihistamines
C. Single application of topical capsaicin has been shown to have significant improvement in perception of itch
D. Topical calcineurin inhibitors are slow acting and typically relief of pruritus only occurs many weeks after initiation of treatment
E. Phototherapy has been shown to be effective in relief of pruritus and ultraviolet-A1 (UVA-1) appears to be more efficacious than narrow-band ultraviolet B

***Answer**: The correct answer is **A**.*

Single studies have demonstrated that newer generation non-sedating antihistamines have little to no relief of pruritus in atopic dermatitis [9, 10], whereas first-generation antihistamines may have a beneficial effect on sleep structure. Topical antihistamines have no effect on itch beyond the cooling effect from the compound vehicle [7].

Topical capsaicin releases neuropeptides within unmyelinated, polymodal C-type cutaneous nerves. Repeated application rather than single application of topical capsaicin prevents reaccumulation of the neuropeptides and decreases the sensation of pruritus [11]. Topical calcineurin inhibitors significantly relieve pruritus with studies demonstrating improvement after 3 days of topical application of tacrolimus [12] or pimecrolimus [13]. Phototherapy is an effective treatment for pruritus. However, the efficacy of narrow-band ultraviolet B (NBUVB) has been shown to be superior to UVA1 [14].

Q4. Which of the following treatment options would be considered the most appropriate for this patient?

A. Topical moisturizers only
B. Low potency topical steroid e.g. hydrocortisone 1% cream with liberal use of moisturizers
C. Phototherapy using NB-UVB
D. Oral corticosteroids at 1 mg/kg/day tapered slowly over 6 months
E. Oral cyclosporine

Answer: *The correct answer is* ***E***.

The patient above has severe eczema as evidenced by the extensive body-surface-area (BSA) involvement.

Moisturizers have been demonstrated to have a short-term and long-term steroid sparing effect [15]. However, the sole use of moisturizers without topical anti-inflammatory therapy is not adequate in moderate to severe eczema and carries a considerable risk of disseminated bacterial and viral infections [16].

Topical glucocorticoids are first-line anti-inflammatory treatment and have been demonstrated to have a significant effect on improving skin lesions compared to placebo [6]. However, given the extent and severity of the patient's skin condition, a low potency steroid such as hydrocortisone cream is unlikely to bring significant relief.

NBUVB has been indicated for chronic moderate forms of eczema with improvement and clearance of the condition [17]. However, phototherapy, with the exception of ultraviolet-A1, is poorly tolerated in acute eczema and is not indicated for treatment in this setting.

Oral glucocorticoids are an option for short-term treatment of acute eczema flares. Long term use in atopic eczema patients, particularly in children, is not recommended [18].

Oral cyclosporine is effective in childhood and adolescence atopic eczema to reduce the BSA involvement, erythema, sleep loss, and glucocorticoid use [19]. Though the use of cyclosporine in children and adolescents is considered "off-label", given the severity of this patient's disease, cyclosporine represents the most appropriate treatment option amongst those listed.

Q5. When using cyclosporine for the treatment of atopic eczema in adults and children, all of the followings are known adverse effect, <u>except</u>:

A. Hypertension
B. Hypermagnesemia
C. Hyperkalemia
D. Hyperuricemia
E. Increased risk of non-melanoma skin cancers

Answer: *The correct answer is* ***B***.

Cyclosporine acts by binding to cyclophilin, which blocks the dephosphorylation of the nuclear factor of activated T cells (NFAT). This prevents the upregulation of IL-2 and IL-2 receptors, resulting in a decrease of $CD4^+$ and $CD8^+$ T cells in the epidermis. The resulting immunosuppression can result in increased risk of infections as well as non-melanoma skin cancers.

In addition to the immunological actions, cyclosporine has multiple side-effects on the kidney, including hypertension due to direct vasoconstriction of the renal vasculature, hyperkalemia due to impairment of urinary potassium excretion [20], and hyperuricemia from decreased urate clearance [21]. Hypomagnesemia rather than hypermagnesemia is a known complication of cyclosporine use and is thought to result from intracellular shift of magnesium [22].

Practical Points

- Severe and recalcitrant eczema can be a cutaneous manifestation of multiple syndromes such as HIES, SCID, A-T and Netherton syndrome
- Adequate prescription of topical steroids is important in management of atopic dermatitis and use of the fingertip unit gives a good estimation of the amount required
- To relief excessive pruritus in atopic dermatitis, first-generation, sedating antihistamines work better than new, non-sedating antihistamines
- Oral cyclosporine is effective in severe, treatment refractory atopic dermatitis
- Side-effects such as hypertension, hyperkalemia and hypomagnesemia should be monitored when using cyclosporine

References

1. Grimbacher B, Holland SM, Gallin JI, Greenberg F, Hill SC, Malech HL, Miller JA, O'Connell AC, Puck JM. Hyper-IgE syndrome with recurrent infections--an autosomal dominant multisystem disorder. N Engl J Med. 1999;340(9):692–702.
2. Eberting CL, Davis J, Puck JM, Holland SM, Turner ML. Dermatitis and the newborn rash of hyper-IgE syndrome. Arch Dermatol. 2004;140(9):1119–25.
3. Buckley RH. The multiple causes of human SCID. J Clin Invest. 2004;114(10):1409–11.
4. Bolognia J, Jorizzo JL, Schaffer JV. Dermatology. Edinburgh: Elsevier/Saunders; 2012.
5. Wilkinson RD, Curtis GH, Hawk WA. Netherton's disease; trichorrhexis invaginata (bamboo hair), congenital ichthyosiform erythroderma and the atopic diathesis. A histopathologic study. Arch Dermatol. 1964;89:46–54.
6. Hanifin J, Gupta AK, Rajagopalan R. Intermittent dosing of fluticasone propionate cream for reducing the risk of relapse in atopic dermatitis patients. Br J Dermatol. 2002;147(3):528–37.
7. Ring J, Alomar A, Bieber T, Deleuran M, Fink-Wagner A, Gelmetti C, Gieler U, Lipozencic J, Luger T, Oranje AP, Schafer T, Schwennesen T, Seidenari S, Simon D, Stander S, Stingl G, Szalai S, Szepietowski JC, Taieb A, Werfel T, Wollenberg A, Darsow U. Guidelines for treatment of atopic eczema (atopic dermatitis) part I. J Eur Acad Dermatol Venereol. 2012;26(8):1045–60.
8. Nelson AA, Miller AD, Fleischer AB, Balkrishnan R, Feldman SR. How much of a topical agent should be prescribed for children of different sizes? J Dermatolog Treat. 2006;17(4):224–8.

9. Chunharas A, Wisuthsarewong W, Wananukul S, Viravan S. Therapeutic efficacy and safety of loratadine syrup in childhood atopic dermatitis treated with mometasone furoate 0.1 per cent cream. J Med Assoc Thai. 2002;85(4):482–7.
10. Hannuksela M, Kalimo K, Lammintausta K, Mattila T, Turjanmaa K, Varjonen E, Coulie PJ. Dose ranging study: cetirizine in the treatment of atopic dermatitis in adults. Ann Allergy. 1993;70(2):127–33.
11. Weisshaar E, Heyer G, Forster C, Handwerker HO. Effect of topical capsaicin on the cutaneous reactions and itching to histamine in atopic eczema compared to healthy skin. Arch Dermatol Res. 1998;290(6):306–11.
12. Boguniewicz M, Fiedler VC, Raimer S, Lawrence ID, Leung DY, Hanifin JM. A randomized, vehicle-controlled trial of tacrolimus ointment for treatment of atopic dermatitis in children. Pediatric Tacrolimus Study Group. J Allergy Clin Immunol. 1998;102(4 Pt 1):637–44.
13. Eichenfield LF, Thaci D, de Prost Y, Puig L, Paul C. Clinical management of atopic eczema with pimecrolimus cream 1% (Elidel) in paediatric patients. Dermatology. 2007;215(Suppl 1):3–17.
14. Reynolds NJ, Franklin V, Gray JC, Diffey BL, Farr PM. Narrow-band ultraviolet B and broad-band ultraviolet A phototherapy in adult atopic eczema: a randomised controlled trial. Lancet. 2001;357(9273):2012–6.
15. Eberlein B, Eicke C, Reinhardt HW, Ring J. Adjuvant treatment of atopic eczema: assessment of an emollient containing N-palmitoylethanolamine (ATOPA study). J Eur Acad Dermatol Venereol. 2008;22(1):73–82.
16. Wollenberg A, Wetzel S, Burgdorf WH, Haas J. Viral infections in atopic dermatitis: pathogenic aspects and clinical management. J Allergy Clin Immunol. 2003;112(4):667–74.
17. Kunz B, Oranje AP, Labreze L, Stalder JF, Ring J, Taieb A. Clinical validation and guidelines for the SCORAD index: consensus report of the European Task Force on Atopic Dermatitis. Dermatology. 1997;195(1):10–9.
18. Ring J, Alomar A, Bieber T, Deleuran M, Fink-Wagner A, Gelmetti C, Gieler U, Lipozencic J, Luger T, Oranje AP, Schafer T, Schwennesen T, Seidenari S, Simon D, Stander S, Stingl G, Szalai S, Szepietowski JC, Taieb A, Werfel T, Wollenberg A, Darsow U. Guidelines for treatment of atopic eczema (atopic dermatitis) Part II. J Eur Acad Dermatol Venereol. 2012;26(9):1176–93.
19. Hoare C, Li Wan Po A, Williams H. Systematic review of treatments for atopic eczema. Health Technol Assess (Winch Eng). 2000;4(37):1–191.
20. Lee CH, Kim GH. Electrolyte and Acid-base disturbances induced by calcineurin inhibitors. Electrol Blood Press. 2007;5(2):126–30.
21. Lin HY, Rocher LL, McQuillan MA, Schmaltz S, Palella TD, Fox IH. Cyclosporine-induced hyperuricemia and gout. N Engl J Med. 1989;321(5):287–92.
22. Nozue T, Kobayashi A, Kodama T, Uemasu F, Endoh H, Sako A, Takagi Y. Pathogenesis of cyclosporine-induced hypomagnesemia. J Pediatr. 1992;120(4 Pt 1):638–40.

Chapter 27
Severe Itchy Rashes

Brian K. Y. Chia and Emily Y. Gan

A 5-month old girl presented with a 4-month history of itchy rashes affecting the face, trunk and the limbs. Her hands and feet as well as the buttocks and intertriginous sites were not affected (Fig. 27.1a, b). She had visited general practitioners on two separate occasions and was treated with miconazole 1% cream and hydrocortisone 1% cream, with no significant improvement. Her parents had a history of atopic dermatitis. She had no significant history of allergic rhinitis or asthma. Her developmental milestones were normal and she had been breastfed with recent introduction of fruit and vegetable puree into her diet. The patient was otherwise healthy, with no oral thrush, nail changes, petechiae, ecchymosis or bleeding diathesis. Estimated body surface area involvement was 10%.

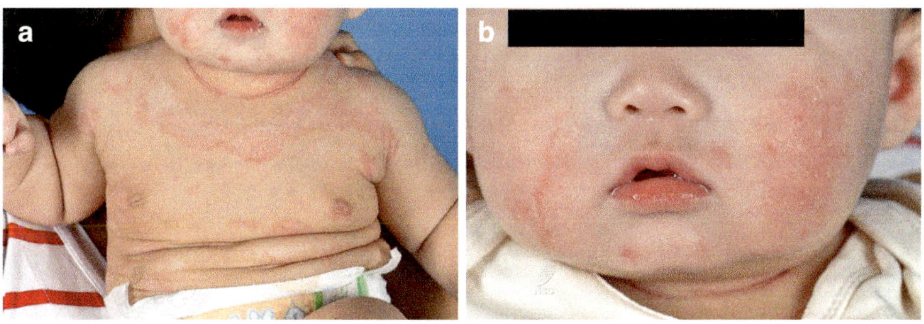

Fig. 27.1 (**a**, **b**) Itchy rashes affecting the face, trunk and the limbs of a 5-months-old girl

B. K. Y. Chia (✉)
National Skin Centre, Singapore, Singapore
e-mail: brian.chia@mohh.com.sg

E. Y. Gan
Department of Dermatology, KK Women's and Children's Hospital, Singapore, Singapore

N. Rezaei (ed.), *Pediatric Allergy*, https://doi.org/10.1007/978-3-030-18282-3_27

Q1. Which one of the following genetic mutations or histocompatibility antigens (HLA) is most likely associated with this condition?

A. *FLG* gene mutation
B. HLA-Cw6 allele
C. *AIRE* gene mutation
D. *SLC39A4* gene mutation
E. *WAS* gene

Answer*: The correct answer is* ***A****.*

Atopic dermatitis is a chronic, pruritic, inflammatory skin dermatosis, often occurring with other atopic diseases such as bronchial asthma and allergic rhinoconjunctivitis [1]. Lesions in atopic dermatitis (AD) can be classified into acute, subacute and chronic stages. Edematous, erythematous papules and plaques with vesiculation, oozing and serous crusting predominate in the acute phase whereas lichenification and prurigo-like lesions are found in the chronic phase. In the first 6 months of life, the face and neck are affected in over 90% of patients [2], whereas classical flexural eczema tends to affect young children between 2 and 12 years of age. The filaggrin gene (*FLG*) encodes a protein that aggregates keratin filaments during terminal differentiation of the epidermis and mutation of this protein represents a major predisposing factor towards atopic dermatitis. Presence of *FLG* mutation variants correlates with early-onset, relatively severe atopic dermatitis that tends to persist into adulthood [3]. The HLA-Cw6 allele is strongly associated with early-onset psoriasis. Compared to atopic dermatitis, chronic plaque psoriasis tends to present with more sharply demarcated and erythematous papulosquamous lesions in addition to nail, scalp and joint involvement [4]. The *AIRE* gene is mutated in autoimmune polyendocrinopathy–candidiasis–ectodermal dystrophy syndrome (APECED) [5]. Patients with this condition suffer from recurrent, treatment-resistant thrush. Skin manifestations may range from a few erythematous scaly plaques and dystrophic nails to severe, generalized, crusted granulomatous plaques. The *SLC39A4* gene mutation occurs in acrodermatitis enteropathica. Clinical manifestations usually appear within 1–2 weeks after weaning from breast milk, or at 4–10 weeks of age if bottle-fed, and include erythema, scale-crusts and erosions especially in the perioral, acral and perineal sites [4]. Wiskott-Aldrich syndrome (WAS) is caused by a loss-of-function mutation in the *WAS* gene. The first clinical signs often include petechiae and ecchymosis of the skin and oral mucosa. Dermatitis typically develops within the first few months of life with the face, scalp and flexural areas most commonly affected [4].

Q2. Which of the following would be the most appropriate topical treatment to initiate for this patient?

A. Clobetasol propionate 0.05% cream with moisturizers twice a day to affected areas
B. Tacrolimus 0.1% ointment with moisturizers twice a day to affected areas
C. Betamethasone valerate 0.025% cream with moisturizers twice a day to affected areas

D. Urea 10% cream only twice a day to affected areas
E. Coal tar 15% in aqueous cream twice a day to affected areas

***Answer**: The correct answer is **C**.*

Topical glucocorticoids are the first-line anti-inflammatory treatment for atopic dermatitis and have a significant effect on improving skin lesions compared to placebo [6]. For the face and body folds, lower potency steroids e.g. Desonide 0.05% cream or Betamethasone valerate 0.025% creams are more appropriate and prolonged use of high potency steroids e.g. Clobetasol propionate should generally be avoided due to the risk of cutaneous atrophy.

The efficacy of tacrolimus and pimecrolimus ointments for atopic dermatitis have been demonstrated in clinical trials [7], but their use in those aged less than 2 years has not been approved. The use of moisturizers is important and has been demonstrated to have a steroid sparing effect in mild to moderate atopic dermatitis in both children [8] and adults [9]. Coal tar based topical therapies are used in the treatment of psoriasis vulgaris.

Q3. With regards to maintenance therapy, which of the following constitutes the *most appropriate* treatment strategy to reduce relapses?

A. Stop topical steroids and continue liberal use of moisturizers twice daily only
B. Use of a low potency topical steroid e.g. betamethasone valerate 0.025% cream twice-weekly to previously inflamed areas with liberal use of moisturizers
C. Use of a medium potency steroid e.g. mometasone furoate 0.1% cream twice-weekly to previously inflamed areas with liberal use of moisturizers
D. Use of topical antibiotics e.g. tetracycline ointment to previously inflamed areas
E. Use of topical antiseptics e.g. chlorhexidine wash as maintenance treatment

***Answer**: The correct answer is **B**.*

Proactive treatment, is defined as a combination of pre-defined, long-term, low-dose, anti-inflammatory treatment applied to previously affected areas of skin in combination with liberal use of moisturizers on the entire body. This reduces the risk of relapses of eczema as compared to a moisturizer-only strategy [10]. This can be accomplished with the use of a low potency topical steroid or a topical calcineurin inhibitor such as tacrolimus 0.03% ointment or pimecrolimus 1% cream in patients older than 2 years [11]. It is inappropriate to use a medium potency steroid such as mometasone furoate as proactive treatment as it carries a significant risk of skin atrophy. Long term topical antibiotic use does not improve the severity of eczema and bears the risk of antibiotic resistance [12]. A Cochrane review failed to demonstrate any benefit with topical antiseptics in patients with AD [13].

Q4. As the infant approaches her age for initiation of complementary feeding, her parents ask about the type of food that might exacerbate her condition. With regard to food allergies in AD, which of the following is the most accurate?

A. The gold standard for diagnosis of a food allergy is skin prick testing
B. Cow's milk, hen's egg, wheat, soy, tree nuts and peanuts are frequently responsible for eczema or exacerbation in older children, but not in infancy
C. Milk and egg free elimination diets are helpful in patients with severe eczema, even when patients have no clinical symptoms upon ingestion
D. Personal history is often not helpful in predicting late reactions to food compared to immediate reactions
E. Compared to serum specific IgE testing, skin prick testing has the benefit of giving quantitative data about the grade of sensitization

***Answer**: The correct answer is **D**.*

Personal history is often not helpful in predicting late reactions to food compared to immediate reactions with a positive predictive value of 30% in the former compared to 80% in the latter [14]. The gold standard for the diagnosis of food allergies is a double-blind placebo-controlled food challenge, i.e. double-blind oral food challenge (OFC) [15].

Among food allergens, cow's milk, hen's egg, wheat, soy, tree nuts and peanuts are most frequently responsible for eczema or exacerbation in infancy [16]. In older children, adolescents and adults, pollen related food allergy should also be taken into account [17].

A systematic review showed no convincing evidence that a milk or egg-free elimination diet is beneficial when unselected AD patients were studied [18]. However, a single prospective controlled study supported the notion that a direct elimination diet of egg may be beneficial for AD patients who have clinical symptoms on ingestion of eggs [19].

Serum specific IgE (sIgE) testing is helpful when skin prick test cannot be applied, e.g. in patients with dermographism, UV and drug induced skin hyporeactivity, eczema at test site and lack of compliance in infancy, and also gives better quantitative data for the grade of sensitization.

Q5. With regard to comorbidities in atopic dermatitis, which of the following best characterizes the "atopic march"?

A. Development of AD followed by, allergic rhinitis and asthma
B. Development of allergic rhinitis, followed by AD and asthma
C. Development of asthma, followed by AD and allergic rhinitis
D. Development of asthma, followed by AD and food allergy
E. Development of AD, followed by allergic rhinitis and food allergy

***Answer**: The correct answer is **A**.*

Atopic dermatitis is a complex genetic disease and is commonly accompanied by asthma and rhinoconjunctivitis. It has been estimated that approximately one-third of patients with AD develop asthma and two-thirds develop allergic rhinitis, although the probabilities could be higher in those with severe atopic dermatitis [20]. These conditions may appear simultaneously or in succession. Atopic dermatitis has a predilection for infants and young children whilst asthma and allergic rhinitis favours older children and adolescents respectively [21]. Given that the "atopic march" starts with atopic dermatitis, treatment should be directed not only at the acute flares but also at improving the epidermal barrier dysfunction thereby potentially reducing epicutaneous sensitization and the driving forward of the atopic march [22].

Practical Points

- Mutation of the *FLG* gene predisposes to early-onset, severe atopic dermatitis that tends to persist into adulthood
- Use of topical steroids over the face and flexures should be limited to those with mild potency
- Proactive treatment reduces the risk of relapses as compared to a moisturizer-only strategy
- Treatment of atopic dermatitis should be directed at improving the epidermal barrier dysfunction to reduce epicutaneous sensitization and preventing the atopic march to forward

References

1. Johansson SG, Hourihane JO, Bousquet J, Bruijnzeel-Koomen C, Dreborg S, Haahtela T, Kowalski ML, Mygind N, Ring J, van Cauwenberge P, van Hage-Hamsten M, Wuthrich B. A revised nomenclature for allergy. An EAACI position statement from the EAACI nomenclature task force. Allergy. 2001;56(9):813–24.
2. Eller E, Kjaer HF, Host A, Andersen KE, Bindslev-Jensen C. Development of atopic dermatitis in the DARC birth cohort. Pediatr Allergy Immunol. 2010;21(2 Pt 1):307–14.
3. Palmer CN, Irvine AD, Terron-Kwiatkowski A, Zhao Y, Liao H, Lee SP, Goudie DR, Sandilands A, Campbell LE, Smith FJ, O'Regan GM, Watson RM, Cecil JE, Bale SJ, Compton JG, DiGiovanna JJ, Fleckman P, Lewis-Jones S, Arseculeratne G, Sergeant A, Munro CS, El Houate B, McElreavey K, Halkjaer LB, Bisgaard H, Mukhopadhyay S, McLean WH. Common loss-of-function variants of the epidermal barrier protein filaggrin are a major predisposing factor for atopic dermatitis. Nat Genet. 2006;38(4):441–6.
4. Bolognia J, Jorizzo JL, Schaffer JV. Dermatology. Edinburgh: Elsevier/Saunders; 2012.
5. Finnish-German APECED Consortium. An autoimmune disease, APECED, caused by mutations in a novel gene featuring two PHD-type zinc-finger domains. Nat Genet. 1997;17(4):399–403.
6. Ring J, Alomar A, Bieber T, Deleuran M, Fink-Wagner A, Gelmetti C, Gieler U, Lipozencic J, Luger T, Oranje AP, Schafer T, Schwennesen T, Seidenari S, Simon D, Stander S, Stingl G, Szalai S, Szepietowski JC, Taieb A, Werfel T, Wollenberg A, Darsow U. Guidelines

for treatment of atopic eczema (atopic dermatitis) part I. J Eur Acad Dermatol Venereol. 2012;26(8):1045–60.
7. Ruzicka T, Bieber T, Schopf E, Rubins A, Dobozy A, Bos JD, Jablonska S, Ahmed I, Thestrup-Pedersen K, Daniel F, Finzi A, Reitamo S. A short-term trial of tacrolimus ointment for atopic dermatitis. European Tacrolimus Multicenter Atopic Dermatitis Study Group. N Engl J Med. 1997;337(12):816–21.
8. Grimalt R, Mengeaud V, Cambazard F. The steroid-sparing effect of an emollient therapy in infants with atopic dermatitis: a randomized controlled study. Dermatology. 2007;214(1):61–7.
9. Eberlein B, Eicke C, Reinhardt HW, Ring J. Adjuvant treatment of atopic eczema: assessment of an emollient containing N-palmitoylethanolamine (ATOPA study). J Eur Acad Dermatol Venereol. 2008;22(1):73–82.
10. Berth-Jones J, Damstra RJ, Golsch S, Livden JK, Van Hooteghem O, Allegra F, Parker CA. Twice weekly fluticasone propionate added to emollient maintenance treatment to reduce risk of relapse in atopic dermatitis: randomised, double blind, parallel group study. BMJ. 2003;326(7403):1367.
11. Thaci D, Reitamo S, Gonzalez Ensenat MA, Moss C, Boccaletti V, Cainelli T, van der Valk P, Buckova H, Sebastian M, Schuttelaar ML, Ruzicka T. Proactive disease management with 0.03% tacrolimus ointment for children with atopic dermatitis: results of a randomized, multicentre, comparative study. Br J Dermatol. 2008;159(6):1348–56.
12. Mitra A, Mohanraj M, Shah M. High levels of fusidic acid-resistant Staphylococcus aureus despite restrictions on antibiotic use. Clin Exp Dermatol. 2009;34(2):136–9.
13. Birnie AJ, Bath-Hextall FJ, Ravenscroft JC, Williams HC. Interventions to reduce Staphylococcus aureus in the management of atopic eczema. Cochrane Database Syst Rev. 2008;(3):CD003871.
14. Breuer K, Heratizadeh A, Wulf A, Baumann U, Constien A, Tetau D, Kapp A, Werfel T. Late eczematous reactions to food in children with atopic dermatitis. Clin Exp Allergy. 2004;34(5):817–24.
15. Bindslev-Jensen C. Standardization of double-blind, placebo-controlled food challenges. Allergy. 2001;56(Suppl 67):75–7.
16. Werfel T, Breuer K. Role of food allergy in atopic dermatitis. Curr Opin Allergy Clin Immunol. 2004;4(5):379–85.
17. Breuer K, Wulf A, Constien A, Tetau D, Kapp A, Werfel T. Birch pollen-related food as a provocation factor of allergic symptoms in children with atopic eczema/dermatitis syndrome. Allergy. 2004;59(9):988–94.
18. Hoare C, Li Wan Po A, Williams H. Systematic review of treatments for atopic eczema. Health Technol Assess (Winch Eng). 2000;4(37):1–191.
19. Bath-Hextall F, Delamere FM, Williams HC. Dietary exclusions for improving established atopic eczema in adults and children: systematic review. Allergy. 2009;64(2):258–64.
20. Dharmage SC, Lowe AJ, Matheson MC, Burgess JA, Allen KJ, Abramson MJ. Atopic dermatitis and the atopic march revisited. Allergy. 2014;69(1):17–27.
21. Spergel JM, Paller AS. Atopic dermatitis and the atopic march. J Allergy Clin Immunol. 2003;112(6 Suppl):S118–27.
22. Bieber T. Atopic dermatitis. N Engl J Med. 2008;358(14):1483–94.

Chapter 28
Skin Dryness on Outer Upper Arms and Thighs

Milagros Lázaro, Sonia de Arriba-Méndez, and Ignacio Dávila

A 4-year-old girl was evaluated in our outpatient clinic for skin dryness particularly on the outer upper arms and thighs, and eczema of antecubital and popliteal folds since she was 3 months of age. She had no family history of allergy and was breast-fed for only 3 months. In addition, she had facial eruptions with palpebral edema after ingestion of chocolate or walnuts. Fruits, foods with cereals and beans were well tolerated. She also had wheezing, cough and shortness of breath when she was near horses. Her parents denied rhinoconjunctival or bronchial symptoms with seasonal pattern.

Skin prick test (SPT) with a locally adapted battery of aeroallergens and foods (including mites, molds, pollens, animal dander and different foods) was positive for grass pollen, horse dander, peach, walnut and hazelnut. Mild nasal symptoms that had appeared since the last spring also suggested a symptomatic pollen allergy.

Total serum IgE was 159 IU/mL and specific IgE to grass pollen and horse dander were 1.94 UA/mL and 2.83 UA/mL respectively. Finally, specific IgE (sIgE) to hazelnut was 60 UA/mL, 7.41 UA/mL to peach, and 4.15 UA/mL to walnut (reference range for sIgE: <0.35 UA/mL). According to her clinical symptoms, she was diagnosed with atopic dermatitis (AD), rhinitis induced by grass pollen, and asthma due to sensitization to horses, and nut allergy.

M. Lázaro
Allergy Department, University Hospital of Salamanca, Salamanca, Spain

S. de Arriba-Méndez (✉)
Pediatric Service, University Hospital Salamanca, Salamanca, Spain
e-mail: sdearriba@usal.es

I. Dávila
Allergy Department, University Hospital of Salamanca, Salamanca, Spain

Allergy Service, Department of Biomedical and Diagnostic Sciences, Biosanitary Institute of Investigation, University Hospital of Salamanca, Salamanca, Spain

N. Rezaei (ed.), *Pediatric Allergy*, https://doi.org/10.1007/978-3-030-18282-3_28

A treatment with moisturizers was recommended, which initially worked well. But after a few months, the girl suffered from moderate xerosis and eczema on intertriginous areas and eyelids and a moderate nocturnal pruritus (SCORAD index was 24). Protopic (tacrolimus) ointment 0.03% in a proactive regimen (twice a week) and, if acute eczema lesions appeared, a topic corticosteroid (methylprednisolone aceponate) were added.

During the following 2–3 years, her parents reported an acceptable control of the atopic dermatitis, with mild or moderate exacerbations that were controlled with the prescribed treatment regimen. However, 1 year before the current visit, the severity of her atopic dermatitis increased (with eczema lesions on eyelids, folds and thoracic region, SCORAD: 52). She was treated with oral prednisone and topical corticosteroids (TCSs), but the disease remained uncontrolled. CsA (3 mg/kg/day) was administrated for 12 months, which worked for the following months stopping the treatment and leaving only xerosis in physical examination. Exacerbating factors implicated in the severe atopic dermatitis, especially food allergens, were ruled out. There were no signs of active cutaneous infections.

Avoiding horse exposure was recommended according to the previous allergic workup. A short-acting bronchodilator as a rescue treatment was added to the management plan. Pulmonary function tests showed normal results on several occasions.

To prevent allergic reactions to foods, a diet without hazelnut, walnut and peach was recommended. However, a few months after that, the patient accidentally ingested a small amount of hazelnut and immediately experienced edema on her eyelids associated with dyspepsia. After this reaction, an adrenaline autoinjector was recommended.

The patient also underwent clinical workup for familial hypercholesterolemia. A mutation in the low-density lipoprotein receptor was found (M236; c.1691 A>G; protein: p.Asn543Ser) using Lipochip platform (Progenika Biopharma, Spain). Treatment with a cholestyramine resin was initiated, and after 6 months total cholesterol and low-density lipoprotein (LDL) reduced from 258 mg/dl and 182 mg/dl to 223 mg/dl and 155 mg/dl, respectively.

Q1. About the progression from atopic dermatitis to other allergic disorders (atopic march), please specify which of the following statements is true?

A. The impaired skin barrier allows an epicutaneous sensitization to allergens
B. Early AD and food sensitization is considered a risk factor on other allergic diseases
C. The atopic march could be considered as the natural history of allergic diseases
D. All the statements are true

Answer*: The correct answer is* ***D****.*

Prevalence of IgE-mediated food allergy is about 35% in children with atopic dermatitis [1]. Skin barrier defects facilitate the entry for allergens and they are considered one of the primary pathomechanisms of atopic dermatitis [2–5]. Children with atopic dermatitis sensitized to several foods at an early age appear to be at additional risk of developing other allergic diseases [6]. This evolution is known as the "atopic march".

The concept of atopic march has been supported by epidemiological studies and further confirmed by experimental evidence from mouse models. In a recent study, two-thirds of children with atopic dermatitis developed allergic rhinitis, and one-third had developed asthma at preschool age. An early onset of atopic dermatitis and food allergy were considered risk factors of an early onset asthma. Nevertheless, almost half of children with atopic dermatitis experience complete remission by school age [7].

In our patient, the early onset of atopic dermatitis is a risk factor for the subsequent development food allergy and the sensitization to pollens and horse dander. Her clinical course is suggestive of an early-onset persistent atopic dermatitis phenotype [8], which is more strongly associated with asthma and food allergy.

Q2. Which statement is correct regarding atopic dermatitis treatment?

A. Emollients represent the first step to improve skin barrier function in AD and reduce skin susceptibility to irritants
B. Tacrolimus is not useful as proactive treatment
C. Topical corticosteroids must be applied only as reactive therapy
D. Systemic immunosuppression with CsA is only a treatment options to adults

Answer*: The correct answer is* ***A****.*

According to guidelines, emollients are the mainstay of maintenance therapy in atopic dermatitis. Hydration of the skin should be maintained by at least twice daily application of moisturizers [9]

In our patient, the recommended topical treatment for the AD worked initially well. TCSs are the most widely used anti-inflammatory treatments, applied on inflammatory skin lesions as needed, if the patient present with pruritus, sleeplessness or new flare. Topical calcineurin inhibitors (TCIs) show good anti-inflammatory and antipruritic effects, with less skin atrophy than TCS.

The proactive treatment (twice weekly) of the previously affected areas, together with emollient therapy for both previously affected and unaffected skin is considered an option in therapy of atopic dermatitis. Clinical trial studies have shown efficacy for TCSs and TCIs, both [10]. In our case, the proactive application of TCIs was effective, reducing the needs of TCSs for several years.

Systemic immunosuppression with CsA (3 mg/kg/day), methotrexate, azathioprine, and mycophenolate mofetil has been implemented for children with severe atopic dermatitis [11, 12]. CsA is usually considered as the first-line option for patients requiring immunosuppressive treatment [13]. Due to the narrow therapeutic index of CsA, its use requires a close follow-up for blood pressure and renal function. Fortunately, severe rashes in our patient were controlled with CsA and no adverse effects were observed with this drug.

Q3. All of the following statements regarding genetic studies of atopic dermatitis are correct, except:

A. Results of studies suggest that a skin barrier pathway is important
B. Results of genetic studies do not involve a LDL receptor mutation on atopic dermatitis
C. Mutations of the *FLG* gene are not the most significant risk factor for atopic dermatitis
D. Results of studies suggest that innate and adaptive immune pathways are involved in atopic dermatitis

Answer*: The correct answer is* ***C****.*

Over 30 genes have been linked to atopic dermatitis, with loss-of-function mutations of the gene encoding FLG being the most significant genetic risk factors [14]. Two major systems that are implicated in atopic dermatitis are skin epithelial function and innate/adaptive immune responses. Unfortunately, at that moment, genetic diagnosis on atopic dermatitis could not be performed in our hospital for this patient.

In an update of autosomal dominant genetic, published 1 year before to carrying out the girl's genetic study [15], no study had reported association of LDL receptor mutation and atopic dermatitis. A recent review summarizing the genetic studies from 2009 to 2016 and association studies did not report an association between LDL receptor mutations and atopic dermatitis [14]. Atopic dermatitis is a systemic disease with increased cardiovascular risk [16]. Atopic dermatitis is associated with increases in inflammatory and cardiovascular risk proteins. It is important to assess whether these biomarkers are modifiable, as suggested by their reduction with CsA treatment in severe chronic atopic dermatitis [17].

Both atopic dermatitis and familiar hyperlipidemia could increase the cardiovascular risk in our patient. Therefore, a close follow-up and treatment is essential to prevent further comorbidities.

Q4. Concerning the diagnosis and severity assessment please indicate the correct answer:

A. The diagnosis of atopic dermatitis is based on clinical criteria
B. Serum biomarkers have been validated in the diagnosis of atopic dermatitis
C. The SCORAD index is used to assess the quality of life in atopic dermatitis
D. An SCORAD index lower than 40 indicates that the patient has a mild atopic dermatitis

Answer*: The correct answer is* ***A****.*

The diagnosis of atopic dermatitis should be established on the basis of history and physical examination. To date, no serum biomarkers have not been validated for diagnosis. Once the diagnosis is established, an assessment of severity, persistence and impact on quality of life is essential as a guide for treatment decisions [18].

The SCORAD index includes the general activity of the disease (objective signs and subjective symptoms) and is widely used. A mild atopic dermatitis corresponds to score levels below 25, while a severe disease scores equal or above 50.

Practical Points

- One third of patients with atopic dermatitis have comorbid IgE-mediated food allergy
- Atopic dermatitis and food allergy together increase the risk for progression to asthma
- Emollients are the mainstay of maintenance therapy in atopic dermatitis
- Topical corticosteroids and topical calcineurin inhibitors have shown equal efficacy in eliminating pruritus and symptomatic therapy of the disease

References

1. Eigenmann PA, Sicherer SH, Borkowski TA, Cohen BA, Sampson HA. Prevalence of IgE-mediated food allergy among children with atopic dermatitis. Pediatrics. 1998;101(3):E8.
2. Cork MJ, Robinson DA, Vasilopoulos Y, Ferguson A, Moustafa M, MacGowan A, Duff GW, Ward SJ, Tazi-Ahnini R. New perspectives on epidermal barrier dysfunction in atopic dermatitis: gene-environment interactions. J Allergy Clin Immunol. 2006;118(1):3–21. quiz 2–3.
3. Bantz SK, Zhu Z, Zheng T. The atopic march: progression from atopic dermatitis to allergic rhinitis and asthma. J Clin Cell Immunol. 2014;5(2):202.
4. Weidinger S, Rodriguez E, Stahl C, Wagenpfeil S, Klopp N, Illig T, Novak N. Filaggrin mutations strongly predispose to early-onset and extrinsic atopic dermatitis. J Invest Dermatol. 2007;127(3):724–6.
5. Filipiak-Pittroff B, Schnopp C, Berdel D, Naumann A, Sedlmeier S, Onken A, Rodriguez E, Folster-Holst R, Baurecht H, Ollert M, Ring J, Cramer C, von Berg A, Bauer CP, Herbarth O, Lehmann I, Schaaf B, Koletzko S, Wichmann HE, Heinrich J, Weidinger S. Giniplus, groups LIs. Predictive value of food sensitization and filaggrin mutations in children with eczema. J Allergy Clin Immunol. 2011;128(6):1235–41.e5.
6. Dharma C, Lefebvre DL, Tran MM, Lou WYW, Subbarao P, Becker AB, Mandhane PJ, Turvey SE, Sears MR, investigators CS. Patterns of allergic sensitization and atopic dermatitis from 1 to 3 years: effects on allergic diseases. Clin Exp Allergy. 2018;48:48.
7. Somanunt S, Chinratanapisit S, Pacharn P, Visitsunthorn N, Jirapongsananuruk O. The natural history of atopic dermatitis and its association with Atopic March. Asian Pac J Allergy Immunol. 2017;35(3):137–43.
8. Roduit C, Frei R, Depner M, Karvonen AM, Renz H, Braun-Fahrlander C, Schmausser-Hechfellner E, Pekkanen J, Riedler J, Dalphin JC, von Mutius E, Lauener RP, the Psg, Hyvarinen A, Kirjavainen P, Remes S, Roponen M, Dalphin ML, Kaulek V, Ege M, Genuneit J, Illi S, Kabesch M, Schaub B, Pfefferle PI, Doekes G. Phenotypes of atopic dermatitis depending on the timing of onset and progression in childhood. JAMA Pediatr. 2017;171(7):655–62.
9. Ring J, Alomar A, Bieber T, Deleuran M, Fink-Wagner A, Gelmetti C, Gieler U, Lipozencic J, Luger T, Oranje AP, Schafer T, Schwennesen T, Seidenari S, Simon D, Stander S, Stingl G, Szalai S, Szepietowski JC, Taieb A, Werfel T, Wollenberg A, Darsow U, European Dermatology F, European Academy of D, Venereology, European Federation of A, European Task Force on Atopic D, European Society of Pediatric D, Global A, Asthma European N. Guidelines

for treatment of atopic eczema (atopic dermatitis). Part I. J Eur Acad Dermatol Venereol. 2012;26(8):1045–60.
10. Wollenberg A, Oranje A, Deleuran M, Simon D, Szalai Z, Kunz B, Svensson A, Barbarot S, von Kobyletzki L, Taieb A, de Bruin-Weller M, Werfel T, Trzeciak M, Vestergard C, Ring J, Darsow U. European Task Force on Atopic Dermatitis EETF. ETFAD/EADV Eczema task force 2015 position paper on diagnosis and treatment of atopic dermatitis in adult and paediatric patients. J Eur Acad Dermatol Venereol. 2016;30(5):729–47.
11. Sidbury R, Davis DM, Cohen DE, Cordoro KM, Berger TG, Bergman JN, Chamlin SL, Cooper KD, Feldman SR, Hanifin JM, Krol A, Margolis DJ, Paller AS, Schwarzenberger K, Silverman RA, Simpson EL, Tom WL, Williams HC, Elmets CA, Block J, Harrod CG, Begolka WS, Eichenfield LF. American Academy of D. Guidelines of care for the management of atopic dermatitis: section 3. Management and treatment with phototherapy and systemic agents. J Am Acad Dermatol. 2014;71(2):327–49.
12. Schmitt J, Schakel K, Schmitt N, Meurer M. Systemic treatment of severe atopic eczema: a systematic review. Acta Derm Venereol. 2007;87(2):100–11.
13. Ring J, Alomar A, Bieber T, Deleuran M, Fink-Wagner A, Gelmetti C, Gieler U, Lipozencic J, Luger T, Oranje AP, Schafer T, Schwennesen T, Seidenari S, Simon D, Stander S, Stingl G, Szalai S, Szepietowski JC, Taieb A, Werfel T, Wollenberg A, Darsow U, European Dermatology F, European Academy of D, Venereology, European Task Force on Atopic D, European Federation of A, European Society of Pediatric D, Global A, Asthma European N. Guidelines for treatment of atopic eczema (atopic dermatitis). Part II. J Eur Acad Dermatol Venereol. 2012;26(9):1176–93.
14. Bin L, Leung DY. Genetic and epigenetic studies of atopic dermatitis. Allergy Asthma Clin Immunol. 2016;12:52.
15. Barnes KC. An update on the genetics of atopic dermatitis: scratching the surface in 2009. J Allergy Clin Immunol. 2010;125(1):16–29.e1-11. quiz 30–1.
16. Brunner PM, Suarez-Farinas M, He H, Malik K, Wen HC, Gonzalez J, Chan TC, Estrada Y, Zheng X, Khattri S, Dattola N, Krueger JG, Guttman-Yassky E. The atopic dermatitis blood signature is characterized by increases in inflammatory and cardiovascular risk proteins. Sci Rep. 2017;7(1):8707.
17. Ungar B, Garcet S, Gonzalez J, Dhingra N, Correa da Rosa J, Shemer A, Krueger JG, Suarez-Farinas M, Guttman-Yassky E. An Integrated Model of Atopic Dermatitis Biomarkers Highlights the Systemic Nature of the Disease. J Invest Dermatol. 2017;137(3):603–13.
18. Eichenfield LF, Stein Gold LF. Practical strategies for the diagnosis and assessment of atopic dermatitis. Semin Cutan Med Surg. 2017;36(2 Suppl 2):S36–S8.

Chapter 29
Wheezing Attacks and Itchy Skin Rashes on Cheeks

Sakine Işık and Suna Asilsoy

A 3-years-old boy presented with recurrent wheezing attacks and itchy skin rashes on different body regions. His clinical history included five wheezing attacks since 6-months-old and he was hospitalized once for a severe wheezing attack at 1 year-old. His wheezing attacks are responsive to treatment of short-acting beta-2 adrenergic agonist (SABA) and inhaled corticosteroid (ICS). His itchy skin rashes had started at 2-months-old and it was confined largely to his cheeks and flexural surfaces of his elbows and knees. Family history was positive for atopy. Laboratory studies on admission revealed elevated total IgE levels (total IgE level was 1200 IU/mL, reference value <100 IU/mL) and eosinophilia (total eosinophil count was 900/μL). Chest radiography was normal.

Q1. What is the possible diagnosis?

A. Primary immunodeficiency
B. Cystic fibrosis
C. Food and/or aeroallergen allergy
D. Congenital pulmonary diseases

Answer: *The correct answer is **C**.*

The patient had history of early-onset of wheezing attacks and itchy skin rashes. His physical examination revealed atopic dermatitis with normal chest examination. Atopic dermatitis is a chronic inflammatory skin disease characterized by pruritic skin lesions, disrupted skin barrier function, dysregulation of the immune system, and allergic reactions to food and environmental allergens. Scratching at the area of

S. Işık (✉)
Department of Pediatric Allergy and Immunology, Süreyyapaşa Chest Diseases and Thoracic Surgery Training Hospital, Istanbul, Turkey

S. Asilsoy
Department of Pediatric Allergy and Immunology, Dokuz Eylul University, İzmir, Turkey

N. Rezaei (ed.), *Pediatric Allergy*, https://doi.org/10.1007/978-3-030-18282-3_29

pruritus leads to redness, cracking, scaling and potential superinfection of the skin. Fifty-five percent of patients with atopic dermatitis have a positive family history of atopy (allergic rhinitis, atopic dermatitis, asthma and food allergy) [1]. This patient had recurrent wheezing attacks which improved after nebulized B2 adrenergic agonist and steroid therapy. His mother had a history of allergic asthma and allergic rhinitis. Allergic asthma and atopic dermatitis due to food and/or aeroallergens were considered as a preliminary diagnosis.

Q2. Which one of the following is the most appropriate next step in the evaluation and management of this patient's condition?

A. Bronchoscopy
B. Measurement of serum Immunoglobulin levels
C. Skin prick test and serum specific IgE levels
D. Sweat test

Answer: *The correct answer is* ***C***.

Exacerbation of atopic dermatitis by foods is classically a delayed T-cell-mediated hypersensitivity reaction. Common foods that cause flares in atopic dermatitis are cow's milk protein, egg, soybean, and wheat [2]. Total IgE concentration is frequently high in patients with atopic dermatitis, which might lead to clinically non-relevant positive allergen-specific IgE [3].

There is general consensus that atopy should be evaluated in children when there is a suspicion or diagnosis of asthma. Identification of specific allergic sensitizations can support the diagnosis of asthma, point-out avoidable disease triggers and have prognostic value for disease persistence [4].

Our patient's history and basic laboratory tests revealed atopy, i.e. elevated total IgE and eosinophil levels. In the next step, the patient underwent skin prick test (SPT) and specific IgE (sIgE) tests for foods and aeroallergens which were positive for cow's milk (32 IU/mL), and house dust mite (*Dermatophagoides pteronyssinus* and *Dermatophagoides farinae*, both being >100 IU/mL).

Q3. All of the following treatments are most likely to benefit this patient, <u>except</u>:

A. Regular inhaled corticosteroid therapy
B. Avoiding from allergens
C. Prophylactic antibiotherapy
D. Regular use of moisturizers and topical corticosteroids, if needed.

Answer: *The correct answer is* ***C***.

Patients and families education is mandatory in treatment of atopic dermatitis. Avoidance of irritants and allergens, skin barrier repair, and use of anti-inflammatory and antimicrobial agents is important in preventing exacerbations. If food-induced flares are suspected, a 4-week period of dietary avoidance should be followed by a trial of food reintroduction to confirm the diagnosis. Proven allergies to cow's milk often resolve with age, thereby necessitating reintroduction of the food at 6- to 12-month intervals to determine if tolerance has developed or not. Regular use of moisturizers and topical steroids, if needed, are preferred over systemic anti-inflammatory treatment, allergen specific immunotherapy and phototherapy, which are all indicated in management of refractory cases of atopic dermatitis [5].

Infantile atopic dermatitis typically presents with erythematous papules and papulovesicles on the cheeks, forehead or scalp and extensor surfaces of the extremities. In childhood, usually by 2 years, lesions are less commonly noted on cheeks and become focused on skin folds including eyelids, neck, antecubital space, wrists, popliteal areas, ankles, and buttock regions [6].

Atopic March is a term coined for progression of atopic diseases. Patients with atopic dermatitis in infancy have an increased risk of food and respiratory allergy (allergic rhinitis and asthma) in late childhood [7, 8]. Severe and early-onset forms of atopic dermatitis is the strongest risk predictor for persistent disease and are associated with respiratory allergy such as asthma and allergic rhinitis in late childhood [9, 10], hence mandating follow-up by pediatric allergy and immunology specialist.

Our patient had recurrent wheezing attacks which got better after ICS therapy. He also needed regular ICS therapy because of frequent wheezing attacks.

Q4. Which one of the following can make suspicious of primary immunodeficiency?

A. History of two episodes of otitis media
B. Positive skin prick test
C. Good response to dietary restriction for dairy products
D. Elevated serum total IgE level of more than 2000 IU/L

Answer: *The correct answer is* ***D***.

More serious differential diagnoses like primary immunodeficiencies (PID) should be considered in children with atypical manifestation of atopic dermatitis in combination with recurrent infections. Hyper IgE syndrome (HIES) and atopic dermatitis with elevated IgE, are two distinct entities both with eczematous skin lesions. AD forms of HIES or Job's syndrome is associated with *STAT3* mutation, severe primary immunodeficiency, increased serum IgE levels (>2000 IU/L), recurrent infections and atopic dermatitis-like skin lesions. Positive SPT or elevated total and sIgE levels for allergens might be present in patients with HIES especially in autosomal recessive DOCK8 deficiency [11, 12]. Patients with severe AD merit evaluation for PID with assessment of serum immunoglobulin levels, even in the presence of positive SPT and/or elevated specific IgE levels for allergens.

There are also other phenotypes of patients having both manifestations of atopic dermatitis and a raised IgE, namely Immunodysregulation polyendocrinopathy enteropathy X-linked (IPEX) syndrome, Wiskott-Aldrich syndrome (WAS), or phosphoglucomutase 3 deficiency.

Q5. On the basis of the clinical diagnosis, which one of the following would be the most appropriate recommendation for the patient's parents?

A. Avoiding allergens
B. Good adherence to topical and inhaled corticosteroid therapy
C. Education of patients and families about disease
D. Regular following of patient by a pediatric allergy specialist
E. All of the above

Answer: *The correct answers is **E**.*

Patients and family education is one of the most effective treatments for atopic dermatitis and asthma.

Education should be tailored according to the socio-cultural background of the family [13]. Information about avoidance of irritants and allergens is important in preventing atopic dermatitis exacerbations. Asthma symptoms and exacerbations are triggered by a variety of specific and non-specific stimuli as well. Due to their pleiotropic anti-inflammatory activity, initiation of ICS therapy constitutes the first step of treatment [14].

Importantly, education should highlight the importance of treatment adherence to prescribed medication such as moisturizes and ICS therapy even in the absence of symptoms of asthma and AD.

Practical Points

- Patients with early-onset of wheezing attacks and itchy skin rashes should be investigated for food and aeroallergen sensitization
- Patients with infancy-onset atopic dermatitis are at increased risk of food allergy
- Patients and families should be educated on avoidance of allergens and irritants and good adherence to treatment
- Patients with severe atopic dermatitis should be evaluated for primary immunodeficiency diseases

References

1. Somanunt S, Chinratanapisit S, Pacharn P, Visitsunthorn N, Jirapongsananuruk O. The natural history of atopic dermatitis and its association with Atopic March. Asian Pac J Allergy Immunol. 2017;35(3):137–43.
2. Fleischer DM, Bock SA, Spears GC, Wilson CG, Miyazawa NK, Gleason MC, Gyorkos EA, Murphy JR, Atkins D, Leung DY. Oral food challenges in children with a diagnosis of food allergy. J Pediatr. 2011;158(4):578–83 e1.
3. Schneider L, Tilles S, Lio P, Boguniewicz M, Beck L, LeBovidge J, Novak N, Bernstein D, Blessing-Moore J, Khan D, Lang D, Nicklas R, Oppenheimer J, Portnoy J, Randolph C, Schuller D, Spector S, Tilles S, Wallace D. Atopic dermatitis: a practice parameter update 2012. J Allergy Clin Immunol. 2013;131(2):295–9 e1-27.

4. Illi S, von Mutius E, Lau S, Niggemann B, Gruber C, Wahn U. Multicentre Allergy Study g. Perennial allergen sensitisation early in life and chronic asthma in children: a birth cohort study. Lancet. 2006;368(9537):763–70.
5. Spergel JM. From atopic dermatitis to asthma: the atopic march. Ann Allergy Asthma Immunol. 2010;105(2):99–106; quiz 7–9, 17.
6. Samochocki Z, Dejewska J. A comparison of criteria for diagnosis of atopic dermatitis in children. World J Pediatr. 2012;8(4):355–8.
7. Shaker M. New insights into the allergic march. Curr Opin Pediatr. 2014;26(4):516–20.
8. Illi S, von Mutius E, Lau S, Nickel R, Gruber C, Niggemann B, Wahn U, Multicenter Allergy Study Group. The natural course of atopic dermatitis from birth to age 7 years and the association with asthma. J Allergy Clin Immunol. 2004;113(5):925–31.
9. Quah PL, Loo EX, Lee GN, Kuo IC, Gerez I, Llanora GV, Chan YH, Aw M, Shek LP, Lee BW. Clinical phenotype and allergen sensitization in the first 2 years as predictors of atopic disorders at age 5 years. World Allergy Organ J. 2015;8(1):33.
10. Mocsai G, Gaspar K, Dajnoki Z, Toth B, Gyimesi E, Biro T, Marodi L, Szegedi A. Investigation of skin barrier functions and allergic sensitization in patients with hyper-IgE syndrome. J Clin Immunol. 2015;35(7):681–8.
11. Grimbacher B, Holland SM, Puck JM. Hyper-IgE syndromes. Immunol Rev. 2005;203:244–50.
12. Joshi AY, Iyer VN, Boyce TG, Hagan JB, Park MA, Abraham RS. Elevated serum immunoglobulin E (IgE): when to suspect hyper-IgE syndrome-a 10-year pediatric tertiary care center experience. Allergy Asthma Proc. 2009;30(1):23–7.
13. Andrade WC, Camargos P, Lasmar L, Bousquet J. A pediatric asthma management program in a low-income setting resulting in reduced use of health service for acute asthma. Allergy. 2010;65(11):1472–7.
14. Barnes PJ. Inhaled glucocorticoids for asthma. N Engl J Med. 1995;332(13):868–75.

Chapter 30
Red Lesions on Face and Body and Fever

Hossein Esmaeilzadeh

An 18-month-old boy with fever was referred to our clinic with irritability and itchy lesions on face and trunk from 5 days ago. Some of the lesions were blisters that were crusted after itching.

In her past medical history dry and itchy skin was reported for which topical steroid and emollients had been ordered that were applied only intermittently and dropped after 1–2 months. Recurrent episodes of itchy red lesions in face and extensors from 1 month of age, followed by similar lesions in face and flexors was also reported. He was exclusively breast fed until 4 months old and cow's milk avoidance in mother's diet had not resulted in any improvement (Fig. 30.1a–c).

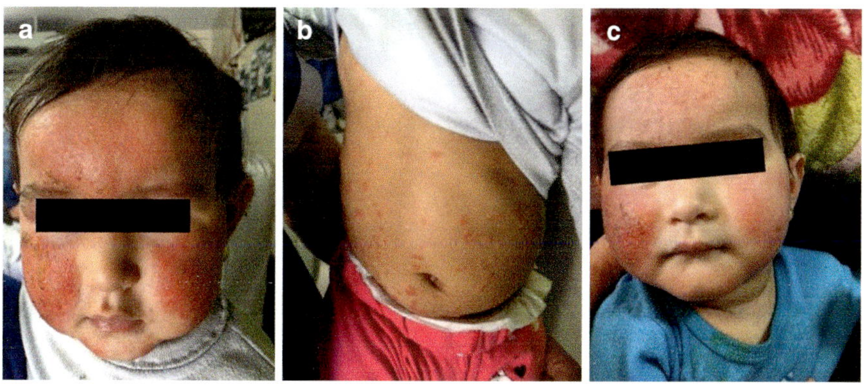

Fig. 30.1 Blisters with itching on day 1 before starting treatment (**a**, **b**), and 7 days after start treatment (**c**), in an 18-month-old boy

H. Esmaeilzadeh (✉)
Allergy Research Center, Namazi Hospital, Shiraz University of Medical Sciences, Shiraz, Iran
e-mail: esmaeilzadeh_ho@sums.ac.ir

N. Rezaei (ed.), *Pediatric Allergy*, https://doi.org/10.1007/978-3-030-18282-3_30

Q1. What is most likely diagnosis?

A. Eczema herpeticum
B. Eczema infantum
C. Impetigo
D. Cellulitis

***Answer**: The correct answer is **A**.*

Eczema herpeticum, caused by infiltration of herpes simplex virus (HSV), starts with clusters of red, itchy lesions with or without painful blisters or vesicles. It may affect any site but is most often seen on face and neck. Lesions occur in sites actively or previously affected by atopic dermatitis or other predisposing skin conditions [1]. Lesions tend to spread over a period of 7–10 days. Fever and swollen local lymph nodes can also be present. Viral infection is confirmed by viral swabs taken by scraping the base of a fresh blister. Tzanck smear showing epithelial multinucleated giant cells and acantholysis, i.e. cell separation, confirms the diagnosis [2]

Q2. Which of the following do you speculate to be his baseline condition?

A. Seborrheic dermatitis
B. Atopic dermatitis
C. Scabies
D. Contact dermatitis

***Answer**: The correct answer is **B**.*

Atopic dermatitis (AD), also known as atopic eczema, is a chronic relapsing inflammation of skin [3, 4]. Patients with AD have increased susceptibility to infection or colonization with a variety of organisms. These include viral infections with HSV, *Molluscum contagiosum*, and human papillomavirus (HPV), as well as bacterial infections with *Staphylococcus aureus* [5, 6]. Fever work up revealed normal CBC and normal physical examination. Tzanck smear showed epithelial multinucleated giant cells and acantholysis and blood PCR for herpes was negative.

Q3. Based on the clinical diagnosis which one of the following would be the most appropriate treatment for patient?

A. Topical corticosteroid
B. Systemic corticosteroid
C. Acyclovir
D. B-lactam antibiotic

***Answer**: The correct answer is **C**.*

Eczema herpeticum is considered as one of the few dermatological emergencies. Oral acyclovir 400–800 mg five times daily, or if available, valacyclovir 1 g twice daily, for 10–14 days or upon fading of the lesions, are considered standards of therapy. Intravenous acyclovir is prescribed if the patient is too ill to take tablets, or if clinical status is deteriorating despite treatment. Secondary bacterial skin infection should be watched for and in case of severe and extensive skin lesions, prevented by systemic prophylactic antibiotics. Topical steroids are not generally recommended, but may be necessary to alleviate symptoms of active atopic dermatitis [6].

Twenty-four hours after the initiation of systemic treatment, his fever had stopped and 4 days later his lesions showed significant improvement. Daily Eucerin emollient and skin hydration were ordered, while discharging the patient with low-potency, daily TCS.

Practical Points

- Viral and bacterial pathogens especially HSV and *Staphylococcus* can superimpose atopic dermatitis lesions
- Eczema herpeticum is a disseminated HSV-1 infection, appearing in patients with underlying skin condition, commonly atopic dermatitis
- Extensive cutaneous vesicular eruptions and superimposed bacterial infections are features of eczema herpeticum that prove to be fatal if untreated

References

1. Wollenberg A, Zoch C, Wetzel S, Plewig G, Przybilla B. Predisposing factors and clinical features of eczema herpeticum: a retrospective analysis of 100 cases. J Am Acad Dermatol. 2003;49(2):198–205.
2. Leung DY, Gao PS, Grigoryev DN, Rafaels NM, Streib JE, Howell MD, Taylor PA, Boguniewicz M, Canniff J, Armstrong B, Zaccaro DJ, Schneider LC, Hata TR, Hanifin JM, Beck LA, Weinberg A, Barnes KC. Human atopic dermatitis complicated by eczema herpeticum is associated with abnormalities in IFN-gamma response. J Allergy Clin Immunol. 2011;127(4):965–73.e1-5.
3. Boguniewicz M, Leung DY. Atopic dermatitis: a disease of altered skin barrier and immune dysregulation. Immunol Rev. 2011;242(1):233–46.
4. Stalder JF, Barbarot S, Wollenberg A, Holm EA, De Raeve L, Seidenari S, Oranje A, Deleuran M, Cambazard F, Svensson A, Simon D, Benfeldt E, Reunala T, Mazereeuv J, Boralevi F, Kunz B, Misery L, Mortz CG, Darsow U, Gelmetti C, Diepgen T, Ring J, Moehrenschlager M, Gieler U, Taieb A. Patient-oriented SCORAD (PO-SCORAD): a new self-assessment scale in atopic dermatitis validated in Europe. Allergy. 2011;66(8):1114–21.
5. Boguniewicz M, Leung DY. Recent insights into atopic dermatitis and implications for management of infectious complications. J Allergy Clin Immunol. 2010;125(1):4–13; quiz 4-5.
6. Leung DY, Guttman-Yassky E. Deciphering the complexities of atopic dermatitis: shifting paradigms in treatment approaches. J Allergy Clin Immunol. 2014;134(4):769–79.

Chapter 31
Eczematous Plaques after Bathing

Sara Manti, Caterina Cuppari, and Carmelo Damiano Salpietro

An 8-month-old Indian girl, presented with, itching, desquamative patterns, eczematous plaques and severe exfoliation on her lower extremities (Fig. 31.1). She was afebrile, had no regional adenopathy, no personal history of allergies, and no family history of atopy and/or atopic diseases. Symptoms resolved spontaneously after 10 days.

It turned out that, after bathing, the mother generally hydrated skin of our patient with a Chinese mixture. During hospitalization, mother discontinued the use of the cream and a spontaneous clinical remission occurred. However, due to the persistent itching, the baby was treated with cetirizine and "non-Chinese" emollients. Moreover, patient did not present specific allergen sensitization, as shown by the absence of both total and specific IgE and negative skin prick test (SPT). Conversely, patch tests for herbal extracts of were positive.

Based on clinical presentation and symptoms as well as results of laboratory test, a diagnosis of ichthyosiform dermatitis was hypothesized. Although a skin biopsy could have helped make a clear diagnosis of the baby's condition, her parents refused it.

Q1. Which diagnostic investigation is most appropriate for this patient?

A. Serum total IgE levels
B. Serum specific IgE levels
C. Skin prick test
D. Skin patch test

Answer: *The correct answer is* ***D****.*

Total and/or specific serum IgE levels can only discriminate children with and without atopy. SPT may be less sensitive than patch tests, as SPT evaluates

S. Manti (✉) · C. Cuppari · C. D. Salpietro
Unit of Pediatric, Department of Pediatrics, University of Messina, Messina, Italy

N. Rezaei (ed.), *Pediatric Allergy*, https://doi.org/10.1007/978-3-030-18282-3_31

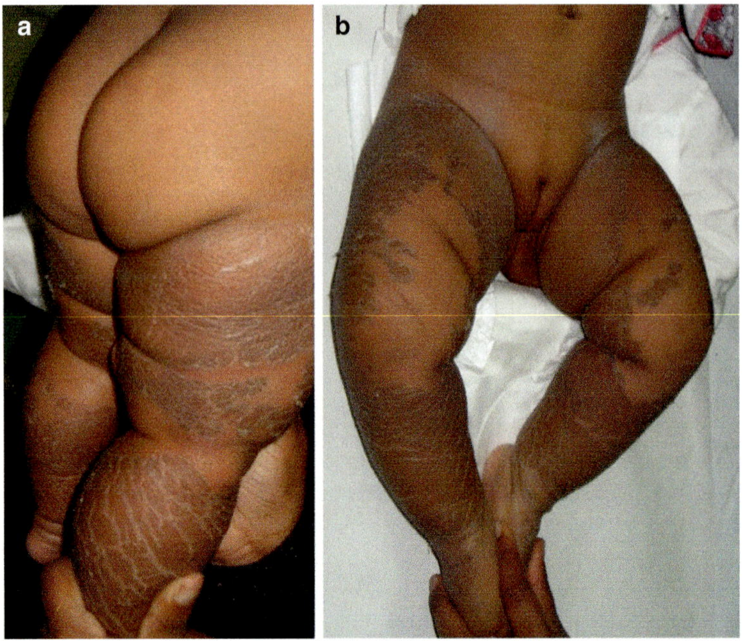

Fig. 31.1 Desquamative and ichthyosiform patterns, and eczematous plaques

mostly the immediate type of hypersensitivity, but the patch test is based on delayed type hypersensitivity. Patch testing for Chinese topical medications (CTMs) would be helpful using a regional standard series and topical traditional Chinese medicament. In fact, negative patch testing results for extracts of herbs and allergens infers the diagnosis of irritant contact dermatitis (ICD). Another major concern is that the active components in most CTMs formulae and their underlying mechanism of action remain unidentified, leading to diagnostic difficulties [1]. Even the same type of CTMs formula might contain complex combinations of individual ingredients, thus limiting the scope of clinical investigation [1]. In addition, studies on CTMs are also problematic because of the limited number of commercially available standardised patch test substances and the danger of acute sensitisation when testing with botanic and active components. Even after determining the composition of a CTMs it may be extremely difficult to obtain the exact ingredients for patch testing. Notwithstanding the fact that CTMs also contain chemical substances that probably cross-react with the standardized compounds of a patch test series. Therefore, it is imperative to perform patch testing on an adequate number of controls in serial dilutions, to exclude false-positive results.

Skin biopsy is not mandatory to make the diagnosis of ICD. Skin biopsy might show spongiotic dermatitis with eosinophils, acanthosis and intercellular edema [2].

Q2. Which type of clinical picture do you suspect to be caused by Chinese medicaments?

A. Local diseases
B. Systemic diseases
C. Local and systemic disease
D. None of the above

Answer: *The correct answer is* ***C****.*

Among the most common diseases associated to CTMs are: Stevens-Johnson syndrome (SJS) [3], generalized maculopapular eruption [4], acute urticaria [5], exanthematous eruption [6]. Patients with hypersensitivity myocarditis [7] and acute bronchospasm [8] from oral and inhaled preparations, respectively, have been also described. CTMs can also result in other adverse reactions, such as herb-herb and herb-drug interactions [9].

Q3. Which one is the principal causative agents of Chinese topical medicaments-mediated adverse reactions?

A. Steroid components
B. Aloe
C. Henna
D. Terpenes and essential-oil extracts

Answer: *The correct answer is* ***D****.*

CTMs are the result of a complex combination of individual ingredients from multiple herbal plant constituents, both in crude and galenic extracted forms [10]. Thus, the specific components in the CTMs causing disease are usually difficult to establish. The most common causative agents of CTMs-mediated adverse reactions are notably terpenes (e.g. camphor and menthol) and essential-oil extracts (e.g. eucalyptus and cinnamon) [11]. Furthermore, it has been reported that CTMs can be adulterated with steroid creams and Ayurvedic medicines, containing also arsenic or mercury [11]. Other popular remedies that can potentially cause side effects include St John's Wort, kava, aloe vera, henna, yohimbine, myrrh and chamomile. Hops and licorice root may also be responsible of CTMs-mediated adverse reactions [11, 12] (Table 31.1). Particularly, the allergic contact dermatitis is caused, more frequently, by Myrrh/mo yao; followed by photosensitivity from St. John's wort, hypersensitivity vasculitis from passion flower, allergic skin reaction from echinacea and hops, bronchospasm from royal jelly and lupus-like syndrome from yohimbine [12].

Q4. Based on the history and clinical features, what is the most likely diagnosis?

A. Irritant contact dermatitis
B. Allergic contact dermatitis

Table 31.1 The most common components of traditional Chinese topical medicaments (CTMs)

CTMs	Components	Uses	Common adverse reactions
Medicated oils (wind-oils)	Menthol Camphor Cinnamon Oil of olive Cassia oil Citronella oil Oil of lavender Cajeput oil	Headaches Insect bite Skin injuries Abdominal pain	Allergic contact dermatitis Positive patch test to fragrance mix, balsam of Peru
Oils for orthopedic injuries (balm for tendons and bones)	Camphor Menthol Essential oils Methyl salicylates Extracts of herbs Mastic Wine Honey Myrrh	Bruised and contused muscle	Severe and purpuric allergic contact dermatitis
Rheumatism oils	Camphor Menthol Essential oils	Rheumatism pains	Irritant contact dermatitis
Miscellaneous	Salicylic acid	Ringworm	Contact dermatitis

C. Ichthyosiform dermatitis
D. Atopic dermatitis

Answer: *The correct answer is **A**.*

Skin is the most common route of exposure among children. Chemicals, such as CTMs, are readily absorbed through thin skin especially in children which show a high ratio skin surface area/body weight [13]. CTMs use is still a popular treatment for dermatological and non-dermatological diseases. CTMs generally constitute a mixture of several components (e.g. essential-oil, herbal plant extracts, corticosteroid, and metals) in which the chemical composition and the dosage of each are often unknown [1].

ICD due to CTMs is an unusual and unique event. ICD develops as a result of a direct insult to the stratum corneum that causes a change in pH or cellular lipids leading to cell activation and an inflammatory response [2, 12]. Hypersensitivity, irritant or allergic contact dermatitis, urticaria, angioedema, anaphylaxis, and SJS have been described as possible adverse effects secondary to the use of herbal drugs [2, 12].

Q5. What is the most appropriate treatment?

A. Suspected topical medicaments should be discontinued
B. Emollients
C. Cetirizine and corticosteroid therapy
D. All of the above

Answer: *The correct answer is **D**.*

When ICD is hypothesized, use of topical medicaments should be discontinued. Treatment includes emollients to reduce water loss from the skin and facilitate barrier repair. Antihistamines can relieve intense itching. Topical steroid therapy should be reserved for severe symptoms and when the lesions involve extensive areas of the skin, systemic steroid therapy would resolve symptoms within 12–24 hours [14]. Some patients may experience complications of contact dermatitis, such as severe infections and therefor require proper antibiotic therapy [13].

Practical Points

- A common misconception is that CTMs have no adverse effects as a result of their natural composition
- Complementary and alternative medications should be included in the differential diagnosis of any allergic reaction
- Molecular and pharmacologic studies are warranted to determine the safety and efficacy of CTMs

References

1. Ng TP, Tan CH, Kua EH. The use of Chinese herbal medicines and their correlates in Chinese older adults: the Singapore Chinese Longitudinal Aging Study. Age Ageing. 2004;33(2):135–42.
2. Sen P, Ho MS, Ng SK, Yosipovitch G. Contact dermatitis: a common adverse reaction to topical traditional Chinese medicine. Int J Dermatol. 2010;49(11):1255–60.
3. Dega H, Laporte JL, Frances C, Herson S, Chosidow O. Ginseng as a cause for Stevens-Johnson syndrome? Lancet. 1996;347(9011):1344.
4. Wong HCG. Generalized allergic maculopapular eruption associated with prostate gland pills, a Chinese proprietary medicine of herbal origin. Ann R Coll Phys Surg Can. 2000;33:104–6.
5. Wong HCG. Acute urticaria associated with Chinese herbal medicine used for atopic dermatitis. Can J Allergy Clin Immunol. 2001;6:77–9.
6. Li LF, Zhao J, Li SY. Exanthematous drug eruption due to Chinese herbal medicines sanjieling capsule and huoxuexiaoyan pill. Contact Dermat. 1994;30(4):252–3.
7. Zaacks SM, Klein L, Tan CD, Rodriguez ER, Leikin JB. Hypersensitivity myocarditis associated with ephedra use. J Toxicol Clin Toxicol. 1999;37(4):485–9.
8. George HC, Wong M. Allergic contact dermatitis from topical Chinese herbal medicine and generalized urticaria and angioedema. BCMJ. 2002;44(4):184–7.
9. Miller LG. Herbal medicinals: selected clinical considerations focusing on known or potential drug-herb interactions. Arch Internal Med. 1998;158(20):2200–11.
10. Lim KS, Tang MB, Goon AT, Leow YH. The role of topical traditional Chinese medicaments as contact sensitisers in chronic venous leg ulcer patients. Ann Acad Med. 2007;36(11):942–6.
11. Leow Y-H, Ng S-K, Wong W-K, Goh C-L. Contact allergic potential of topical traditional Chinese medicaments in Singapore. Am J Contact Dermat. 1995;6(1):4–8.
12. Ernst E. Adverse effects of herbal drugs in dermatology. Br J Dermatol. 2000;143(5):923–9.
13. American Academy of Allergy, Asthma and Immunology; American College of Allergy, Asthma and Immunology. Contact dermatitis: a practice parameter. Ann Allergy Asthma Immunol. 2006;97(3 Suppl 2):S1–38.
14. Usatine RP, Riojas M. Diagnosis and management of contact dermatitis. Am Fam Phys. 2010;82(3):249–55.

Chapter 32
Multiple Blisters Over the Dorsum of the Hand

Wojciech Baran and Jacek Szepietowski

An 8-year-old girl presented with multiple blisters on the erythematous background on the dorsum of her hand. Five days ago, during her holiday trip to Bulgaria she had a temporary black henna tattoo (TBHT) on her right hand. Two days after itchy blisters reflecting the tattoo design had appeared. Her past medical history and familial history did not reveal any dermatological disorders including atopy or allergy. She once had TBHT in last summer vacations, without any complications. On examination multiple blisters under the tattoo were present, with erythrodermic background and moderate itching (Numeric Rating Scale; i.e. Itch NRS = 6) (Fig. 32.1). Laboratory data did not reveal any significant abnormalities.

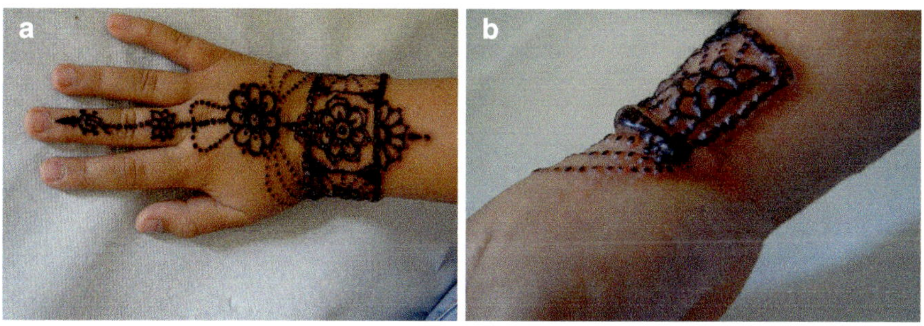

Fig. 32.1 Temporary black henna tattoo on the right hand of an 8-year-old girl (**a**), and formation of blisters on the erythematous background under the tattoo (**b**)

W. Baran (✉) · J. Szepietowski
Department of Dermatology, Venereology and Allergology, Wroclaw Medical University, Wroclaw, Poland
e-mail: wojciech.baran@umed.wroc.pl

N. Rezaei (ed.), *Pediatric Allergy*, https://doi.org/10.1007/978-3-030-18282-3_32

Q1. Which of the following immunological mechanisms is responsible for the development of the skin lesions?

A. Type I immune reaction
B. Type II immune reaction
C. Type III immune reaction
D. Type IV immune reaction

Answer: *The correct answer is* ***D****.*

Allergic contact dermatitis is a disease caused by the type IV delayed hypersensitivity reaction. In the first phase called an induction phase, contact allergens cross the horny layer of the epidermis and form hapten-protein conjugates. Langerhans cells recognize them as a foreign body and present the complex to T-lymphocytes in the regional lymph nodes. Some of the activated T cells evolve into skin memory T cells and trigger acute immune system reaction after next contact with the allergen, in the so called elicitation phase [1]. In our case probably the first TBHT was responsible for the induction phase, and in the subsequent contact, the elicitation phase was responsible for acute flare of allergic contact dermatitis.

Q2. Which of the following diagnostic tests is the gold-standard for this condition?

A. Skin prick test
B. Serum total IgE level
C. Skin patch test
D. Serum specific IgE level

Answer: *The correct answer is* ***C****.*

Patch testing for chemical substances is the gold standard in the diagnosis of allergic contact dermatitis [2]. In our patient it was conducted using the True Test for Skin Allergy Patch Testing with re-evaluation at 48 h and 72 h after application. After 48 h, reaction to the para-phenylenediamine (PPD) 1% solution showed a vesicular lesion (++), and after 72 h erosions (+++) emerged. Other substances were negative. The clinical suspicion of a PPD sensitization was confirmed.

Q3. Which substance in the TBHT is the most suspected sensitizer?

A. Balsam of Peru
B. Para-phenylenediamine
C. Mercaptobenzothiazole
D. Thiuram mix

Answer: *The correct answer is* ***B****.*

Black henna is derived from red henna pigment of *Lawsonia inermis* plants, mixed with various substances. The PPD is essential to make the henna darker and longer lasting. Low concentrations of oxidized PPD form do not have sensitizing effects. Black henna is prepared without any standardization and probably higher concentrations of PPD in non-oxidized may be used. European Union prohibits the use of PPD in any topical product, with the exception of hair dyes, which may contain up to 6% of PPD [3].

Practical Points

- Allergic contact dermatitis is caused by type IV delayed hypersensitivity reaction
- In the induction phase, contact allergens cross the horny layer of the epidermis and form hapten-protein conjugates, which are presented to T cells by Langerhans cells
- Activated T cells evolve into dermal memory T cells and trigger acute immune system reaction after next exposure to the allergen, in the elicitation phase

References

1. Kaplan DH. Early events in the induction of allergic contact dermatitis. Nat Rev Immunol. 2012;12(2):114–24.
2. Spornraft-Ragaller P, Schnuch A, Uter W. Extreme patch test reactivity to p-phenylenediamine but not to other allergens in children. Contact dermat. 2011;65(4):220–6.
3. Panfili E, Esposito S, Di Cara G. Temporary Black Henna Tattoos and Sensitization to para-Phenylenediamine (PPD): two paediatric case reports and a review of the literature. Int J Environ Res Public Health. 2017;14(4):pii:E421.

Chapter 33
Recurrent White Papules on Her Palm

Sara Manti, Valeria Dipasquale, Andrea Barbalace, and Caterina Cuppari

An 11-year-old girl presented with recurrent white papules on her palms. The papules spontaneously resolved, leaving no residual mark (Fig. 33.1a, b).

There was no history of atopy and/or atopic diseases, and she was not taking any medications. The physical examination revealed no other abnormalities. Both hot and cold water induced a prodrome of skin pruritus and development of papules on the palms of the hands approximately 5–6 min after the initial contact. Each episode lasted for 20–30 min. Results from laboratory tests, including a CBC including circulating eosinophils, LFT, electrolytes, serum total IgE values, and autoimmune blood testing were normal.

A water-challenge test revealed similar results. Also, an exercise test, a pressure test, and ice cube test were performed to rule out physical urticaria, all resulting negative.

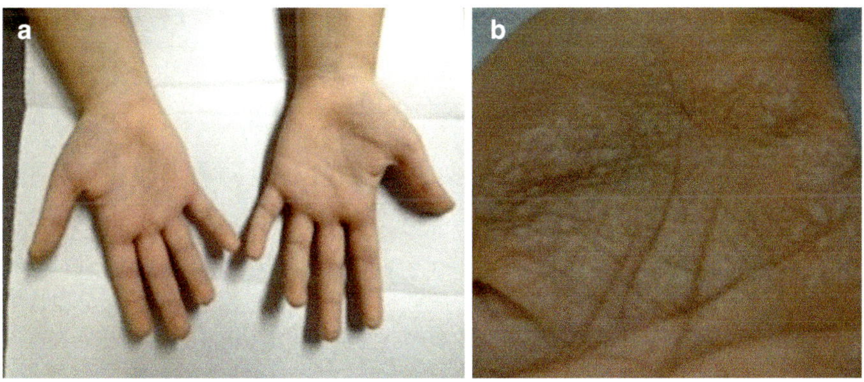

Fig. 33.1 (**a**, **b**) Wheals were exclusively present on the palms of the hands

S. Manti (✉) · V. Dipasquale · A. Barbalace · C. Cuppari
Unit of Pediatric, Department of Pediatrics, University of Messina, Messina, Italy
e-mail: smanti@unime.it

N. Rezaei (ed.), *Pediatric Allergy*, https://doi.org/10.1007/978-3-030-18282-3_33

Q1. Which one of the following categories is most likely the case in this patient?

A. Physical urticaria
B. Cholinergic urticaria
C. Aquagenic palmar keratoderma
D. Contact dermatitis

Answer: *The correct answer is* ***C****.*

Aquagenic palmar keratoderma (APK) is the diagnosis. APK is an acquired condition characterized by formation of edematous, translucent papules and plaques on the palms after 2–5 min of immersion in water, i.e. "hand in bucket sign": patients arrive in their physician's office with their hand in a bucket of water to more readily demonstrate their lesions. Several unusual presentations have been also reported in the literature, including a localized form on the heel and involvement of the dorsum of fingers, sparing of the palms, and also a unilateral type [1].

APK shows a predilection for adolescents and women. This disorder has been reported under many different names including aquagenic palmoplantar keratoderma, aquagenic syringeal acrokeratoderma, acquired aquagenic papulotranslucent acrokeratoderma, and aquagenic wrinkling of the palms [1].

Q2. Which of the following category of differential diagnoses does APK belong to?

A. Hereditary papulotranslucent acrokeratoderma
B. Physical urticaria
C. Contact dermatitis
D. Cholinergic urticaria

Answer: *The correct answer is* ***A****.*

One important differential diagnosis is hereditary papulotranslucent acrokeratoderma (HPA), which appears soon after puberty and persists throughout the patient's life. In histology, focal hyperkeratosis and acanthosis with normal eccrine ducts are seen [2].

APK is an acquired palmoplantar keratoderma that predominantly affects adolescent and young adult women. No cases of affected male patients have yet been documented. APK manifests with burning and translucent to whitish papules and plaques after exposure to water, involving hands and occasionally feet. Some APK patients experience an atopic diathesis, others do not.

HPA is a congenital palmoplantar keratoderma with probably autosomal dominant inheritance. In contrast to APK, men and women are similarly affected. HPA manifests with asymptomatic translucent yellow-white papules and plaques, involving both hands and feet and is more frequently associated to atopic diathesis [3].

Q3. What is the hallmark pathophysiology of APK?

A. Cystic fibrosis
B. Atopy

C. Autoimmune diseases
D. All of the above

Answer: *The correct answer is **D**.*

Generally, APK is observed in healthy subjects, yet a predilection has been described in patients with cystic fibrosis (CF) and as an adverse effect of selective cyclooxygenase-2 inhibitor therapy. Most cases are sporadic, however, familial aggregation has been reported in the literature [4]. In particular, the majority of "reported cases" were associated with CF. In fact, APK affects 40% of patients with CF. Interestingly, APK risk has been related to the same mutations found in CF, e.g. the homozygous or heterozygous ΔF508 mutation of the *CFTR* gene.

The pathophysiology of APK remains unclear, while several causative mechanisms including: (1) aberration of the sweat glands, (2) barrier defect in the stratum corneum due to keratin defect, and (3) defective chloride channels which induce an osmotic gradient and hypertonic sweat. The elevated skin sodium levels increased the water-binding capacity of keratin and caused APK [1].

Other associations include atopy (i.e. asthma, rhinitis, urticaria), hyperhidrosis, hepatitis C, osteomyelitis, melanoma, Behçet disease, nail psoriasis and medications like aspirin [5]. Moreover, an association of APK with familial lactose intolerance has also been reported [6]. Our patient underwent a sweat chloride test to rule out subclinical cystic fibrosis.

Q4. Which of the following treatment is the best therapeutic option for this clinical entity?

A. Ammonium lactate
B. Aluminum chloride
C. Gloves
D. Petroleum jelly

Answer: *The correct answer is **B**.*

Although the action mechanism of topical aluminium chloride is not still clear, it is currently the most widely employed therapy [1]. Other treatment options include barrier creams, glycerol emollients, 5–20% salicylic lotion, 10 % urea cream, iontophoresis, TCS, formalin in alcohol solution, antihistamines, topical erythromycin, and botulinum toxin [7].

Botulinum toxin is effective in hyperhidrosis, affecting preganglionic sympathetic and parasympathetic and postganglionic parasympathetic nerves. Authors recommend botulinum toxin for cases not responding to topical treatment, as second-line therapy [8].

Treatments involving the application of 12% ammonium lactate creams or petroleum jelly or the use of gloves have not shown to be effective [9].

Q5. Which option best describes the clinical course of patients with APK?

A. APK has a good prognosis
B. APK has a poor prognosis

C. APK has a variable prognosis
D. There are poor available literature data on this matter

Answer: *The correct answer is* ***C.***

Because of its transient nature, APK is probably more prevalent than reported in the literature. Several cases of spontaneous remission have been described [10], however, in most patients, APK tends to persist and cause significant physical and psychological discomfort.

Whenever possible, the triggering agent must be removed. Prolonged water exposure and temperature of the water affects the rate and intensity of lesion development. Treatment is variable and tailored to the individual, which makes a gold-standard management algorithm difficult to design. In our case, the manifestations progressively diminished in our patient and faded completely after 12 months.

Practical Points

- The "hand-in-the-bucket sign" for the diagnosis of aquagenic palmar keratoderma (APK) means that lesions appear more readily when the patients puts hands in water
- The natural history, clinical features, and histology provide the "key points" to differentiate APK from other diagnoses
- APK can be an alarm for underlying cystic fibrosis

References

1. Lee H-C TT-F. Aquagenic syringeal acrokeratoderma. Dermatol Sinica. 2008;26:632.
2. Onwukwe MF, Mihm MC Jr, Toda K. Hereditary papulotranslucent acrokeratoderma. A new variant of familial punctate keratoderma? Arch Dermatol. 1973;108(1):108–10.
3. Yagerman SE, Lager M, Soter NA. Acquired aquagenic papulotranslucent acrokeratoderma. Dermatol Online J. 2016;22(12):pii:13030/qt7kw3c23w.
4. Garcon-Michel N, Roguedas-Contios AM, Rault G, Le Bihan J, Ramel S, Revert K, Dirou A, Misery L. Frequency of aquagenic palmoplantar keratoderma in cystic fibrosis: a new sign of cystic fibrosis? Br J Dermatol. 2010;163(1):162–6.
5. Luo DQ, Zhao YK, Zhang WJ, Wu LC. Aquagenic acrokeratoderma. Int J Dermatol. 2010;49(5):526–31.
6. Treudler R, Tebbe B, Steinhoff M, Orfanos CE. Familial aquagenic urticaria associated with familial lactose intolerance. J Am Acad Dermatol. 2002;47(4):611–3.
7. Adisen E, Karaca F, Gurer MA. Transient reactive papulotranslucent acrokeratoderma in a 50-year-old woman: case report and review of the literature. Am J Clin Dermatol. 2008;9(6):404–9.
8. Bagazgoitia L, Perez-Carmona L, Salguero I, Harto A, Jaen P. Letter: aquagenic keratoderma: successful treatment with botulinum toxin. Dermatol Surg. 2010;36(3):434–6.
9. Syed Z, Wanner M, Ibrahimi OA. Aquagenic wrinkling of the palms: a case report and literature review. Dermatol Online J. 2010;16(7):7.
10. Coelho-Macias V, Fernandes S, Lamarao P, Assis-Pacheco F, Cardoso J. Aquagenic keratoderma associated with a mutation of the cystic fibrosis gene. Rev Portug Pneumol. 2013;19(3):125–8.

Chapter 34
Refractory Urticaria Over Exposed Areas

Federica Porcaro, Lucia Caminiti, Stefania Arasi, and Giovanni Battista Pajno

A 16-year-old Caucasian girl was admitted at our Allergy Unit with an 18-month history of recurrent urticaria. She reported erythema, followed by intense itching, swelling and hives only in the sun exposed areas of body after about 15 min of minimal sunlight exposition. A complete spontaneous resolution occurred after about 30–60 min of sun exposure [1]. In her past medical history she had mildly disturbing allergic rhinitis to grass and *Alternaria*. Her quality of life had been seriously compromised by urticaria and her past medical history was otherwise unremarkable.

Antinuclear antibody, anti-thyroid antibodies, serology for celiac disease and *Helicobacter pylori* fecal antigen were negative. ESR, liver and renal function panel, WBC count, hepatitis C virus serology and ferritin and heme metabolites were normal. Phototest [2] was positive for ultraviolet (UV) B (UVB) (>1.2 J/cm^2).

Q1. What is the most likely diagnosis?

A. Photodermatosis induced through a photoallergic or phototoxic mechanism.
B. Common polymorphic light eruption with transitory wheals
C. Solar urticaria
D. None of the above

Answer: *The correct answer is* ***C.***

F. Porcaro (✉)
Respiratory Unit, Academic Department of Pediatrics, Bambino Gesù Children's Hospital, IRCCS, Rome, Italy
e-mail: federica.porcaro@opbg.net

L. Caminiti · S. Arasi · G. B. Pajno
Allergy Unit, Department of Pediatrics, University of Messina, Messina, Italy

N. Rezaei (ed.), *Pediatric Allergy*, https://doi.org/10.1007/978-3-030-18282-3_34

Even if the patient had personal history of atopy, appearance of urticaria only after sunlight exposition is pathognomonic for Solar Urticaria (SU), which was confirmed by phototest.

Exclusion of other conditions such as food allergy, adverse drug reaction, assumption of topical or systemic drugs related to chronic urticaria (e.g. contraceptives, antibiotics, furosemide, etc.), infectious diseases and immunological or lymphoproliferative disorders, is necessary [3].

Solar urticaria is characterized by wheal and flare that usually occur within 5–10 min of exposure to ultraviolet radiation, however, rare instances of delayed onset solar urticaria have been described. Common polymorphic light eruptions usually emerge as itchy, burning rash after exposure to sunlight or artificial UV light with a delayed onset. Direct light exposure is necessary, which might occur even through thin clothing [4].

Q2. Which statement is true with regards to the SU?

A. Ultraviolet radiation, UVB and more frequently UVA, induced urticarial skin lesions at the photo exposed sites
B. It is burdened by the risk of anaphylactic shock after whole-body exposure
C. Both A and B
D. None of the above

Answer: *The correct answer is* ***C***.

The absorption of light by one or more chromophores in the skin or serum of patients with solar urticaria produces a photoproduct capable of binding to IgE and to the mast cell membrane. The ensuing degranulation of mast cell would lead to an inflammatory wheal-type response.

As a consequence, most patients with solar urticaria describe a sensation of itching or burning at photoexposed sites. Systemic symptoms, including headache, nausea, wheezing, dizziness, syncope and anaphylactic shock have also been reported [4].

Q3. What is the most appropriate next step in management of the described condition?

A. Avoidance of sunlight, protective clothing, broadband sunscreens
B. Short course of oral steroid for severe exacerbations especially when associated with angioedema
C. Both A and B
D. None of the above

Answer: *The correct answer is* ***C***.

In our patient, avoidance of sunlight and protective clothing were insufficient to control the symptoms. Combination of three types of H1-antihistamines at standard dose (cetirizine 10 mg/day, desloratadine 5 mg/day and hydroxyzine 25 mg/day) as well as combination of H1-antihistamine at double dose (cetirizine 20 mg/day) with

H2-antihistamine at standard dose (ranitidine 150 mg/day) and leukotriene receptor antagonists (LTRAs) (montelukast 10 mg), were all ineffective. Short courses of prednisone tablets (25 mg daily, over 5 days) were also poorly effective and the patient still had urticaria with sunlight exposure.

Treatment of SU is highly challenging and often unsatisfactory with specific guidelines lacking. Avoidance of known provoking stimuli should be the primary strategy in any treatment protocol. Antihistamines are the mainstay of treatment for children with SU and combinations of antihistamines (two different second-generation antihistamines or the combination of a second and first generation antihistamine) may improve symptom control. In non-responsive patients doubling the dose of antihistamines, is an effective treatment option. LTRAs should only be used as a second and add-on therapy. Short-term use of oral corticosteroids should be reserved to gain control in children who remain poorly responsive to maximal doses of H1 antihistamines in combination with H2 antihistamines receptor blockade and LTRAs [3].

Q4. Which one of the following treatments would be considered in the long-term treatment of our patients?

A. Oral corticosteroids
B. Cyclosporine A
C. Omalizumab
D. None of the above

Answer: *The correct answer is* ***C****.*

After the failure of conventional therapies, the patient was started experimental therapy with omalizumab (Xolair, Novartis Europharm). On the basis of her initial serum IgE level (moderately elevated, 228 IU/mL) and her body weight (57.7 kg), a calculated dose of 375 mg of omalizumab every 2 weeks was given subcutaneously. Cyclosporine A may be considered in patients with severe unremitting disease uncontrolled by antihistamines. Besides suppression of T-cell-mediated mechanisms, it has been proposed that cyclosporine A inhibits basophil and mast cell degranulation. Systemic corticosteroids can be used only as a short course during acute exacerbations.

Therapeutic response of this patient was promptly seen already at first administration and improvement persisted with maintenance doses. Six months later, we reduced the dose, in agreement with the recent indication for CSU up to suspension. Phototest was negative both for UVA and for UVB at the end of this period. The patient is still in follow up with ongoing omalizumab treatment.

Additional immune modifiers and experimental therapy should be limited for use in difficult cases and limited centers. In refractory patients, the guidelines recommend addition of omalizumab, cyclosporine A or montelukast. Because of the frequent renal function monitoring and the significant increase of adverse events related to prolonged use of cyclosporine A, attention is now focused on omalizumab that has shown a good efficacy and optimal safety in treated patients, even though data on long-term side effects related to its use are not yet available [3].

Practical Points

- We describe the case of a girl affected by solar urticaria induced by visible light
- Although light provocation test is difficult to perform, it is essential for the correct diagnosis and management of solar urticaria
- Avoidance of sunlight exposure and antihistamines are the mainstay of treatment in children with solar urticaria
- Short-term use of oral steroids should be reserved for disease flares
- Third line therapy, e.g. omalizumab, should be considered only in patients with solar urticaria refractory to conventional treatment

References

1. Arasi S, Crisafulli G, Caminiti L, Guarneri F, Aversa T, Porcaro F, Pajno GB. Treatment with omalizumab in a 16-year-old Caucasian girl with refractory solar urticaria. Pediatr Allergy Immunol. 2015;26(6):583–5.
2. De Argila D, Aguilera J, Sanchez J, Garcia-Diez A. Study of idiopathic, exogenous photodermatoses, part II: photobiologic testing. Acta Dermo-sifiliogr. 2014;105(3):233–42.
3. Powell RJ, Du Toit GL, Siddique N, Leech SC, Dixon TA, Clark AT, Mirakian R, Walker SM, Huber PA, Nasser SM. BSACI guidelines for the management of chronic urticaria and angio-oedema. Clin Exp Allergy. 2007;37(5):631–50.
4. Botto NC, Warshaw EM. Solar urticaria. J Am Acad Dermatol. 2008;59(6):909–20. quiz 21-2

Chapter 35
Chronic Urticaria

Irena Ivkovic-Jurekovic, Marta Navratil, and Iva Topalusic

A 15-year-old girl was referred to allergologist for assessment of a possible allergy due to a 6-month history of intermittent hives, and a description of symptoms corresponding to the definition of chronic urticaria. She had no family history of urticaria or atopy.

Physical examination was unremarkable except for the few hives on her abdomen and legs. Workup results showed sensitization to nuts with positive skin prick test (SPT), and elevated total IgE and specific IgE (sIgE) against peanut, hazelnut and walnut. However, the sensitization was not clinically significant and she has been eating nuts without showing any symptoms of allergy.

Our experience confirms that chronic urticaria may be associated with celiac disease. Evidence suggests that the duration of exposure to gluten in patients with celiac disease is related to the risk of developing other autoimmune diseases [1, 2].

Acute infection and chronic inflammatory diseases were ruled out. Her thyroid hormone concentrations were normal but the thyroid peroxidase antibody level (TPO-Ab) was slightly elevated. Thyroid ultrasound revealed chronic lymphocytic thyroiditis with normal thyroid function. Her stool was negative for parasites, yet positive for *Candida spp*. However, antibodies against *Candida albicans* in the patient's serum could not be detected. The patient had positive autologous serum skin test (ASST) [3], but circulating auto-antibodies against IgE and against the Fc subunit of high-affinity IgE receptor (FcεRIα) were negative [4]. Non-sedating

I. Ivkovic-Jurekovic (✉) · M. Navratil
Children's Hospital Zagreb, Zagreb, Croatia

Faculty of Dental Medicine and Healthcare, University of Osijek, Osijek, Croatia
e-mail: irena.ivkovic-jurekovic@kdb.hr

I. Topalusic
Children's Hospital Zagreb, Zagreb, Croatia

N. Rezaei (ed.), *Pediatric Allergy*, https://doi.org/10.1007/978-3-030-18282-3_35

H1-antihistamine levocetirizine was introduced and after 2 weeks of persistence of symptoms, the dose was increased fourfold [5]. Her symptoms subsided thereafter, but did not disappear completely. She was advised by her nutritionist to adhere to gluten-free diet. After a month she reported no remaining signs of urticaria.

Q1. Which one of the following is the most likely cause of chronic urticaria in this patient?

A. Food allergy
B. *Candida* in stool
C. Chronic lymphocytic thyroiditis
D. Celiac disease

Answer: *The correct answer is* ***D.***

Food allergy is only a very rare cause of chronic urticaria. Although the patient has showed sensitization to nuts with positive SPT and sIgE, she had been eating nuts without showing any symptoms of allergy.

There have been some reports showing that intestinal colonisation of *Candida spp.* could be a cause of chronic urticaria. Our patient had no detectable specific antibodies against *Candida albicans*. Therefore we excluded *Candida* as a possible cause of chronic urticaria.

Recently published data show that chronic lymphocytic thyroiditis is associated with increased risk of chronic spontaneous urticaria (CSU), especially in females [6, 7]. Pathogenic mechanisms in patients with CSU and thyroid autoimmunity may include IgE against autoantigens, immune complexes, and activation of complement system. Total resolution of symptoms in our patient following introduction of gluten-free diet led us to conclusion that celiac disease was the trigger for chronic urticaria in this case. In the meantime we have obtained positive results to both anti-tissue transglutaminase (anti-tTG) IgG and anti-endomysium (EmA) IgA autoantibodies. The girl had no recurrence of chronic urticaria so far.

Q2. Skin prick test with a standard panel of common inhalant and food allergens should be performed:

A. In all patients with chronic urticaria
B. Only in patients with chronic spontaneous urticaria
C. In patients with chronic spontaneous urticaria and medical history suggestive of atopy
D. Should not be performed at all.

Answer: *The correct answer is* ***C.***

According to the recommendations for diagnosis and management of chronic urticaria, SPT is not mandatory in all patients with chronic urticaria since allergy is very rarely a cause of this condition [5]. SPT may be performed in suspected cases and is used to confirm the diagnosis of food or drug allergy caused by IgE-mediated hypersensitivity reaction. Positive SPT indicates allergic sensitization and is accompanied by allergen-specific IgE in serum, yet this might not always be clinically relevant.

Q3. All of the following should be suspected as an associated condition of chronic urticaria, except:

A. Autoimmune disease
B. Helicobacter pylori infection
C. Malignancies
D. Hereditary angioedema

Answer: *The correct answer is* ***D.***

Detailed medical history and physical examination to identify causes and precipitating factors are important for diagnosis in chronic urticaria [5]. *Helicobacter pylori* infection and malignancies have been reported to be only rare causes of chronic urticaria [5]. Autoimmune diseases have to be excluded as they may share the same pathogenic mechanism as chronic spontaneous urticaria. Hereditary angioedema is not accompanied by hives.

Q4. Which one is the first-line therapy for chronic urticaria?

A. Low dose oral corticosteroid
B. Combination of H1- and H2-antihistamine
C. Non-sedating H1-antihistamine
D. Omalizumab

Answer: *The correct answer is* ***C.***

Non-sedating, second-generation H1-antihistamines are first line treatment for chronic urticaria while the second step is raising the dose of the same drug. In refractory patients, the guidelines recommend addition of omalizumab or cyclosporine A [8]. Systemic corticosteroids can be introduced in short courses during acute exacerbations [8].

Practical Points

- Chronic urticaria is defined by the presence of wheals, angioedema, or both during most days of the week, for a duration of more than 6 weeks
- Chronic urticaria may be inducible or spontaneous
- The therapeutic approach comprises two main steps: (1) avoidance of the cause or trigger, and (2) symptomatic pharmacological treatment by reducing mast cell mediator release or reducing the effect of these mediators on the target organ

References

1. Ludvigsson JF, Lindelof B, Rashtak S, Rubio-Tapia A, Murray JA. Does urticaria risk increase in patients with celiac disease? A large population-based cohort study. Eur J Dermatol. 2013;23(5):681–7.
2. Sategna Guidetti C, Solerio E, Scaglione N, Aimo G, Mengozzi G. Duration of gluten exposure in adult coeliac disease does not correlate with the risk for autoimmune disorders. Gut. 2001;49(4):502–5.
3. Konstantinou GN, Asero R, Maurer M, Sabroe RA, Schmid-Grendelmeier P, Grattan CE. EAACI/GA(2)LEN task force consensus report: the autologous serum skin test in urticaria. Allergy. 2009;64(9):1256–68.
4. Platzer MH, Grattan CE, Poulsen LK, Skov PS. Validation of basophil histamine release against the autologous serum skin test and outcome of serum-induced basophil histamine release studies in a large population of chronic urticaria patients. Allergy. 2005;60(9):1152–6.
5. Zuberbier T, Aberer W, Asero R, Bindslev-Jensen C, Brzoza Z, Canonica GW, Church MK, Ensina LF, Gimenez-Arnau A, Godse K, Goncalo M, Grattan C, Hebert J, Hide M, Kaplan A, Kapp A, Abdul Latiff AH, Mathelier-Fusade P, Metz M, Nast A, Saini SS, Sanchez-Borges M, Schmid-Grendelmeier P, Simons FE, Staubach P, Sussman G, Toubi E, Vena GA, Wedi B, Zhu XJ, Maurer M, European Academy of A, Clinical I, Global A, Asthma European N, European Dermatology F, World Allergy O. The EAACI/GA(2) LEN/EDF/WAO Guideline for the definition, classification, diagnosis, and management of urticaria: the 2013 revision and update. Allergy. 2014;69(7):868–87.
6. Kim YS, Han K, Lee JH, Kim NI, Roh JY, Seo SJ, Song HJ, Lee MG, Choi JH, Park YM. Increased risk of chronic spontaneous urticaria in patients with autoimmune thyroid diseases: a nationwide, population-based study. Allergy Asthma Immunol Res. 2017;9(4):373–7.
7. Kolkhir P, Pogorelov D, Olisova O, Maurer M. Comorbidity and pathogenic links of chronic spontaneous urticaria and systemic lupus erythematosus—a systematic review. Clin Exp Allergy. 2016;46(2):275–87.
8. Maurer M, Vena GA, Cassano N, Zuberbier T. Current and future therapies for treating chronic spontaneous urticaria. Expert Opin Pharmacother. 2016;17(8):1131–9.

Chapter 36
Exacerbation of Eczema and History of Food Allergy

Elena Camelia Berghea

A 6-year-old boy was seen for the first time by an allergist at the age of 2 years with a history of recurrent episodes of urticaria and angioedema after ingestion of grilled fish (cod) or grilled chicken meat, with no symptoms between the episodes. Physical examination was unremarkable during current assessment.

Laboratory data showed elevated levels of serum total IgE (489.7 IU/mL) and eosinophilia (950 μL^{-1}), positive specific IgE (sIgE) for cod fish (8.9 IU/mL), white egg (0.89 IU/mL), egg yolk (0.54 IU/mL), and negative sIgE for chicken meat, cow's milk proteins, wheat, peanut, nuts or soy. Oral food challenge (OFC) tests were positive for fish (cod, salmon, trout) and negative for chicken meat or egg, regardless of preparation type.

The parents were advised to avoid fish in the child's diet and to be careful about food contamination in the preparation process.

After a long symptom-free period, the patient came in with a severe eczema at the age of 4 years and 8 months, not improved by emollients and topical corticosteroids. He also reported a history of intermittent wheezing, respiratory distress, cough induced by viral respiratory infections, and persistent blocked and itchy nose. Examination revealed severe xerosis, eczematous lesions, and papular dermatitis affecting the flexural areas, especially the antecubital and popliteal fossae. There were thickened, lichenified plaques with excoriation and keratosis pilaris on the arms.

Q1. With the above descriptions about the skin condition, the <u>least</u> likely possible disease is?

A. Scabies
B. Ichthyosis
C. Psoriasis

E. C. Berghea (✉)
Emergency Clinical Hospital for Children M.S. Curie, Bucharest, Romania

University of Medicine and Pharmacy Carol Davila, Bucharest, Romania

N. Rezaei (ed.), *Pediatric Allergy*, https://doi.org/10.1007/978-3-030-18282-3_36

D. Wiskott-Aldrich syndrome
E. Cutaneous T cell lymphoma

Answer: *The correct answer is* ***D.***

Normal count for thrombocytes excludes Wiskott-Aldrich syndrome. Relevant laboratory data revealed elevated serum level of total IgE (5334 IU/mL). Specific IgE panel was positive for food and inhalant allergens presented in Table 36.1.

Q2. The reason of eczema exacerbation might be:

A. Late reaction induced by a food
B. Skin exposure to pollens
C. Skin exposure to dust mite
D. All of the above

Answer*: The correct answer is* ***D****.*

Q3. In the light of clinical symptoms of the boy, which statement is correct?

A. Exclusion of all food proteins with a positive specific IgE result
B. No evictions because the polisensitization in atopic dermatitis has no clinical significance
C. The clinical history of the patient is the only way to decide if and what food to be excluded

Table 36.1 Specific IgE levels to inhalant and food allergens in a 6-year-old boy

	Actual value, U/mL	Normal range, U/mL
Food allergens		
Cow's milk proteins	28.8	<0.35
Egg white	30.2	<0.35
Egg yolk	10.2	<0.35
Wheat	14.8	<0.35
Gluten	3.64	<0.35
Peanuts	14.7	<0.35
Hazelnuts	15.4	<0.35
Fish	27.1	<0.35
Soy	10.07	<0.35
Inhalant allergens		
Dermatophagoides pteronyssinus	>100	<0.35
Dermatophagoides farinae	>100	<0.35
Phleum pratense	54.16	<0.35
Betulla verrucosa	5.73	<0.35
Ambrosia elatior	4.35	<0.35
Artemisia	3.12	<0.35

D. Flares of eczema are mostly non-IgE mediated food allergy such that the specific IgE does not help to drive the diet
E. A stepwise procedure addressing individual factors is recommended

***Answer**: The correct answer is **E**.*

A diagnosis of food allergy should be considered in children with atopic eczema with a history of previous adverse reaction to food or in infants and young children with moderate or severe atopic eczema that has not been controlled by optimum management [1].

Due to multiple food and inhalant allergens sensitivities, we looked for molecular diagnosis (IgE Multiplex—FABER test), and the results were:

- Food allergens:
  - Peanuts:
    - Ara h 1 (7S Vicilin; CCD-bearing Protein (XF) Ara h 1-NT)—5.07
    - Ara h 2, 3, 6, 9—negative
  - Hazelnuts:
    - Cor a 1, 8, 9, 14—negative
  - Egg:
    - Gal d 1 (ovomucoid)—17.02
    - Gal d 5 (ovalbumin)—2.48
  - Soy:
    - Gly m1 (Hydrophobic Seed Protein)—negative
    - Agglutinin—negative
    - Gly m TI—2.91
  - Cow's milk proteins:
    - alpha-lactalbumin (Bos d 4)—6.07
    - beta-lactoglobulin (Bos d 5)—11.53
    - casein (Bos d 8)—12.4
    - bovine serum albumin (Bos d 6)—15.02
  - Wheat:
    - Tri a 7k-LTP—negative
    - Tri a 18 (Hevein-like; Agglutinin; Lectin)—negative
    - Tri a Gliadin—negative
    - Tri a 28 (alpha-Amylase Inhibitor)—negative
  - Fish:
    - Mer mr 1 (Parvalbumin)—37.03

- Inhalant allergens:
  - Dust mites:
    - Der p 1—12.62
    - Der p 2—80.02
    - Der p 10—negative
    - Der f 1—10.3
    - Der f 2—58.41
  - Birch:
    - Bet v1—negative
    - Bet v2—6.39
  - Grasses:
    - Phl p 1—15.3
    - Phl p 5—23.8
    - Phl p 2, 6, 7—negative
  - Weeds:
    - Art v 1—negative
    - Amb a 1—8.54

Q4. The positive value of specific IgE for molecular components are highly suggestive of clinical relevant allergy for the following food allergens, except?

A. Baked cow's milk proteins
B. Raw and baked egg proteins
C. Raw but not baked egg proteins
D. Fish
E. Possible cow meat

***Answer**: The correct answer is **C**.*

We advised the mother to exclude from the boy's diet the relevant foods for 2–4 weeks and followed up for the improvement of the eczema scores, with complete remission only after 2 weeks of the start of the diet. The guidelines recommend the oral provocation test as the only diagnostic tool instrument to differentiate between clinically relevant food allergy and silent sensitization [2]. Due to multiple food exclusions from the diet, we performed oral provocation tests in order to avoid unnecessary evictions. The result were positive for cow's milk proteins and egg proteins. The avoiding diet was therefore continued for 9–12 month. After 12 months, the oral challenge provocation tests with cow's milk proteins and egg proteins were still positive and the exclusion diet was recommended for another 6–12 months.

Year after year, in the season of grasses pollens, the child started to experience moderate/severe allergic rhinitis symptoms, wheezing, dyspnea and cough all over the season, also associated with upper respiratory tract infections. Under appropriate symptomatic treatment, including antihistamines H1, topical nasal corticosteroids, inhaled corticosteroids (ICS), short-acting beta-agonists (SABA), leukotriene receptor antagonists (LTRAs), and prophylaxis of exposure to inhaled allergens, the child's respiratory disease was well controlled.

Practical Points

- Primary food allergy mainly affects young children
- Primary food allergy is caused by class I food allergens which are heat-stable and resistant to degradation or proteolytic digestion, having the potential to induce severe reactions
- Adults frequently develop food allergy as a consequence of an inhalant sensitization with class II allergens
- Class II allergens are easily degradable food allergens that tend to induce milder reactions, often limited to oral allergy symptoms
- The presented case was an example of polysensitivity to food and respiratory allergens in a child with atopic dermatitis
- Molecular component diagnosis is useful in identifying sensitization to major and minor allergens and possible cross-reactivity, when several food and respiratory allergies are present

References

1. Kelly JP, Hourihane J. Dietary intervention in eczema. Paediatr Child Health. 2011;21(9):406.
2. Muraro A, Werfel T, Hoffmann-Sommergruber K, Roberts G, Beyer K, Bindslev-Jensen C, Cardona V, Dubois A, duToit G, Eigenmann P, Fernandez Rivas M, Halken S, Hickstein L, Host A, Knol E, Lack G, Marchisotto MJ, Niggemann B, Nwaru BI, Papadopoulos NG, Poulsen LK, Santos AF, Skypala I, Schoepfer A, Van Ree R, Venter C, Worm M, Vlieg-Boerstra B, Panesar S, de Silva D, Soares-Weiser K, Sheikh A, Ballmer-Weber BK, Nilsson C, de Jong NW, Akdis CA. EAACI food allergy and anaphylaxis guidelines: diagnosis and management of food allergy. Allergy. 2014;69(8):1008–25.

Chapter 37
Shortness of Breath, Chest Tightness, and Wheezing

Taher Cheraghi

A 10-year-old boy is brought to hospital with a complaint of shortness of breath, chronic cough, chest tightness and episodic wheezing. His Symptoms get worse at night and often awaken the child. He experiences the above signs and symptoms approximately 4 days a week and 10 nights a month. He also complains of easy fatigability and exercise intolerance when playing. The symptoms worsen on exposure to house dust, tobacco smoke, strong perfumes and weather changes. On physical examination, he has no fever. Chest auscultation is normal, but there is a report of wheezing in three previous hospital records. Eczematous rashes are visible over his antecubital and popliteal fossae. In view of family history, his mother suffers from runny nose, and his sister has had similar episodes of wheezing during winter months and on contact to cold, wind, and molds. CXR shows hyperinflation and prominent bronchovascular markings. Complete blood count shows 8% eosinophilia. Total serum IgE level is 950 IU/mL.

Q1. Regarding the above presenting signs and symptoms, what is the most likely diagnosis?

A. Chronic bronchitis
B. Bronchiolitis
C. Pneumonia
D. Asthma

Answer: *The correct answer is* ***D.***

Wheezing during dyspnea episodes, nocturnal coughs, exercise intolerance, episodic but not constant nature of clinical features, positive personal and family history of atopy, and worsening of symptoms upon exposure to viral infections, inhalant

T. Cheraghi (✉)
Department of Pediatrics, 17th Shahrivar Children's Hospital, School of Medicine, Guilan University of Medical Sciences, Rasht, Iran
e-mail: tcheraghi@gums.ac.ir

N. Rezaei (ed.), *Pediatric Allergy*, https://doi.org/10.1007/978-3-030-18282-3_37

allergens and irritants, absence of fever or pulmonary consolidation, are all in line with a diagnosis of asthma [1–4]. There are also some clinical manifestations that are absent in this patient and incompatible with diagnosis of asthma. These are: occurrence of wheezing soon after birth, constant nature of symptoms, association of symptoms with failure to thrive, absence of temporality of worsening of symptoms with typical asthma triggers, and poor response to asthma medications [5]. It is noteworthy that absence of wheezing at the time of examination, as in this case, does not rule out asthma: because the wheezing in most asthmatic patients is episodic. Moreover, wheezing might be absent in very severe asthma exacerbations due to absence of air exchange [1]. Considering the temporal variability of asthma symptoms over months, weeks, days, and even different hours of a day, normal physical examination at the time of examination does not exclude asthma [6].

Q2. To confirm the diagnosis of asthma and exclude other differential diagnoses, which of the following procedures do you order first?

A. Arterial blood gasses
B. Computerized tomography scan
C. Pulmonary function test
D. Chest X-Ray

Answer: *The correct answer is* ***C.***

In non- emergency situations, after taking comprehensive history and making physical examination, diagnosis of asthma is confirmed when airflow obstruction is present and this obstruction is reversible and of course when possible differential diagnoses are excluded. A pulmonary function test (PFT) is mandatory to demonstrate airflow obstruction [1, 7, 8].

There is no way to determine the severity and reversibility of airflow obstruction or differentiate it precisely from other differential diagnoses, without performing objective measurements with spirometry [5, 9]. Additionally, while it is a common saying that asthma is underdiagnosed, there are some instances of over-diagnosis of asthma in which diagnosis of asthma has been made based on clinical interview. Putting all of the above together, performing PFT for patients 5 year old or older is necessary for definitive asthma diagnosis [1, 9].

Spirometry of the patient showed forced vital capacity (FVC), forced expiratory volume in 1 second (FEV1), FEV1/FVC, and forced expiratory flow at 25–75% (FEF25%–FEF75%), to be all within normal limits.

Q3. Which of the below options can be used to detect asthma in a bronchoprovocation test in these patients?

A. Cold air
B. Methacholine
C. Exercise
D. All of the above

Answer: *The correct answer is* ***D.***

Patients with asthma, who have not been exposed to asthma triggers, usually have normal spirometry and peak expiratory flow rate (PEF) [4, 9]. In these cases, provocation tests should be performed using methacholine, exercise or cold air by experienced personnel in a suitable setting to uncover the silent asthma. A fall in FEV1 by 15% or more following bronchoprovocation, is diagnostic for bronchial hyperreactivity. Remember that airway hyperresponsiveness is not specific for asthma and less frequently may be present in other diseases such as cystic fibrosis (CF), allergic rhinitis, or chronic obstructive pulmonary disease (COPD). Negative predictive value of provocation test to exclude asthma is on the other hand, higher. It is prudent that provocation challenge is not performed when FEV1 is less than 65% of predicted value for that person.

Q4. Which of the following medications is prescribed for the patient?

A. Combination of short acting and long acting beta-2 agonists
B. Maintenance monotherapy with long acting beta-2 agonist
C. Combination of maintenance inhaled corticosteroid and as needed short acting beta-2 agonist
D. Maintenance therapy with short acting beta-2 agonist

Answer: *The correct answer is* ***C.***

Short-acting beta-agonists (SABA) are administered as needed for a short time when the patient is symptomatic. Long-acting beta-agonists (LABA) are prescribed only in combination with inhaled corticosteroids (ICS) in moderate to severe asthma to help control asthma in children 4 years and older and adults. Monotherapy of this medication (LABA), is contraindicated in asthma [1, 4, 10].

The patient has taken part in a birthday party during which he has been exposed to strong perfumes and other triggers. Next morning, he is brought to the emergency department of a hospital with respiratory distress, drowsiness, cyanosis, tachycardia, and tachypnea. O2 saturation is 55%, FEV1 is 35%, and peak flow meter shows 38% of his personal best.

Q5. All of the following medications may be used in this condition, except:

A. Short acting beta agonist
B. Cromolyn Sodium
C. Systemic corticosteroids
D. Magnesium Sulfate

Answer: *The correct answer is* ***B.***

Oxygen supplementation and SABA are the two most crucial measures to mitigate asthma exacerbations. The next step treatments are ipratropium bromide and systemic corticosteroids. If, despite using the above measures, the patient remains ill and in danger of respiratory failure, assisted ventilation may be needed. Assisted ventilation may be associated with complications like pneumothorax and pneumomediastinum, hence, every action must be taken to resolve the exacerbation without using ventilators. Adjunctive medications like subcutaneous epinephrine, parenteral magnesium sulfate, beta-2 agonists, and methylxanthines, as well as heliox are of benefit on these occasions. Cromolyn Sodium may be used as an alternative medicine to inhaled corticosteroids in mild persistent asthma for maintenance therapy, not for emergency management. It is noteworthy that mucolytics and chest physiotherapy are not helpful on this condition and even may aggravate bronchospasm [4].

Q6. Beta-2 agonist is administered before repeating the pulmonary function test. What percentage of reversibility in FEV1 -from baseline level- is significant and diagnostic for asthma?

A. 6%
B. 8%
C. 10%
D. 12%

Answer: *The correct answer is* ***D.***

According to joint task force of American thoracic society and European respiratory society [11], 12% or more of positive change in FEV1 from the baseline spirometry after inhalation of SABA is a significant change to approve reversibility of airway obstruction. Reversibility is not specific for asthma and other diseases may be associated with this pattern. Instead, asthma diagnosis is based on detailed history, physical examination, confirmation of reversible obstruction by spirometry, and exclusion of other differential diagnoses [1].

Q7. Which of the following statements is true regarding criteria to discharge the patient from hospital?

A. Resolution of signs and symptoms of asthma exacerbation is sufficient to discharge the patient
B. A stable PEF more than 65% and O_2 saturation more than 90% for more than 2 h in room air, is sufficient to discharge the patient
C. Disappearance of signs and symptoms, PEF more than 70% and O_2 saturation more than 92% for at least 4 h in room air, is sufficient to discharge the patient
D. Resolution of asthma exacerbation and PEF more than 68%, and O_2 saturation more than 90% on supplemental oxygen, is sufficient to discharge the patient

Answer: *The correct answer is* ***C.***

In order to discharge the patient from emergency department, patient not only should have recovered from asthma exacerbation, but also should have stable vital signs for at least 4 h, breathing room air. Objective measurements by peak expiratory flow meters and pulse oximeters is mandatory to discharge the patient. Patients should not have required bronchodilators for at least a 3 h interval [4].

Q8. Before discharging the patient from hospital, which actions should be taken to prevent possible future exacerbations?

A. Provide the patient with "written asthma action plan"
B. Prescribe short acting beta-2 agonist to control asthma signs and symptoms
C. Prescribe "inhaled corticosteroids" to control inflammation and prevent subsequent exacerbations
D. All of the above

Answer: *The correct answer is* ***D.***

Patients should be counseled and instructed, according to a "written asthma action plan", on:

1. How to use daily medications
2. The correct inhaler technique
3. How to recognize the early signs and symptoms of asthma exacerbation
4. How to take prompt actions with available medications to combat the exacerbations and refer to the medical center
5. Provision of an emergency telephone number to contact in emergency situations and receive help
6. Avoiding exposure to triggers of asthma and withdraw from factors that aggravate asthma
7. Reinforcing adherence to treatment

Administering a peak flow meter is an important element to adhere to the "written asthma action plan". Health care providers should educate the patient and family members or caregivers how to use it to monitor asthma and what to do when they are in RED, YELLOW, and GREEN zones [4, 5, 10]. The optimal controlling dose of ICS should be obtained [4], prior to discharge.

Q9. How often the patient should be revisited by a physician after discharge from hospital?

A. Every 1–4 weeks
B. Every 6–8 weeks
C. Every 2 months
D. Every 3 months

Answer: *The correct answer is* ***A.***

Patients should be visited by an asthma specialist or health care provider within 1-4 weeks after discharge from hospital to ensure that the asthma is under control, review the asthma action plan, inhaler techniques, triggers of exacerbations, risk factors and adhernece of the patient [10].

Q10. On follow-up visit 4 months later, the patient is not well-controlled and unsatisfied with medications. Which of the following actions should be taken?

A. Double the dose of current medications
B. Add a drug from another category to previous medications
C. Add oral corticosteroid to previous medications
D. Check the inhaler technique and patients adherence to therapy

Answer: *The correct answer is* ***D.***

Stepping up the medications, while diagnosis is inaccurate, or inhaler technique is wrong or patient adherence to medications is poor, or when there is incomplete avoidance of environmental asthma triggers, adds nothing to patient but drug side effects [1].

Q11. Which one of the following classifications are applicable in asthma?

A. Classification based on severity of asthma
B. Classification based on level of control of asthma
C. Classification of asthma exacerbation
D. All of the above

Answer: *The correct answer is* ***D.***

All of the above classifications are applicable in asthma, but in different situations. **Classification based on severity** is useful **before the start of treatment** and is based on five items in patients less than 4 years and on six items in those above 4 years [1]. These items are:

1. Frequency of symptoms per week.
2. Frequency of nocturnal symptoms per month.
3. Frequency of using SABA per week to control symptoms.
4. Interference of asthma to daily activities, school or work attendance.
5. Number of exacerbations in recent year.
6. Pulmonary function parameters which are only applicable in patients 5 year old or older who are able to perform pulmonary function tests.

According to this classification, asthma is classified into two main categories: intermittent, and persistent. Persistent asthma is further subclassified into three degrees of severity: mild, moderate, and severe persistent [1, 4].

Classification based on level of control is applicable after starting treatment and is based on following factors to be considered in the past 4 weeks:

1. Frequency of daily symptoms more than 2 day per week
2. Every limitation of activities including exercise caused by asthma
3. Requiring SABA more than 2 day per week
4. Any nocturnal cough or awakening during sleep

If the patient does not fulfil any of the above items, he/she has well controlled asthma, when having 1–2 of these items, asthma is partly controlled, and if the patient has 3–4 of these items, has uncontrolled asthma.

The third classification is used for assessing the **severity of asthma exacerbation** and is based on short history of the patient, physical examination including auscultation, use of accessory respiratory muscles, respiratory rate, pulse rate, level of consciousness, speech condition, patient posture in bed, pulse oximetry, and if not in severe exacerbation and impending arrest, PEF or FEV1. When the patient is stable, you could take comprehensive history or perform pulmonary function test to assess the response to treatment objectively and thereafter monitor patient's response to treatment [1, 4].

Q12. Which one of the following features defines the airway remodeling in asthma?

A. Hypertrophy and hyperplasia of smooth muscle cells
B. Subepithelial fibrosis and sub-basement membrane thickening
C. Angiogenesis and mucus hypersecretion
D. All of the above

Answer: *The correct answer is* ***D.***

Remodeling is a permanent structural change in airway wall elements that leads to hyporesponsiveness of the airway to environmental allergens and irritants or even asthma medications. The end result of remodeling is airway wall thickness and luminal narrowing [1].

Practical Points

- Episodic wheezing and dyspnea, nocturnal coughs, positive family history of atopy, worsening of symptoms following respiratory viral infections, and after exposure to inhalant allergens point to a diagnosis of asthma
- Wheezing appearing soon after birth with constant nature, associated with failure to thrive, pulmonary consolidation, and poor response to asthma medications, are against a diagnosis of asthma
- Wheezing is not a constant feature of asthma and patients might present with an essentially normal clinical picture between episodes of exacerbation
- Oxygen supplementation and administration of SABA are the two most crucial measures to mitigate asthma exacerbations
- A fall in forced expiratory volume in 1 second (FEV1) by 15% or more following bronchoprovocation, or rise in FEV1 by 12% or 200ml after inhalation of short acting beta agonist is diagnostic for bronchial hyperreactivity

References

1. National Asthma E, Prevention P. Expert panel report 3-guidelines for the diagnosis and management of asthma full report. 2007. https://www.nhlbi.nih.gov/health-pro/guidelines/current/asthma-guidelines/full-report.
2. Strunk LBBRC. Asthma in older children: special considerations. In: Leung DY, Szefler SJ, Akdis CA, Bonilla FA, Sampson H, editors. Pediatric allergy: principles and practice: Elsevier Health Sciences; 2016. p. 311–28.
3. GINA-2017-main-report-final_V2.pdf. 2017. www.ginasthma.org.
4. Andrew H, Joseph D, Spahn SHS. Childhood asthma. In: Kliegman RM, Blum NJ, Shah SS, ST Geme JW, Tasker RC, Wilson KM, editors. Nelson textbook of pediatrics. 2-volume set. Medicine. 21st ed. Philadelphia: Elsevier; 2020. p. 1932–57.
5. Sheikh A, O'Hehir R, Holgate S, editors. Middleton's allergy essential. Amsterdam: Elsevier; 2016.
6. Adkinson NF Jr, Bochner BS, Burks AW, Busse WW, Holgate ST, Lemanske RF, O'Hehir RE. Middleton's allergy E-book: principles and practice. Amsterdam: Elsevier; 2013.
7. Ali Altalag JR, Wilcox P. Pulmonary function tests in clinical practice. New York, NY: Springer; 2009.
8. Gold WM, Koth LL. Pulmonary Function Testing. In: Murray JF, Nadel JA, editors. Textbook of respiratory medincine. 6th ed. Philadelphia: Saunders; 2016.
9. Thomas M, Wilkinson T. Asthma diagnosis in the community—time for a change? Clin Exp Allergy. 2014;44(10):1206–9.
10. Brozek JL, Bousquet J, Agache I, Agarwal A, Bachert C, Bosnic-Anticevich S, Brignardello-Petersen R, Canonica GW, Casale T, Chavannes NH, Correia de Sousa J, Cruz AA, Cuello-Garcia CA, Demoly P, Dykewicz M, Etxeandia-Ikobaltzeta I, Florez ID, Fokkens W, Fonseca J, Hellings PW, Klimek L, Kowalski S, Kuna P, Laisaar KT, Larenas-Linnemann DE, Lodrup Carlsen KC, Manning PJ, Meltzer E, Mullol J, Muraro A, O'Hehir R, Ohta K, Panzner P, Papadopoulos N, Park HS, Passalacqua G, Pawankar R, Price D, Riva JJ, Roldan Y, Ryan D, Sadeghirad B, Samolinski B, Schmid-Grendelmeier P, Sheikh A, Togias A, Valero A, Valiulis A, Valovirta E, Ventresca M, Wallace D, Waserman S, Wickman M, Wiercioch W, Yepes-Nunez JJ, Zhang L, Zhang Y, Zidarn M, Zuberbier T, Schunemann HJ. Allergic rhinitis and its impact on asthma (ARIA) guidelines—2016 revision. J Allergy Clin Immunol. 2017;140(4):950–8.
11. Pellegrino R, Viegi G, Brusasco V, Crapo RO, Burgos F, Casaburi R, Coates A, van der Grinten CPM, Gustafsson P, Hankinson J, Jensen R, Johnson DC, MacIntyre N, McKay R, Miller MR, Navajas D, Pedersen OF, Wanger J. Interpretative strategies for lung function tests. Eur Respir J. 2005;26(5):948–68.

Chapter 38
Chronic Cough and Acute Wheezing

Juan J. L. Sienra-Monge, Jaime M. Del-Rio-Chivardi, and Elsy M. Navarrete-Rodríguez

A 5-year-old girl presented with a 3-months history of wet cough, wheezing and dyspnea that got worse during the night. Sneezing and nasal congestion were common throughout the day. In the last 4 days these symptoms had worsened and dysphonia and rhinorrhea have added. She also has history of hospitalization at 2 years old due to the same condition, which her parents recall that was not associated with the use of mechanical ventilation. Both parents have allergic rhinitis.

On physical examination we found distal cyanosis, tachypnea, irritability, oral hyperemia, postnasal drip, hypertrophic turbinates' and wheeze.

Q1. What is your most likely differential diagnosis?

A. Gastroesophageal reflux.
B. Pneumonia
C. Primary immunodeficiency
D. Acute asthma
E. Croup

Answer: *The correct answer is* ***D.***

Asthmatic patients who begin in the first 3 years of life, regularly have parents or close relatives with rhinitis, asthma or atopy. In the absence of positive family history, viral infections are the usual triggers and the symptoms typically disappear after 18–36 months. According to Global Initiative for asthma (GINA) [1], this crisis is classified as moderate.

Q2. A common differential diagnosis to exclude is:

A. Chronic sinusitis.
B. Laryngomalacia.

J. J. L. Sienra-Monge · J. M. Del-Rio-Chivardi · E. M. Navarrete-Rodríguez (✉)
Hospital Infantil de México Federico Gómez, Ciudad de México, Mexico

N. Rezaei (ed.), *Pediatric Allergy*, https://doi.org/10.1007/978-3-030-18282-3_38

C. Alpha 1 antitrypsin deficiency.
D. Foreign body in the airway.
E. Unstable thorax.

Answer: *The correct answer is* ***A.***

Differential diagnoses of wheezing are established based on the age of the patient and the medical history. Our patient is 5 years old, and the cough started progressively since 3 months ago. This discards congenital problems such as laryngomalacia, as well as sudden-onset events, such as foreign body aspiration. A chronic infectious disease such as rhinosinusitis is often associated with this condition and is a trigger for a new crisis.

Q3. The severity of asthma crisis is established based on?

A. Peripheral cyanosis with SaO_2 90%
B. Heart rate with QT segment elevation
C. Heart rate, respiratory rate and pulse oximetry
D. Respiratory frequency and wheezing
E. Blood gas with $PaO_2 > 90\%$

Answer: *The correct answer is* ***C.***

International asthma guidelines have suggested that assessment of exacerbation severity should be based on the degree of dyspnea, respiratory rate, pulse rate, oxygen saturation and lung function.

Q4. The initial management of this patient should include:

A. Magnesium sulfate and montelukast
B. Short acting beta-2 agonist and systemic steroid
C. Long-acting bronchodilator and ipratropium
D. Aminophylline and IV salbutamol
E. Systemic steroid and oxygen at high concentrations

Answer: *The correct answer is* ***B.***

The initial management of all patients includes repeated administration of short-acting beta-2 adrenergic agonist, oxygen at concentrations greater than 40% if available, and early introduction of oral corticosteroids.

Q5. Once the acute event has been overcome, what will be the next best treatment?

A. Budesonide 200 μg plus montelukast 4 mg
B. Salmeterol plus budesonide 500/100
C. Vilanterol plus fluticasone 25/100
D. Salbutamol plus ipratropium
E. Salbutamol as needed plus montelukast 4 mg

Answer: *The correct answer is* ***A.***

The patient has more than 3 months of uncontrolled asthma and the symptoms suggest a mild to moderate persistent asthma, therefore, the treatment is established in the international management guidelines (global initiative for asthma) GINA [1], step 3. The first option is to use a medium dose of steroid or combine a lower dose with another controller drug, such as montelukast. The use of long-acting beta agonist with topical steroids is recommended in patients above 6 years of age or in children under 6 years old and severe disease. Symptomatic management with salbutamol is insufficient when the inflammation is persistent.

Practical Points

- Asthma is the most frequent chronic inflammatory lung disease of childhood
- Exacerbations should be treated with short acting beta-2 agonist and systemic steroids
- Long-term control should be based on the symptoms prior to the crisis
- When the patient first presents with acute exacerbation with no history of disease severity prior to the attack, treatment should at least start on level 3 [1–4]

References

1. Tebo AE, Jaskowski T, Davis KW, Whiting A, Clifford B, Zeft A, McNally B, Hill HR, Bohnsack J, Prahalad S. Profiling anti-cyclic citrullinated peptide antibodies in patients with juvenile idiopathic arthritis. Pediatr Rheumatol Online J. 2012;10:29.
2. Adkinson NF, Middleton E. Middleton's allergy: principles and practice. 8th ed. Amsterdam: Elsevier; 2013.
3. Castro-Rodriguez JA, Holberg CJ, Wright AL, Martinez FD. A clinical index to define risk of asthma in young children with recurrent wheezing. Am J Respir Crit Care Med. 2000;162(4. Pt 1):1403–6.
4. Larenas-Linnemann D, Salas-Hernandez J, Vazquez-Garcia JC, Ortiz-Aldana I, Fernandez-Vega M, Del Rio-Navarro BE, MDC C-S, Luna-Pech JA, Ortega-Martell JA, Romero-Lombard J, EDC L-E, Villaverde-Rosas J, Mayorga-Butron JL, Vargas-Becerra MH, Bedolla-Barajas M, Rodriguez-Perez N, Aguilar-Aranda A, Jimenez-Gonzalez CA, Garcia-Bolanos C, Garrido-Galindo C, Mendoza-Hernandez DA, Mendoza-Lopez E, Lopez-Perez G, Wakida-Kuzonoki GH, Ruiz-Gutierrez HH, Leon-Molina H, Martinez-De la Lanza H, Stone-Aguilar H, Gomez-Vera J, Olvera-Salinas J, Oyoqui-Flores JJ, Galvez-Romero JL, Lozano-Saenz JS, Salgado-Gama JI, Jimenez-Chobillon MA, Garcia-Aviles MA, Guinto-Balanzar MP, Medina-Avalos MA, Camargo-Angeles R, Garcia-Torrentera R, Toral-Freyre S, Montes-Narvaez G, Solorio-Gomez H, Rosas-Pena J, Romero-Tapia SJ, Reyes-Herrera A, Cuevas-Schacht F, Esquer-Flores J, Sacre-Hazouri JA, Compean-Martinez L, Medina-Sanchez PJ, Garza-Salinas S, Baez-Loyola C, Romero-Alvarado I, Miguel-Reyes JL, Huerta-Espinosa LE, Correa-Flores MA, Castro-Martinez R. Mexican asthma guidelines: GUIMA 2017. Rev Alerg Mex. 2017;64(Suppl 1):s11–s128.

Chapter 39
Wheezing and Shortness of Breath After Viral Pharyngitis

Juan J. L. Sienra-Monge, Elsy M. Navarrete-Rodríguez, and Jaime M. Del-Rio-Chivardi

A 12-year-old boy with a history of asthma, presented to the emergency department with respiratory symptoms such as wheeze, shortness of breath, chest tightness and cough. His parents noticed progressive dyspnea on exertion and cough and started short-acting beta-2 adrenergic agonist (SABA) as need. The boy was not using inhaled corticosteroids (ICS) or other asthma controlling medication and his flare up was related to a viral pharyngitis 5 days ago.

He had a history of hospitalization at 7 years due to the same condition which his parents recall that was not associated with the use of mechanical ventilation. Upon admission, the physical examination reveals respiratory rate 25 min^{-1}, O_2 saturation 94% in room air and wheeze.

Q1. The most effective way to achieve rapid reversal of airflow limitation in urgency department is:

A. Repeated administration of inhaled SABA (up to 4–10 puffs every 3–4 h) via pressurized metered-dose inhalers (pMDI) and spacer
B. Repeated administration of inhaled SABA via nebulizer because delivery of SABA via nebulizer is better than a pMDI and spacer or a dry powder inhaler (DPI)
C. Controlled oxygen supplementation with target saturation of 98%
D. Repeated administration of inhaled SABA (up to 4–10 puffs every 20 min for the first hour) and controlled oxygen supplementation with target saturation of 98%
E. Repeated administration of inhaled SABA (up to 4–10 puffs every 20 min for the first hour)

Answer: *The correct answer is* ***E.***

J. J. L. Sienra-Monge · E. M. Navarrete-Rodríguez (✉) · J. M. Del-Rio-Chivardi
Hospital Infantil de México Federico Gómez, Ciudad de México, Mexico

N. Rezaei (ed.), *Pediatric Allergy*, https://doi.org/10.1007/978-3-030-18282-3_39

For mild to moderate exacerbations, repeated administration of inhaled SABA (up to 4–10 puffs every 20 min for the first hour) is usually the most effective way to achieve rapid reversal of airflow limitation [1]. Nebulizer delivery is not significantly better than [pressurized] metered-dose inhalers (pMDI) delivered by spacer in adults or children during asthma exacerbations [2].

After the first hour, the dose of SABA required varies from 4–10 puffs every 3–4 h up to 6–10 puffs every 1–2 h, or more often [1].

Q2. Which one of the following is a factor that increases the risk of asthma-related death in this patient?

A. Not currently using inhaled corticosteroids
B. Hospitalization or emergency care visit for asthma at 7 years old
C. Use of SABA in the last 15 days
D. Age of the patient
E. History of viral pharyngitis

Answer: *The correct answer is* ***A***.

Factors that increase the risk of asthma-related death include:

1. Over-use of SABAs, especially use of more than one canister of salbutamol (or equivalent) monthly [3]
2. Hospitalization or emergency care visit for asthma in the past year [3]
3. History of intensive care unit admissions and mechanical ventilation due to asthma
4. Not currently using ICS [4]
5. Currently using or having recently stopped using oral corticosteroids or oral theophylline [4].
6. Poor adherence with asthma medications [5]

You decide to start oral corticosteroid (OCS) and continue bronchodilator. The patient's condition improves and it is time for discharge.

Q3. Which of the following is true in relation to home-based management plan?

A. Continue OCS for 3 weeks, start controller treatment, assess inhaler technique and adherence, follow-up appointment about 3 weeks later
B. As needed reliever medication, OCS for 5 days, start controller treatment, assess inhaler technique and adherence. Follow-up appointment about 2–7 days later
C. Continue OCS for 5 days, start controller treatment, assess inhaler technique and adherence, follow-up appointment about 3 weeks later
D. Continue OCS for 5 days, start controller treatment, assess inhaler technique and adherence, follow-up appointment about 2–7 days later and start treatment with omalizumab
E. Discontinue OCS, start controller treatment, assess inhaler technique and adherence, follow-up appointment about 3 weeks later

Answer: *The correct answer is* ***B.***

Discharge plan should include:

1. Provision and education on the use of as needed reliever medication such as SABAs
2. Continue OCS started at hospital
3. Start or continue controller treatment like ICS
4. Review inhaler technique and adherence
5. Follow-up appointment 2–7 days later [1]

Q4. You decide to start ICS/formoterol (80/4.5) as controller every 12 h; in case of worsening symptoms the patient should:

A. Continue with controller and start SABA every 8 h
B. Continue with controller and start SABA as need or a combination of ICS/formoterol inhaler up to a maximum total formoterol dose of 72 μg in a day
C. Continue with controller and start SABA as need or a combination of ICS/formoterol inhaler up to a maximum total formoterol dose of 18 μg in a day
D. Continue with controller and start SABA as need or a combination of ICS/formoterol inhaler up to a maximum total budesonide dose of 2000 μg in a day independently formoterol dose
E. Continue with controller and start SABA as need or a combination of ICS/formoterol inhaler up to a maximum total budesonide dose of 1000 μg in a day independently formoterol dose

Answer: *The correct answer is* ***B.***

The combination of rapid-onset long-acting beta agonist (formoterol) and low dose ICS (budesonide or beclometasone) in a single inhaler, as both the controller and reliever medication, is effective in improving asthma control. The combination ICS/formoterol inhaler may be taken up to a maximum total formoterol dose of 72 μg in a day.

Q5. Which of the following is an indication for starting OCS after completion of short course rescue OCS?

A. Failure to respond to an increase in reliever and controller medication for 7 days
B. Failure to respond to an increase in reliever and controller medication for 14 days
C. PEF <80% of their personal best or predicted value
D. PEF <60% of their personal best or predicted value
E. The asthma plan should not include the option to start OCS

Answer: *The correct answer is* ***D.***

For most patients, the "written asthma action plan" should provide instructions for when and how to commence OCS. Typically, a short course of OCS is used (e.g. 40–50 mg/day usually for 5–7 days, for patients who:

1. Fail to respond to an increase in reliever and controller medications for 2–3 days
2. Deteriorate rapidly or who have a PEF or FEV1 < 60% of their personal best or predicted value
3. Have a history of sudden severe exacerbations

Practical Points

- Short-acting beta-2 agonist administered up to 4–10 puffs every 20 min for the first hour, is the most effective way to break an asthma attack
- Over-use of beta-2 agonists and solo use of beta-2 agonists, history of hospitalization, emergency care visit for asthma, intensive care unit admissions due to asthma in the past year, and poor adherence to medications, predict mortality in asthma

References

1. Tebo AE, Jaskowski T, Davis KW, Whiting A, Clifford B, Zeft A, McNally B, Hill HR, Bohnsack J, Prahalad S. Profiling anti-cyclic citrullinated peptide antibodies in patients with juvenile idiopathic arthritis. Pediatr Rheumatol Online J. 2012;10:29.
2. Abramson MJ, Puy RM, Weiner JM. Injection allergen immunotherapy for asthma. Cochrane Database Syst Rev. 2010;8:CD001186.
3. Suissa S, Blais L, Ernst P. Patterns of increasing beta-agonist use and the risk of fatal or near-fatal asthma. Eur Respir J. 1994;7(9):1602–9.
4. Ernst P, Spitzer WO, Suissa S, Cockcroft D, Habbick B, Horwitz RI, Boivin JF, McNutt M, Buist AS. Risk of fatal and near-fatal asthma in relation to inhaled corticosteroid use. JAMA. 1992;268(24):3462–4.
5. Sturdy PM, Victor CR, Anderson HR, Bland JM, Butland BK, Harrison BD, Peckitt C, Taylor JC, Mortality, Severe Morbidity Working Group of the National Asthma Task F. Psychological, social and health behaviour risk factors for deaths certified as asthma: a national case-control study. Thorax. 2002;57(12):1034–9.

Chapter 40
Cough and Dyspnea

Hossein Esmaeilzadeh

A 9-year-old girl was admitted to our department with sudden-onset cough and fever and exacerbation episodes with dyspnea for the past 2 days. The patient a had history of asthma at 4 years of age and her asthma was properly controlled as "mild persistent" for the past 5 years. She had experienced no asthma attacks in the last year even though she had been medication-free for short periods. Initial physical examination revealed diffuse rales and wheezing over both lungs. Her vitals revealed tachypnea, respiratory rate of 32, pulse rate of 135 bpm, temperature of 38 °C and oxygen saturation levels 80% in room air. The patient was hospitalized with the impression of asthma exacerbation in the context of pneumonia. Asthma attack was controlled and antibiotic therapy was initiated. With the continuation of her fever on routine antibiotic regiment, ceftriaxone and clindamycin, she was switched to meropenem and vancomycin, 3 days after first-dose antibiotics had started. Fever discontinued within 48 h and the symptoms of cough and respiratory distress improved significantly. Laboratory findings on the second day of admission disclosed a WBC count of 10,700/μL with 30% eosinophils. Plain chest radiograph showed diffuse mild ground glass appearance in both lungs.

Q1. All of the following are considered as likely diagnoses, <u>except</u>:

A. Viral infection
B. Eosinophilic pneumonitis
C. Allergic asthma with superimposed viral infection
D. Acute asthma attack

Answer: *The correct answer is* ***B.***

H. Esmaeilzadeh (✉)
Allergy Research Center, Namazi Hospital, Shiraz University of Medical Sciences, Shiraz, Iran
e-mail: esmaeilzadeh_ho@sums.ac.ir

N. Rezaei (ed.), *Pediatric Allergy*, https://doi.org/10.1007/978-3-030-18282-3_40

Acute presentation reveals asthma attack for which the most probable cause is viral infection. Eosinophilic pneumonitis and parasites have chronic presentation. Wheeze, high eosinophilia and history of asthma make viral infection alone less possible.

Q2. Which one of the following is the appropriate approach to eosinophilia?

A. Stool exam
B. ImmunoCap specific IgE and IgG for aspergillosis
C. Total serum IgE
D. Bronchoalveolar lavage
E. All of the above

Answer: *The correct answer is* ***E.***

In case of eosinophilia, stool exam is mandated to look for parasites. Specific IgG and IgE for aspergillosis are necessary to fulfill the diagnostic criteria for probable allergic bronchopulmonary aspergillosis (ABPA). Bronchoalveolar lavage (BAL) can help in the diagnosis of infectious parasites.

IgE level was 1075 IU/mL (reference range: 20–100 IU/mL). Skin prick test was negative for aspergillosis and asthma control was achieved. Airway secretions obtained through BAL were sent for PCR for *Aspergillus*, *Candida*, and *Tuberculosis*. The patient was discharged with desirable asthma control after completion of her antibiotic course.

Five days later the patient was readmitted with the same presentations, cough, dyspnea and diffuse bilateral wheezing sounds, but no fever. IgE levels were 1359 and 1661 IU/mL in second checking. The results of further laboratory tests are summarized in Table 40.1.

On the second day of her admission she developed severe subcutaneous emphysema at anterior and posterior areas of the neck along with dyspnea. Spiral chest CT scan revealed severe pneumomediastinum and severe emphysema in chest wall. Ground glass densities and findings in favor of bronchiectasis were reported in both lungs in CT scan (Fig. 40.1).

Candida albicans was reported in the airway secretions obtained from previous admission. Further tests were negative for *Aspergillus*-specific IgG (18.5 g/L, reference range <50) and IgE (<0.1 IU/mL, reference range <0.1) and *Candida*-specific IgG (4.2 g/L, reference range <113), but positive for *Candida*-specific IgE (0.74 IU/mL, reference range <0.1).

The patient was admitted in intensive care unit due to a decrease in of breath sounds and severe respiratory distress, and thoracic catheter was inserted. Meropenem plus vancomycin were restarted, along with intravenous infusion of methylprednisolone 1 mg/kg/day and IV fluconazole. A week later, the thoracic catheter was removed following a marked improvement of dyspnea and control of asthma symptoms.

Table 40.1 Complete blood count, comprehensive metabolic profile and immunologic test results of a 9-year-old girl with sudden-onset dyspnea

Test	Results	Normal range
WBC	14,950	3500–11,000 μL^{-1}
Neutrophils	81%	
Lymphocytes	14%	
Eosinophils	1%	
Monocyte	4%	
ESR	12 mm/h	Up to 20 mm/h
CRP	1 mg/L	Up to 6 mg/L
Alb	4.3 g/dL	3/5–5/2
IgM	1.55 g/mL	0/24–2/1
IgA	2.7 g/mL	0/34–3/05
IgG	8.68 g/L	5/53–13/07
Anti-tetanus antibody	0.26 IU/mL	<0/1 IU/mL
Dihydrorhodamine test	198	<50
C3	134 mg/dL	90–180 mg/dL
C4	29/2 mg/dL	10–40 mg/dL
CH50	116 mg/dL	
ANA	0/3 U/mL	>10 U/mL
Sweat chloride test (*2)	45 mmol/L 30 mmol/L	>60 mmol/L
P-ANCA	1/1 U/mL	>12 U/mL
C-ANCA	2/6 U/mL	>12 U/mL

P-ANCA perinuclear anti-neutrophil cytoplasmic antibodies, *C-ANCA* cytoplasmic anti-neutrophil cytoplasmic antibodies, *CH50* total complement activity

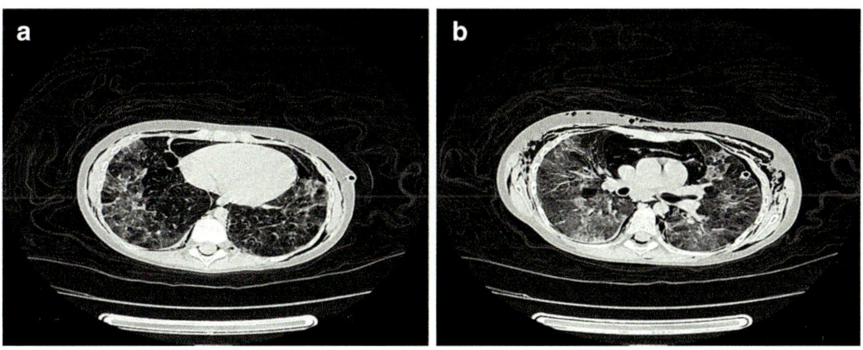

Fig. 40.1 Severe emphysema in chest wall and bronchiectasis in spiral chest CT scan of a 9-year-old girl with sudden onset dyspnea. Ground glass densities are in favor of bronchiectasis

Q3. What is the most likely diagnosis?

A. Allergic bronchopulmonary mycosis
B. Aspergiloma
C. Severe allergic asthma
D. Pulmonary phase of parasites like *Ascaris*

Answer: *The correct answer is* ***A.***

Exposure to indoor and outdoor fungal allergens evokes severe reactions in asthmatic patients (1–3). The most common immunologic reaction is ABPA and a less frequent syndrome in response to other fungal species is allergic bronchopulmonary mycosis (ABPM) [1]. ABPM is characterized by infiltrations in chest radiography, peripheral blood eosinophilia, high total IgE titer and serologic response to fungi other than *Aspergillus* by positive specific IgE (sIgE) [2, 3]. Findings in chest radiography are nonspecific, and high-resolution computed tomography (HRCT) is the modality of choice in ABPM. The findings of HRCT include central bronchiectasis, mucus plugging and bronchocele formation [4, 5]. Aspergiloma is the invasive infiltration of *Aspergillus* with mass induction. Emphysema, bronchiectasis and high specific IgE are not among the usual manifestations of allergic asthma or pulmonary phase of *Ascaris* nematode.

Q4. What would be the most appropriate treatment for the patient?

A. Prednisolone
B. Itraconazole
C. Intravenous fluconazole
D. Answers A and B are correct

Answer: *The correct answer is* ***D****.*

The main treatment of ABPA is high-dose prednisolone, with itraconazole prescribed as corticosteroid sparing agent for at least 8 weeks. ABPM is managed using the same protocol.

Our patient was transferred to ward with final diagnosis of ABPM on high dose itraconazole (200 mg every 12 h) and high dose prednisolone (0.75 mg/kg/day) and discharged after 10 days. In her follow-up a month later her general condition had improved dramatically and she had no need for oxygen supplement. IgE level had decreased to 255 IU/mL and the patient had normal breath sounds. High dose of fluticasone plus salmeterol inhaler spray and oral montelukast were prescribed to control symptoms of severe asthma. After 3 months of follow-up her corticosteroid regiment was tapered to become steroid-free within one month. By then, she reached good asthma control, total IgE level of 86 IU/mL and total eosinophil count dropped to 100/μL. After 6 months of follow-up, her asthma medication was tapered to low dose of fluticasone with mild persistent asthma. She has since achieved good asthma control in follow-up visits.

Practical Points

- Treatment-resistant asthma with eosinophilia and high-titer total IgE points to an important differential diagnosis of asthma which is allergic bronchopulmonary aspergillosis
- Specific IgG and IgE assay and radiologic findings are diagnostic for allergic bronchopulmonary aspergillosis

References

1. Al-Mobeireek AF, El-Rab M, Al-Hedaithy SS, Alasali K, Al-Majed S, Joharjy I. Allergic bronchopulmonary mycosis in patients with asthma: period prevalence at a university hospital in Saudi Arabia. Respir Med. 2001;95(5):341–7.
2. Fukutomi Y, Tanimoto H, Yasueda H, Taniguchi M. Serological diagnosis of allergic bronchopulmonary mycosis: progress and challenges. Allergol Int. 2016;65(1):30–6.
3. Chowdhary A, Agarwal K, Kathuria S, Gaur SN, Randhawa HS, Meis JF. Allergic bronchopulmonary mycosis due to fungi other than Aspergillus: a global overview. Crit Rev Microbiol. 2014;40(1):30–48.
4. Saini SK, Boas SR, Jerath A, Roberts M, Greenberger PA. Allergic bronchopulmonary mycosis to Fusarium vasinfectum in a child. Ann Allergy Asthma Immunol. 1998;80(5):377–80.
5. Kumar R, Poongadan MN, Singh M. Allergic bronchopulmonary aspergillosis presenting as lobar or total lung collapse. Pneumonol Alergol Pol. 2015;83(2):144–50.

Chapter 41
Upper Respiratory Tract Infection and Wheezing

Javad Ghaffari

A 6-year-old boy presented to the emergency department with respiratory distress. His mother reports an upper respiratory tract infection for the last 4 days. He complains of shortness of breath and frequent cough. He has been diagnosed with asthma at the age of 2 and is currently on controller medication with fluticasone 125 μg inhaler, one puff twice a day. On examination, he has moderate intercostal and suprasternal retractions. He maintains a sitting position and cannot utter a complete sentence. He is tachycardic and tachypneic with a respiratory rate of 45 per min. His arterial O_2 saturation is 92% in room air (fraction of inspired oxygen (FiO_2): 21%), blood pressure is 90/60 mmHg and his temperature is 37.2 °C. He has expiratory wheezing throughout all lung fields with scattered rales. Peak expiratory flow (PEF) measured by peak flow meter is 55%.

Q1. How severe would you rate his asthma?

A. Mild
B. Moderate
C. Severe
D. Impending of respiratory arrest

Answer: *The correct answer is* ***B.***

Hallmark manifestations of asthma are wheezing, shortness of breath, chest tightness and cough that varies over time in intensity. Prevalence of asthma is variable ranging from 1% to 18% in different countries: www.ginasthma.org [1]. The most common subtypes of asthma include: *allergic asthma* which is common in children who have a positive family history of allergic disorders such as asthma, allergic rhinitis, atopic dermatitis, and food or drug allergy and *non-allergic asthma*

J. Ghaffari (✉)
Department of Allergy and Clinical Immunology, Mazandaran University of Medical Sciences, Sari, Iran
e-mail: j.ghaffari@mazums.ac.ir

N. Rezaei (ed.), *Pediatric Allergy*, https://doi.org/10.1007/978-3-030-18282-3_41

which is more common in adults: www.ginasthma.org [1]. The natural course of asthma can generally adopt either of the two patterns:

1. Transient non-atopic wheezing which is more common in early childhood and usually resolves at preschool or early school years.
2. Persistent atopic wheezing with the onset in early childhood and high probability of persistence in late childhood or adulthood.

Pulmonary Index Score is a useful tool in assessing the severity of asthma attack. Moderate asthma attack is characterized by breathlessness when talking, talking in short phrases and agitation, increased respiratory rate, use of accessory muscle commonly, loud wheeze throughout expiration, increased pulse rate (100–120 per min), PEF between 60% and 80%, presence of pulsus paradoxus between 10 and 25 mmHg, $PCo_2 < 42$ mmHg with arterial O_2 saturation remaining between 91% and 95% and $PaO_2 > 60$ mmHg at sea level [2], and less commonly, presence of pulsus paradoxus between 10 and 25 mmHg.

Q2. What is the first choice of treatment?

A. Ipratropium bromide
B. Albuterol
C. Inhaler corticosteroid
D. Anti-leukotriene agents

Answer: *The correct answer is* ***B.***

Inhaled short-acting beta-2 adrenergic agonist (SABA) are the first choice treatment in asthma attack. Albuterol nebulizer solution should be administered at a minimum dose of 2.5 mg, as often as every 20 min up to three doses if needed (0.15 mg/kg). Maintenance dose can follow either a 0.15–0.3 mg/kg (max 10 mg) every 1–4 h protocol or up to 0.5 mg/kg/h by continuous nebulization. Albuterol metered dose inhaler (MDI) (90 μg/puff) should be administered at 2–8 puffs up to every 20 min, up to three doses as needed, then every 1–4 h as needed [2]. Repeated administration of inhaled SABA (up to 4–10 puffs every 20 min for the first hour) is usually effective in controlling mild to moderate asthma exacerbations [2]. During the first hour, the dose of SABA required varies from 4 to 10 puffs every 3–4 h up to 6–10 puffs every 1–2 h, or more often. No additional SABA is needed if there is a good response to initial treatment (i.e. PEF >60–80% of predicted or personal best for 3–4 h).

Delivery of SABA via a pMDI and spacer or a DPI leads to a similar improvement in lung function as delivery via nebulizer [2].

Q3. What is the next best management step if the patient is irresponsive to albuterol?

A. Systemic steroid
B. Montelukast

C. Adrenaline
D. Mepolizumab

Answer: *The correct answer is* ***A.***

Mepolizumab (anti-IL-5) has been shown to improve asthma control, but is not approved for use during asthma attacks. Epinephrine should be reserved for extreme circumstances such as impending respiratory failure. Leukotriene receptor antagonists (LTRAs) such as montelukast are not approved to control acute asthma attacks and are less effective than inhaled corticosteroids (ICS) for controller therapy. Anticholinergics such as ipratropium bromide can be added to SABA during exacerbations, but not to be used as first line therapy.

For most patients with acute asthma, exacerbations improve with frequent bronchodilator use and a short course of oral or intravenous systemic corticosteroid. Dosing of systemic steroid administration includes prednisone 0.5–1 mg/kg every 6–8 h for 48 h and then 0.5–1 mg/kg/day twice a day for 3–7 days (max 60 mg/day) [2].

Oral corticosteroids (OCS) are prescribed in severe asthma exacerbations (e.g. PEF or forced expiratory volume in the 1st second (FEV1) less than 60%) and/or when the patient is not responding to treatment with SABA after 1 h. Tapering is not needed if OCS is prescribed for less than 2 weeks [2] or alternatively less than 7 days. Typically, a short course of OCS is recommended (e.g. 40–50 mg/day usually for 5–7 days) to continue home management of patients who:

1. Fail to respond to an increase in reliever and controller medication for 24–48 h
2. Deteriorate rapidly or who have a PEF or FEV1 < 60% of their personal best or predicted value
3. Have a history of sudden severe exacerbations, i.e. more than two episodes within a year

For children 6–11 years, the recommended dose of OCS is 1–2 mg/kg/day (maximum of 40 mg/day) for 3–5 days. Patients should remain in contact with their physician during the OCS course [2].

Practical Points

- Two clinical types of asthma have been conventionally described: transient non-atopic wheezing which is more common in early childhood and persistent atopic wheezing with onset in early childhood and high probability of persistence in late childhood or adulthood
- Pulmonary Index Score is a useful tool in assessing the severity of asthma attack
- Anticholinergics can be used as add-on therapy to short-acting beta-agonists (SABA) during asthma exacerbations
- A short course of oral or systemic corticosteroid should be considered if the patient is irresponsive to short-acting beta-agonist

References

1. The Global Initiative for Asthma (GINA). National Heart, Lung, and Blood Institute, National Institutes of Health, USA, and World Health Organization. 1993. www.ginasthma.org. Accessed 2019.
2. Kliegman R, Behrman RE, Nelson WE. Nelson textbook of pediatrics. 20th ed. Philadelphia, PA: Elsevier; 2016.

Chapter 42
Recurrent Nighttime Awakening Due to Shortness of Breath

Alireza Shafiei

A 5-year-old boy with a history of asthma from 2 years of age is on treatment with daily montelukast since one month ago. His symptoms are not under control and disturb his daily activity and sleep.

Q1. What is the best treatment for him?

A. Add inhaler corticosteroid to montelukast
B. Use inhaler corticosteroid instead of montelukast
C. Add short curse corticosteroid to montelukast
D. Use inhaler corticosteroid and Long acting bronchodilator

Answer: *The correct answer is* ***B.***

According to the Expert Panel Report number 3 (EPR3) on asthma [1], if alternative treatments are used with inadequate response, treatment should discontinue and the preferred treatment should be used before stepping up the initial one.

Q2. With this new treatment, his symptoms are under control for one month. What is your next suggestion?

A. Discontinue his drug and use bronchodilator as needed
B. Decrease his treatment gradually in one month
C. Continue his drug for at least two months
D. Discontinue his drug and use oral corticosteroid as needed

Answer: *The correct answer is* ***C.***

According to EPR3 step-down of asthma medication should be maintained for at least 3 months, if asthma is well controlled.

A. Shafiei (✉)
Department of Allergy and Clinical Immunology, Bahrami Hospital, School of Medicine, Tehran University of Medical Sciences, Tehran, Iran
e-mail: ar-shafiei@tums.ac.ir

N. Rezaei (ed.), *Pediatric Allergy*, https://doi.org/10.1007/978-3-030-18282-3_42

A 28 year old man develops generalized urticaria after bee sting, A couple of years later, he is admitted in the emergency ward, with tong and lips angioedema, urticaria, dyspnea and hypotension after being stung by a honey bee.

Q3. What is the most possible diagnosis?

A. Acute urticaria and angioedema
B. Anaphylaxis
C. Papular Urticaria
D. Hereditary angioedema

Answer: *The correct answer is* ***B.***

Anaphylaxis presents with sudden onset of symptoms in more than one body system: urticaria, angioedema, dyspnea and hypotension in this case.

Q4. What is the best treatment for him?

A. Epinephrine 0.01 mg/kg
B. Normal Saline 20 mL/kg
C. Methylprednisolone 1 mg/kg
D. Diphenhydramine 1 mg/kg

Answer: *The correct answer is* ***A.***

Epinephrine is drug of choice in treatment of anaphylaxis. It sould be injected intramascular in the thigh as soon as possible.

Q5. What is the best possible method to prevent recurrence?

A. Using antihistamines
B. Avoidance of honey bee
C. Epinephrine autoinjector
D. Immunotherapy

Answer: *The correct answer is* ***D.***

Practical Points

- Patients who are symptomatic on alternative treatments of asthma, could benefit from the best preferred treatment before stepping up, according to standard therapy
- Epinephrine is lifesaving in anaphylaxis. It should be injected as soon as possible
- Hymenoptera venom immunotherapy is highly effective, up to 95%, in decreasing the risk for severe anaphylaxis

Reference

1. National Asthma Education and Prevention Program, Third Expert Panel on the Diagnosis and Management of Asthma Bethesda (MD): National Heart, Lung, and Blood Institute (US). 2007. https://www.ncbi.nlm.nih.gov/books/NBK7232/.

Chapter 43
Tachypnea, Fever and Eosinophilia

Kevin S. Gipson, Ryan H. Avery, and Luke A. Wall

An 8-year-old boy with no significant past medical history presents to pulmonology clinic for initial consultation for a chief complaint of tachypnea and fatigue for one week, with an onset of fever (T: 39.4 °C) over the past 3 days [1]. In clinic, he is found to be tachypneic and tachycardic, with a transcutaneous oxygen saturation of 85% in room air. He has a mild cough, but is afebrile. Physical exam demonstrates supraclavicular retraction and coarse rales throughout both lung fields, but is otherwise unremarkable except for signs of onychophagia (Fig. 43.1). The patient has no history of recurrent cough or wheeze, rhinitis, or sinopulmonary infections. Other members of the household are well and there is no family history of chronic pulmonary disease or immunodeficiency. The boy lives with his family on a small farm in a rural region of the southern United States, and helps with chores. There is no tobacco exposure.

The boy was admitted to the hospital for further evaluation and treatment with oxygen supplementation, inhaled bronchodilators, and systemic steroids. At time of admission a CXR demonstrates diffuse reticulonodular lung opacities (Fig. 43.2). CBC demonstrates elevated WBC (32,500 cells/μL) and absolute eosinophilia (12,700 cells/μL, or 39%), and an elevated total serum IgE (11,500 IU/mL). The

K. S. Gipson
Division of Pediatric Pulmonology, Department of Pediatrics, Massachusetts General Hospital, Harvard Medical School, Boston, MA, USA

R. H. Avery
Department of Pathobiological Sciences, Louisiana State University School of Veterinary Medicine, Baton Rouge, LA, USA

L. A. Wall (✉)
Section of Allergy Immunology, Department of Pediatrics, Children's Hospital, Louisiana State University School of Medicine, New Orleans, LA, USA
e-mail: lwall@lsuhsc.edu

N. Rezaei (ed.), *Pediatric Allergy*, https://doi.org/10.1007/978-3-030-18282-3_43

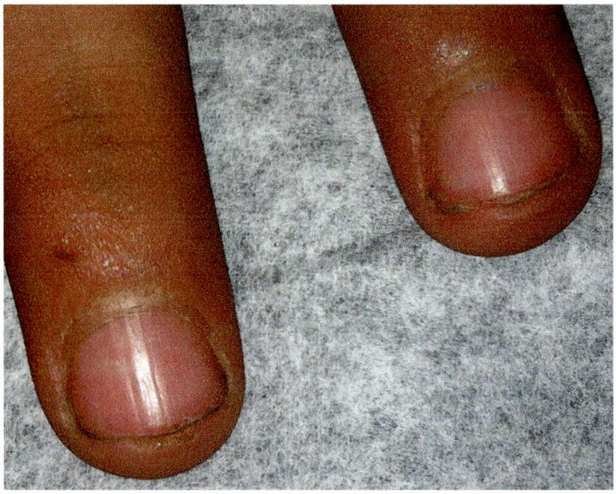

Fig. 43.1 The patient's soiled fingernails demonstrating signs of onychophagia (nail-biting)

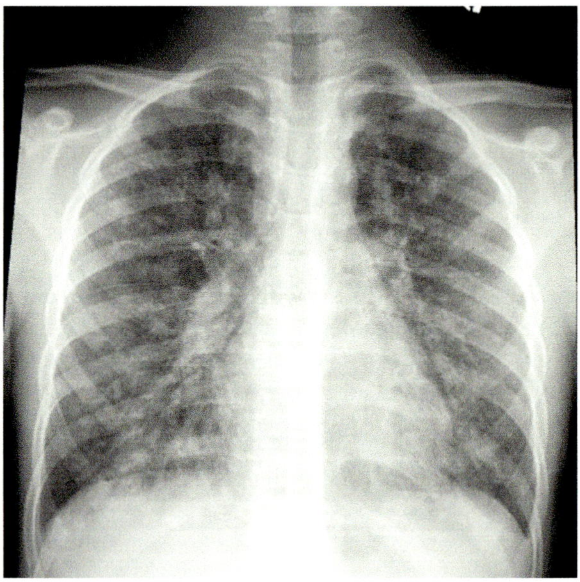

Fig. 43.2 The patient's initial chest radiograph at our facility at time of admission, demonstrating diffuse reticulonodular lung opacities

patient is scheduled for flexible bronchoscopy and BAL, which demonstrates marked pulmonary eosinophilia (86%).

Q1. What is the most likely etiology of this patient's respiratory symptoms?

A. Acute exacerbation of previously undiagnosed asthma
B. Hypersensitivity pneumonitis
C. Eosinophilic granulomatosis with polyangiitis
D. Helminth-associated eosinophilic pneumonitis

Answer: *The correct answer is* ***D.***

While all of the above options are reasonable considerations in the context of this child's presentation, a helminth-associated eosinophilic pneumonitis is the most likely etiology for his respiratory signs and striking peripheral and pulmonary eosinophilia. Though asthma might present for the first time in an 8-year-old patient, absence of wheeze and the presence of rales on pulmonary auscultation, the interstitial pattern on CXR (Fig. 43.2), and the lack of history of atopy are inconsistent with this diagnosis. The acute nature of the patient's symptoms, the presence of fever, rales on chest auscultation, and potential chronic exposure to allergens on the family farm raise the possibility of hypersensitivity pneumonitis (HP), also known as extrinsic allergic alveolitis, as a differential diagnosis. However, during the acute phase of HP the BAL is generally lymphocytic, not eosinophilic [2, 3]. Though a nonspecific finding, the rales in HP are typically bibasilar and not diffuse as are in this case. Similar respiratory symptoms in the setting of increased IgE could be due to allergic bronchopulmonary aspergillosis (ABPA). However, this disease typically occurs in the context of an underlying chronic pulmonary disorder such as asthma or cystic fibrosis. This patient has no history of prior allergic rhinitis or pansinusitis, and has no cutaneous findings or overt signs of systemic vasculitis which would be indicative of eosinophilic granulomatosis with polyangiitis (EGPA).

The patient's condition rapidly improved, and by day 3 of hospitalization his rales and oxygen requirement had completely resolved. A hypersensitivity panel was negative. He was discharged on a course of oral steroid and as needed bronchodilator.

He was seen 3 weeks later in allergy clinic follow-up, where his WBC count remained elevated (22,600 cells/μL) and serum total IgE has increased to 12,700 IU/mL. On further history, the full extent of the child's farm chores is revealed to include the care of livestock, including pigs. An evaluation for parasitic infection was performed on the child, and was notable for a serum *Ascaris*-specific IgE level of 433 kU/L (reference range < 0.35 kU/L). His fecal sample revealed no *Ascaris* eggs.

Q2. Given the finding of elevated serum *Ascaris*-specific IgE, what is this child's most likely diagnosis?

A. Löffler syndrome
B. Visceral larva migrans
C. Hypereosinophilic syndrome
D. Tropical pulmonary eosinophilia

Answer: *The correct answer is* ***A.***

This patient has a classic presentation of Löffler syndrome, a helminth-associated eosinophilic pneumonitis which occurs when *Ascaris* larvae, hatched from orally-ingested eggs in the intestine and brought to the capillary-alveolar interface of the lungs via the portal venous system, transmigrate through the lung parenchyma and airways to the upper airway, where they are subsequently re-ingested and complete their maturation in the host gut [4]. This transmigration provokes a marked eosinophil-mediated inflammatory reaction within the airways and lung parenchyma, yielding a syndrome of ephemeral, migratory pulmonary infiltrates on chest radiograph, respiratory symptoms including cough and hypoxemia, and peripheral blood and pulmonary eosinophilia. While the initial description of this disease was due to ascariasis, the helminths *Ancylostoma duodenale*, *Necator americanus*, and *Strongyloides stercoralis* have similar life cycles in the human host and also elicit an eosinophilic pneumonitis [5]. Visceral larva migrans (VLM) is a syndrome of hematogenous seeding of the larvae of *Toxocara canis*, leading to pulmonary eosinophilic granulomas and visceral involvement including hepatomegaly, without true trans-pulmonary passage of helminths in the human host [5, 6]. The hypereosinophilic syndrome involves end-organ damage due to eosinophilic infiltration without parasitic infection, and tropical pulmonary eosinophilia (TPE) is due to microfilarial pathogens [5].

Löffler syndrome is generally self-limited, resolving gradually upon completion of the trans-pulmonary migratory phase of the *Ascaris* life cycle [7]. Considering the fact that these acute respiratory symptoms are caused during the larval stage of *Ascaris* infection, the individual would not demonstrate *Ascaris* eggs in fecal sample (which are only produced by adult worms). In mild cases, it is often not necessary to treat patients with anthelmintic medications. In our patient, we elected to treat him with anthelmintic after follow-up total serum IgE and WBCs remained elevated despite resolution of pulmonary symptoms. We suspected a chronic reinfection via his ongoing environmental exposures on the farm.

Our patient was treated with Albendazole 400 mg once by mouth approximately 1 month after the resolution of his pulmonary symptoms. This treatment was followed by quick deceleration in his total serum IgE and WBC count.

Q3. Primary or co-infection with which trans-pulmonary migrating helminth is a strong relative contraindication to the use of systemic corticosteroids?

A. *Toxocara canis*
B. *Ascaris suum*
C. *Strongyloides stercoralis*
D. *Necator americanus*

Answer: *The correct answer is* ***C.***

Strongyloides hyperinfection syndrome is a potentially fatal condition of disseminated strongyloidiasis in the context of cell-mediated immunodeficiency or suppression, and a major risk of systemic steroid use in this patient with *Strongyloides* infection [8, 9]. A recent review found over 50 reported cases of hyperinfection since 2000, with the most common risk factor being systemic steroid use, though many of these patients had comorbid immune-modulating diseases, including malignancy and auto-immune disorders [9]. Steroids act to decrease eosinophil survival in the host by suppression of eosinophil survival factors and induction of eosinophil apoptosis, hence permitting fulminant *Strongyloides* infection to proceed unabated [10]. While it is critical to rule out co-infection with other parasites in cases of helminth-associated eosinophilic pneumonitis, parasites other than *Strongyloides* are not typically implicated in hyperinfection syndromes with use of steroids. In addition, specific monoclonal antibodies are now among the approved medications in the treatment of allergic disorders, with the end result being inhibition of IgE or eosinophils. Such biologics could also theoretically lead to *Strongyloides* hyperinfection syndrome in a patient with undiagnosed infection.

When strongyloidiasis is excluded, systemic steroids can be helpful in managing the acute respiratory symptoms of Löffler syndrome. Our patient responded rapidly to systemic steroids, with complete resolution of his respiratory symptoms within 72 h of hospitalization.

Q4. Following resolution of a helminth-associated eosinophilic pneumonitis, which intervention is most likely to minimize further clinical sequelae for this patient?

A. Long-term moderate-dose inhaled corticosteroid
B. Monthly subcutaneous injection of a monoclonal anti-IgE antibody
C. Intermittent dosing of anthelmintics
D. Definitive identification of the source of infection

Answer: *The correct answer is* ***D.***

A rigorous search for the source of the helminth is necessary to prevent reinfection of the patient. Definitive identification of the infectious source facilitates any necessary public health intervention [11]. In our case, a site visit to the family farm revealed *Ascaris suum* eggs in both pig feces and in the soil surrounding the pig enclosures (Fig. 43.3). This young patient was responsible for cleaning pig enclosures using equipment which was soiled with pig feces. We postulated that the patient was chronically inoculated with *Ascaris* eggs via onychophagia of soiled nails. Environmental remediation was undertaken and the patient has remained well thereafter, without evidence of further parasitic infection or pulmonary sequelae.

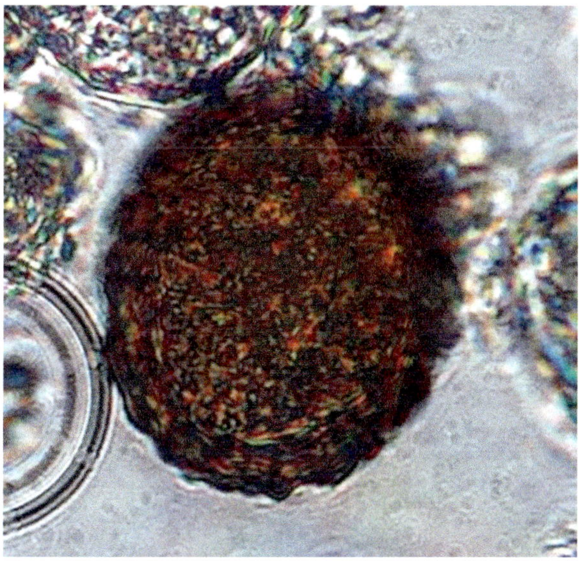

Fig. 43.3 Fecal sample from pig on the patient's farm demonstrating *Ascaris* egg

Practical Points

- Löffler syndrome is a helminth-associated eosinophilic pneumonitis which occurs when helminths transmigrate through the lung parenchyma and airways, provoking a marked eosinophil-mediated inflammatory response
- The clinical picture is a constellation of transient pulmonary infiltrates on CXR, respiratory symptoms including cough and hypoxemia, and peripheral blood and pulmonary eosinophilia
- Supportive care including supplemental oxygen and inhaled bronchodilators is helpful in acute management of Löffler-associated respiratory symptoms
- Anthelmintic treatments may be used in particularly severe or refractory cases of Löffler syndrome, though the condition is generally self-limited
- *Strongyloides* co-infection should be ruled out in patients who have risk factors for helminth exposure before the use of systemic steroids, particularly in otherwise immunosuppressed patients to avoid the potential risk of a disseminated hyperinfection syndrome
- The same cautionary statement applies to monoclonal antibodies which are designed to inhibit IgE or eosinophils
- Helminth infection should be considered in the differential diagnosis for asthma, eosinophilia, or elevated IgE, even in developed countries

References

1. Gipson K, Avery R, Shah H, Pepiak D, Begue RE, Malone J, Wall LA. Loffler syndrome on a Louisiana pig farm. Respir Med Case Rep. 2016;19:128–31.
2. Fan LL. Hypersensitivity pneumonitis in children. Curr Opin Pediatr. 2002;14(3):323–6.
3. Vece TJ, Fan LL. Diagnosis and management of diffuse lung disease in children. Paediatr Respir Rev. 2011;12(4):238–42.
4. Sharma OP, Maheshwari A. Lung disease in the tropics. Ann N Y Acad Sci. 1991.
5. Knutsen APTJ, Wooldridge JL, et al. Environmental exposures in the normal host. In: Bush A, Wilmott RW, Boat TF, Chernick V, editors. Kendig and Chernicks disorders of the respiratory tract in children. 8th ed. Amsterdam: Elsevier; 2012. p. 858–76.
6. Cheepsattayakorn A, Cheepsattayakorn R. Parasitic pneumonia and lung involvement. Biomed Res Int. 2014;2014:874021.
7. Diemert DJ. Ascariasis. In: Walker DH, editor. Tropical infectious diseases: principles, pathogens and practice. Amsterdam: Elsevier; 2011. p. 794–8.
8. Kassalik M, Mönkemüller K. Strongyloides stercoralis hyperinfection syndrome and disseminated disease. Gastroenterol Hepatol. 2011;7(11):766–8.
9. Segarra-Newnham M. Manifestations, diagnosis, and treatment of Strongyloides stercoralis infection. Ann Pharmacother. 2007;41(12):1992–2001.
10. Druilhe A, Letuve S, Pretolani M. Glucocorticoid-induced apoptosis in human eosinophils: mechanisms of action. Apoptosis. 2003;8(5):481–95.
11. Miller LA, Colby K, Manning SE, Hoenig D, McEvoy E, Montgomery S, Mathison B, de Almeida M, Bishop H, Dasilva A, Sears S. Ascariasis in humans and pigs on small-scale farms, Maine, USA, 2010-2013. Emerg Infect Dis. 2015;21(2):332–4.

Chapter 44
Cough and Fever

Nikolaos A. Karantaglis

A 2.5-year-old boy was admitted to the hospital due to cough and fever. The boy was born as a preterm twin at gestational age of 34 weeks and had been hospitalized in the NICU for 10 days. He had a history of atopic dermatitis since early infancy and one hospitalization at the age of 5 months due to bronchiolitis and several episodes of wheezing afterwards. The boy received prophylaxis with inhaled fluticasone 150 μg twice daily, prescribed with a spacer, plus montelukast sachets 4 mg once daily for the last year. He had an IgE level of 196 IU/mL (reference value <60) in a lab test performed a year ago.

His parents revealed that 3 days before the hospitalization he had a mild chocking episode while eating peanuts. His cough persisted for three days, followed by a fever (T: 39 °C) starting few hours before his admission in hospital.

On examination the boy was conscious, febrile, had reduced respiratory sounds in his left lung, rhinitis and a reddish pharynx. Rest of his clinical evaluation was clear with oxygen saturation 98% without any signs of respiratory distress.

Laboratory findings on admission revealed WBC: 21,800 cells/μL with 74% neutrophils and 16% lymphocytes, ESR: 51 mm/h and CRP: 63.8 mg/L. CXR revealed consolidation of the left lower lobe plus hyperinflation of the right lung (Fig. 44.1).

Q1. Which of the following can be listed as a possible differential diagnosis?

A. Pneumonia
B. Episodic viral wheeze
C. Foreign body aspiration
D. All of the above

Answer: *The correct answer is* ***D.***

N. A. Karantaglis (✉)
Pediatric Pulmonology Unit, 3rd Pediatric Department, Hippokrateion Hospital, Aristotle University of Thessaloniki, Thessaloniki, Greece
e-mail: karantaglis@auth.gr

N. Rezaei (ed.), *Pediatric Allergy*, https://doi.org/10.1007/978-3-030-18282-3_44

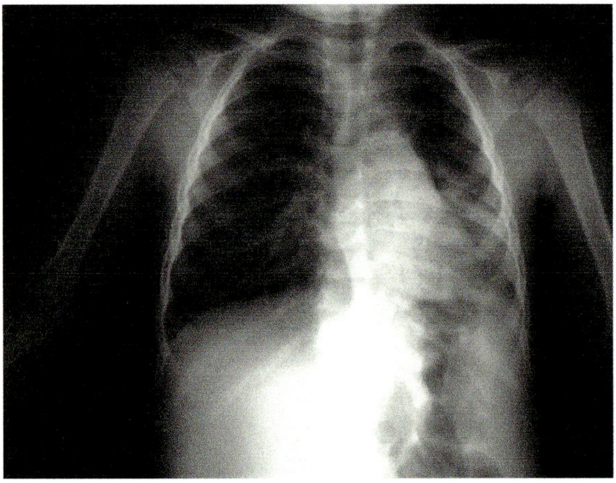

Fig. 44.1 Consolidation of the left lower lobe and subsequent hyperinflation of the right lung of a toddler presenting with cough and fever

Community acquired pneumonia is a common infection in children less than 5 years old and both the laboratory findings and the CXR support this diagnosis for our patient.

Given the boy's medical history with wheezing episodes in preschool years, his symptoms could be due to a viral infection, such as rhinovirus, influenza or RSV, causing an exacerbation of his transient wheezing. Although foreign body aspiration is not generally common, it is supported by the reported incident of chocking and the subsequent cough.

Q2. What would you think as the first-line of treatment for this patient?

A. Antibiotics
B. Oxygen
C. Bronchodilators
D. Oseltamivir

Answer: *The correct answer is* ***A.***

Giving antibiotics in order to empirically treat the present infection is a prudent decision. Since there are no signs of respiratory distress and the patient holds a saturation of 98% there is no need for oxygen supplementation at this time and as the foreign body has not been excluded yet, it is wise not to use bronchodilators unless it is necessary. Finally, oseltamivir has no place as an initial treatment as there are no signs of flu infection. Cefuroxime, a second generation cephalosporin, was initiated. The patient remained febrile, below 38 °C, after admission.

Q3. What would you propose as the next diagnostic test?

A. Spirometry
B. Chest ultrasound
C. CT scan
D. Flexible bronchoscopy

Answer: *The correct answer is* ***D.***

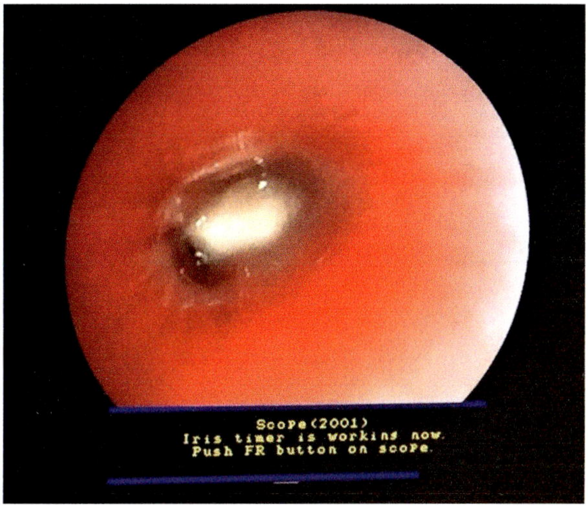

Fig. 44.2 Foreign body (peanut) inside the left main bronchus of a toddler presenting with cough and fever

Spirometry is not possible, as the toddlers age makes it impossible. Chest ultrasound could be useful in case of suspected complicated pneumonia or a pleural effusion but the clinical signs and the X-ray do not support this diagnosis. CT scan has little to add in a case with pneumonia. If the index of suspicion of a foreign body aspiration is high, many physicians forgo CT scanning and proceed with bronchoscopy for a more definite diagnosis. Flexible bronchoscopy is highly successful in detecting foreign body aspiration.

Flexible bronchoscopy was carried out the next day. There was redness and swelling of the trachea and the left main bronchus. A foreign body (peanut) was found in the left main bronchus. A short course of systemic steroids was given and 4 days later the foreign body was removed with rigid bronchoscopy, which was the procedure of choice considering previous localization (Fig. 44.2).

The clinical suspicion was based on the facts that there was no wheezing or signs of significant respiratory distress and the patient's fever literally stopped soon after the hospitalization, and last but not least a history of chocking after eating peanuts 3 days before. A foreign body aspiration must always be included in the differential diagnosis of wheezing in a child at preschool age [1–3].

Practical Points

- Whether localized or associated with consolidation and/or hyperinflation in CXR, foreign body aspiration should always be included in differential diagnosis of wheezing in children
- Fever is not a reliable differentiating symptom, as foreign body aspiration might lead to lobar pneumonia. Alternatively asthma exacerbation might associate a febrile viral infection

References

1. Kann K, Long B, Koyfman A. Clinical mimics: an emergency medicine-focused review of asthma mimics. J Emerg Med. 2017;53(2):195–201.
2. McVea S, Bourke T. Optimising the management of wheeze in preschool children. Practitioner. 2016;260(1794):11–4, 2.
3. Bertelli L, Gentili A, Modolon C, Corsini I, Cazzato S. A foreign body aspiration in a preschool child mimicking a multitrigger wheezing: a case report and review of the literature. Pediatr Emerg Care. 2012;28(12):1382–4.

Chapter 45
Yellow-Colored Facial Skin Rash

Mojgan Kianiamin, Farzaneh Rahmani, and Nima Rezaei

A 10-day-old neonate is referred to the hospital with eczematous yellow-colored skin rash on her face. The baby feeds very well and has normal temperature with normal reflexes. Her conjunctive looks anicteric.

Q1. What is the next step in skin rash evaluation?

A. Taking detailed history and observe the baby
B. Evaluate for phenylketonuria
C. Asking for an immunologist consult
D. Stop giving breast milk

Answer: *The correct answer is* ***A****.*

Facial skin rash is a very important physical finding during neonatal period. It may define an underlying metabolic disorder e.g. phenylketonuria, or unmask a severe infection with *Staphylococci*. On the other side it may be a hallmark of severe combined immunodeficiency in Omenn's syndrome or simply an allergy mark in

M. Kianiamin (✉)
Chamran Medical Hospital, Tehran, Iran

F. Rahmani
Network of Immunity in Infection, Malignancy and Autoimmunity (NIIMA), Universal Scientific Education and Research Network (USERN), Tehran, Iran

NeuroImaging Network (NIN), Universal Scientific Education and Research Network (USERN), Tehran, Iran
e-mail: f-rahmani@alumnus.tums.ac.ir

N. Rezaei
Department of Immunology, School of Medicine, Research Center for Immunodeficiencies (RCID), Children's Medical Center, Tehran University of Medical Sciences (TUMS), Tehran, Iran

Network of Immunity in Infection, Malignancy and Autoimmunity (NIIMA), Universal Scientific Education and Research Network (USERN), Tehran, Iran

N. Rezaei (ed.), *Pediatric Allergy*, https://doi.org/10.1007/978-3-030-18282-3_45

atopic dermatitis [1]. Taking a good history with complete physical examination in neonatal period, plays the fundamental role in the diagnosis.

Her history revealed presentation of mild hyperbilirubinemia 2–3 days after birth. She was taking breast milk with some traditional herbal medicine to control the jaundice. The parents denied giving her any cow's milk formula. Laboratory data revealed leukocytosis with neutrophil predominance and normal bilirubin levels.

Q2. What is the most likely diagnosis?

A. Cow's milk allergy via breast milk
B. Infantile atopic dermatitis
C. Wiskott-Aldrich syndrome
D. Eczematoid rash with herbal medicine

Answer: *The correct answer is* ***D****.*

Cow's milk allergy and atopic dermatitis often develop later on at least 3–4 weeks-old, when cow' milk formula or complementary food is added to the baby's diet [1]. Wiskott Aldrich syndrome (WAS) is an X-linked recessive disorder with thrombocytopenia and eczema. The earliest manifestation of WAS are petechiae and bruises in a male neonate [1]. Eczematoid rash with herbs is not common in early life. According to the baby's history, the rash should subside quickly after stop using the herbal medicine.

Q3. Which one of the following requests will best support this idea?

A. Total leukocyte and platelet count
B. Prick test for cow s milk protein
C. Radioallergosorbent assay for casein and lactalbumin
D. Stop giving herbal medicine

Answer: *The correct answer is* ***D****.*

Allergic disorders are diagnosed clinically and laboratory evaluations are generally aimed at confirming clinical suspicions. Immediate type skin prick test (SPT) or measurement of specific IgE (sIgE) in the serum (Radioallergosorbent assay: RAST), are among useful laboratory investigations in adults that lack sensitivity in neonatal period or in suspected T-cell-mediated reactions. According to this case, eczematoid reactions seen in the baby can be classified as delayed type hypersensitivity reaction, hence, food challenge or patch test appear to be the most useful modalities.

You advise the mother to discontinue the herb and continue exclusive breastfeeding for the next 2 weeks. She is coming back with normal appearance. Her mother was asked to bring in the suspicious herb.

Q4. What the offending herb could be?

A. Chamomile
B. Licorice
C. Purgative manna
D. Caraway

Answer: *The correct answer is* ***C****.*

Purgative manna is a traditional herbal medicine which has been recommended by ancient Iranian medical literature to treat neonatal hyperbilirubinemia. Medicinal plants such as *Fumaria parviflora*, *Cichorium intybus*, *Alhagi pseudalhagi* and *Purgative manna* have been used in the treatment of neonatal jaundice as complementary therapies for many years in Iran and Southeast Asian countries. *Purgative manna* which is produced by the act of an insect on some of plants such as *Cotoneaster discolor*, is known as *Shir-Khesht* in Iran [2]. Its laxative and biliousness effects might interrupt bilirubin enterohepatic circulation and decrease indirect bilirubin levels.

Practical Points

- Purgative manna is a traditional herbal medicine, recommended for neonatal hyperbilirubinemia by ancient Iranian medical literature
- Eczematoid rash with herbs is not common in early life. Taking a detailed medical history and subsiding rash quickly after discontinuation of the herb were in favor of this diagnosis

References

1. Barrett M, Luu M. Differential diagnosis of atopic dermatitis. Immunol Allergy Clin North Am. 2017;37(1):11–34.
2. Fallah R, Fallahzadeh MA, Noori-Shadkam M. Evaluation of safety and efficacy of purgative manna (billinaster drop) and glycerin suppository in icterus of healthy term newborns. Curr Drug Saf. 2014;9(1):29–33.

Chapter 46
Recurrent Angioedema of the Eyes and Lips

Eva Rebelo Gomes and Carmo Abreu

A 13-year-old boy with a personal history of rhinitis and asthma was referred to our clinic for multiple episodes of angioedema of the eyes and lips. In some of these episodes, he presented also generalized pruritus and dyspnea and had been admitted in the emergency department requiring treatment with adrenaline in eight occasions. Most episodes occurred within 1–2 h after a meal, but involvement of any suspected food was not clear.

For 4 years, his paediatrician had performed multiple prick tests and specific IgE (sIgE) for food allergens which were negative for wheat, rye, oat, corn, peanut, almond, walnut, chestnut, soybean, milk, cocoa, strawberry, egg white, egg yolk, codfish, tuna, salmon, shrimp, pea, pork, cheese and tomato. The laboratory tests such as CBC, LFT, renal and thyroid function and tryptase level were all normal. Positive results were only obtained for mites and cat epithelium allergens.

He took daily inhaled budesonide 400 μg and fluticasone nasal spray 27.5 μg twice daily. The patient was instructed to carry an adrenaline autoinjector and he had used it once a month in the last year.

Q1. What is the most likely diagnosis?

A. Panic disorder
B. Chronic urticaria/angioedema
C. Recurrent anaphylaxis
D. Mastocytosis

Answer*: The correct answer is* ***C****.*

E. R. Gomes
Basic and Clinical Immunology Unit, Laboratory of Immunology, Faculty of Medicine, University of Porto, Porto, Portugal

Centro Hospitalar do Porto, Porto, Portugal

C. Abreu (✉)
Centro Hospitalar do Porto, Porto, Portugal
e-mail: mccpereira@chtmad.min-saude.pt

N. Rezaei (ed.), *Pediatric Allergy*, https://doi.org/10.1007/978-3-030-18282-3_46

Suspected anaphylaxis is one of the common chief complaints in patients referred to an allergist. It is often very difficult to differentiate a true anaphylaxis from panic disorders, as patients with panic disorder can be commonly atopic and suffer from asthma, and superimposed acute urticaria/angioedema. When the attack has not been witnessed directly by a clinician, even when compatible with panic attack, the possibility of anaphylaxis something to think about. Usually the patient is observed by allergologist months after the event has taken place and important information might be forgotten or not recorded at the time. Importantly, up to 50% of the allergic patients have mild to severe psychological disorders and 16% have psychological conditions requiring treatment. Importantly, up to 10% of the allergic patients are revealed to have panic disorders [1]. Based on the background and abusive use of the adrenaline autoinjector, panic disorders could be a hypothesis. However, history of observation in the emergency service and therapeutic response to adrenaline in these episodes, increase the likelihood of episodes of true anaphylaxis.

Urticaria is a disease characterized by the development of wheals, angioedema, or both. Urticaria needs to be differentiated from other medical conditions where wheals, angioedema, or both, can occur as a symptom [2]. Our patient had proper asthma control and no history of wheals, yet presented with episodes angioedema of the eyes and lips, associated with objectified bronchospasm in emergent department. Together these symptoms appear to be part of a systemic reaction more than mere urticaria.

Systemic mastocytosis is a clonal disorder of mast cells that may variably present with characteristic skin lesions, episodes of mast cell mediator release, and disturbances of hematopoiesis. Symptoms result from excessive mast cell mediator release, especially histamine, and may include pruritus and flushing, abdominal pain, diarrhea, dyspnea, tachycardia, or profound hypotension [3]. Because of the increased risk of anaphylaxis in mastocytosis, all patients with severe or recurrent anaphylaxis should be analysed for underlying mastocytosis by estimating baseline serum tryptase, which was normal in our patient.

Anaphylaxis has been defined as a severe, life-threatening systemic hypersensitivity reaction [4]. Cutaneous symptoms occur in most cases of anaphylaxis, especially in pediatric patients. Respiratory and/or cardiovascular symptoms, such as stridor, wheezing or hypotension are also frequent [5]. Hypotension and shock are less commonly present as early manifestations of anaphylaxis during childhood [6, 7]. In children, bronchospasm should alert clinicians to the potential severity of the reaction [5].

Anaphylaxis usually occur within 2 h of exposure to an allergen [8]. Food allergy is the most common cause of anaphylaxis in children, followed by drugs and insect's stings, latex, exercise and cold. In about 30% of the cases the cause cannot be identified and the anaphylactic reaction is classified as idiopathic [7].

Q2. Which one of the following should be the initial step in the management of this patient?

A. Skin prick tests with aeroallergens
B. Skin prick tests with food allergens
C. Skin and Intradermic test with hymenoptera venom
D. Written diary of symptoms and reactions

Answer*: The correct answer is* ***D****.*

In a case of multiple episodes of urticaria and anaphylaxis, with no clear trigger identified, the "reaction diary" can be a very useful tool. A reaction diary is a chronological listing of all the events and actions done as well as the symptoms the patient has experienced before and during the reaction. The physician should request the patient to keep a record of specific foods or drugs taken, the practice of physical exercise, exposure to cold environments, stressful events, menstrual cycle in women, etc. The diary should be carefully analysed and consistency is assessed. It is important to note that a diary lacks standardization and is not diagnostic but can be a useful tool as it helps narrowing the potential causes of the problem.

Q3. What is the major risk factor for life-threatening anaphylaxis in this patient?

A. Asthma
B. Atopy
C. Recurrent Angioedema
D. Allergic rhinitis

Answer: *The correct answer is* ***A***.

Patients who have had an anaphylactic reaction have a strong likelihood of having another one, and a history of asthma appears to be a major risk factor for life-threatening anaphylactic reactions to food. In fact, almost all fatal cases of anaphylaxis occur in patients with asthma [9, 10].

Q4. In view of these findings, which one of the following would be the best treatment option at this time?

A. Adrenaline autoinjector
B. Anti-leukotrienes
C. Oral corticosteroids
D. Antihistamines

Answer: *The correct answer is* ***A***.

Adrenaline (epinephrine) is the medication of choice for treatment of anaphylactic episodes. Rapid administration is crucial and can be lifesaving. The α-adrenergic effects of adrenaline cause an increase in peripheral vascular resistance, blood pressure and coronary artery perfusion, while reducing angioedema and urticaria. Whilst the β1-adrenergic effects of adrenaline increase heart rate and contractility, the β2-adrenergic effects mediate bronchodilation and inhibit the release of inflammatory mediators [11]. Early use of adrenaline has been associated with a better outcome [12]. Even after self-administration the patient should be observed in the emergency room and a surveillance of 6–8 h is advised as 6% of the cases of anaphylaxis in children are biphasic, which means that symptoms recur 4–6 h after the first manifestations [13].

After 6 weeks, the patient attended our clinic for the second time. He had two new anaphylactic episodes and used the self-injector twice, besides being observed in the emergency room. The patient and family had done a complete diary of events and from its analysis, it was possible to identify the intake of a tablet of ibuprofen 400 mg 1–2 h before the initial symptoms, which was in both episodes eyelid angioedema. He was asymptomatic between episodes.

The child's parents then reported frequent episodes of headache and that he usually took NSAIDs with meals to avoid gastrointestinal side effects, which explained that reaction occurred almost always after meals. The patient had tolerated paracetamol before, but had switched to ibuprofen which was more effective in treating his headaches. He denied the previous intake of aspirin.

Q5. According to the current European classification of NSAID hypersensitivity, how would classify this patient at this point?

A. NSAID-induced urticaria/angioedema (NIUA)
B. Single-NSAID-induced urticaria/angioedema or anaphylaxis (SNIUAA)
C. NSAID-exacerbated respiratory disease (NERD)
D. NSAID-exacerbated cutaneous disease (NECD)

***Answer**: The correct answer is **B**.*

NSAIDs are widely used to control pain and fever and to treat various inflammatory diseases. By inhibiting the synthesis of prostaglandins, they can induce both beneficial effects and adverse reactions, including drug-induced hypersensitivity reactions, which affect all age groups, including children and adolescents. Paracetamol and ibuprofen are widely used in children and are thus the most frequently implicated drugs in this age group. Ibuprofen is an anti-inflammatory propionic acid derivative, which shares similar characteristics with naproxen, fenoprofen, flurbiprofen, ketoprofen and oxaprozin [14]. In recent case-series of NSAID hypersensitivity in children, ibuprofen was the most frequent implicated drug [15].

Different classification of reactions to NSAIDs and phenotypes have been described over the last years. An updated classification from the European Academy of Allergy and Clinical Immunology (EAACI) grouped the clinical entities induced by hypersensitivity to NSAIDs into five groups**: NSAIDs-exacerbated respiratory disease (NERD)**, induced by aspirin or other NSAIDs manifesting primarily as bronchial obstruction, dyspnea, and nasal congestion/rhinorrhea. NERD occurs in patients with an underlying chronic airway respiratory disease such as asthma, rhinosinusitis or nasal polyps, **NSAIDs-exacerbated cutaneous disease (NECD)**, induced by aspirin or other NSAIDs manifesting as wheals and/or angioedema occurring in patients with a history of chronic spontaneous urticaria, **NSAIDs-induced urticaria/angioedema (NIUA)** induced by aspirin or other NSAIDs manifesting as wheals and/or angioedema occurring in otherwise healthy subjects (without history of chronic spontaneous urticaria). Symptoms should be induced by at least two NSAIDs with different chemical structure. **Single-NSAID-induced urticaria/angioedema or anaphylaxis (SNIUAA)** is defined as immediate reactions to a single NSAID or to several NSAIDs belonging to the same chemical group, manifesting as urticaria, angioedema and/or anaphylaxis. These subjects tolerate other chemically non-related NSAIDs and usually do not have a history of chronic urticaria or asthma. **Single-NSAID-induced delayed hypersensitivity reactions (SNIRD)** refers to reactions to a single NSAID appearing usually within 24–48 h after drug administration and manifesting by either skin symptoms, exanthema, fixed drug eruption, other organ specific symptoms (e.g. renal, pulmonary) or severe cutaneous adverse reactions [16].

To confirm the diagnosis, the patient was challenged with ibuprofen. During the test and after 5 min after 300 mg of ibuprofen there was angioedema of the eye and lip. Bronchospasm with a 20% drop in FEV1 developed after 20 min. The patient was instructed to avoid all NSAIDs and take paracetamol instead until further diagnostic workup. He was also referred for an appointment at Pediatric neurology to investigate the recurrent headaches.

Two months later, the boy presented to the emergency room with pain and intermittent claudication of the right leg, and ketorolac (30 mg IV) was administered. Angioedema of the eyes and dyspnea appeared in 5 min after injection. The reaction was treated with adrenaline and reversed within 30 min. A basophil activation test was performed without degranulation after stimulation with ketorolac (ibuprofen not available).

Q6. Which one of the following is needed next step in the evaluation and management of this patient?

A. Oral challenge with a Cox2 preferential inhibitor
B. Oral challenge with a specific Cox2 inhibitor
C. Oral challenge with aspirin
D. Skin tests with NSAIDs

Answer: *The correct answer is* ***A***.

Oral challenge with NSAID is recommended in three occasions: (1) oral challenge with a culprit drug to confirm hypersensitivity, (2) oral challenge with other than causative NSAIDs (usually challenge test with aspirin) in order to confirm/exclude cross-reactivity, and (3) oral challenge with the most likely tolerated alternative drug. The oral challenge test with the culprit drug remains the gold standard to confirm the diagnosis of NSAIDs hypersensitivity, and all patients with equivocal history should be tested accordingly [16].

In view of the result of the oral challenge test with ibuprofen and subsequent reaction to ketorolac reaction, cross-reactivity to different groups of NSAIDs is confirmed. In order to find an alternative anti-inflammatory drug, and based on the characteristics and indication of the different anti-inflammatories available for pediatric age (specific Cox2 inhibitor is not approved for children under 16 years), we performed oral challenge test with the most likely tolerated alternative drug, Cox2 preferential inhibitor. Nimesulide was shown to be an alternative safe drug in our case, as previously described by other authors [17]. The patient tolerated 175 mg of

Practical Points

- All patients with a suspicion of anaphylaxis attack should be screened for systemic mastocytosis using baseline serum tryptase levels
- Cutaneous symptoms are the most common manifestation of anaphylaxis while hypotension and shock are less common in pediatric patients
- Food allergy is the most common cause of anaphylaxis in children
- A "reaction diary" is a useful tool to identify trigger(s) of the so-called idiopathic anaphylactic reaction
- History of asthma along with a previous episode of anaphylaxis are strong predictors of future life threatening anaphylactic reactions

nimesulide without cutaneous, respiratory or gastrointestinal symptoms. After discontinuation of others NSAIDs there was a resolution of the anaphylaxis episodes.

References

1. Schmidt-Traub S, Bamler KJ. The psychoimmunological association of panic disorder and allergic reaction. Br J Clin Psychol. 1997;36(Pt 1):51–62.
2. Zuberbier T, Aberer W, Asero R, Bindslev-Jensen C, Brzoza Z, Canonica GW, Church MK, Ensina LF, Gimenez-Arnau A, Godse K, Goncalo M, Grattan C, Hebert J, Hide M, Kaplan A, Kapp A, Abdul Latiff AH, Mathelier-Fusade P, Metz M, Nast A, Saini SS, Sanchez-Borges M, Schmid-Grendelmeier P, Simons FE, Staubach P, Sussman G, Toubi E, Vena GA, Wedi B, Zhu XJ, Maurer M, European Academy of Allergy and Clinical Immunology; Global Allergy and Asthma European Network; European Dermatology Forum; World Allergy Organization. The EAACI/GA(2) LEN/EDF/WAO Guideline for the definition, classification, diagnosis, and management of urticaria: the 2013 revision and update. Allergy. 2014;69(7):868–87.
3. Metcalfe DD, Mekori YA. Pathogenesis and pathology of mastocytosis. Annu Rev Pathol. 2017;12:487–514.
4. Johansson SG, Bieber T, Dahl R, Friedmann PS, Lanier BQ, Lockey RF, Motala C, Ortega Martell JA, Platts-Mills TA, Ring J, Thien F, Van Cauwenberge P, Williams HC. Revised nomenclature for allergy for global use: report of the Nomenclature Review Committee of the World Allergy Organization, October 2003. J Allergy Clin Immunol. 2004;113(5):832–6.
5. Muraro A, Roberts G, Clark A, Eigenmann PA, Halken S, Lack G, Moneret-Vautrin A, Niggemann B, Rance F, EAACI Task Force on Anaphylaxis in Children. The management of anaphylaxis in childhood: position paper of the European Academy of Allergology and Clinical Immunology. Allergy. 2007;62(8):857–71.
6. Bohlke K, Davis RL, DeStefano F, Marcy SM, Braun MM, Thompson RS, Vaccine Safety Datalink Team. Epidemiology of anaphylaxis among children and adolescents enrolled in a health maintenance organization. J Allergy Clin Immunol. 2004;113(3):536–42.
7. Braganza SC, Acworth JP, McKinnon DR, Peake JE, Brown AF. Paediatric emergency department anaphylaxis: different patterns from adults. Arch Dis Child. 2006;91(2):159–63.
8. de Silva IL, Mehr SS, Tey D, Tang ML. Paediatric anaphylaxis: a 5 year retrospective review. Allergy. 2008;63(8):1071–6.
9. Sampson HA. Food allergy and the role of immunotherapy. J Allergy Clin Immunol. 1992;90(2):151–2.
10. Pumphrey R. Anaphylaxis: can we tell who is at risk of a fatal reaction? Curr Opin Allergy Clin Immunol. 2004;4(4):285–90.
11. Gu X, Simons FE, Simons KJ. Epinephrine absorption after different routes of administration in an animal model. Biopharm Drug Dispos. 1999;20(8):401–5.
12. Gold MS, Sainsbury R. First aid anaphylaxis management in children who were prescribed an epinephrine autoinjector device (EpiPen). J Allergy Clin Immunol. 2000;106(1 Pt 1):171–6.
13. Dibs SD, Baker MD. Anaphylaxis in children: a 5-year experience. Pediatrics. 1997;99(1):E7.
14. Blanca M, Thong BY. Drug hypersensitivity reactions: more basic and clinical research is needed. Curr Opin Allergy Clin Immunol. 2015;15(4):273–6.
15. Alves C, Romeira AM, Abreu C, Carreiro-Martins P, Gomes E, Leiria-Pinto P. Non-steroidal anti-inflammatory drug hypersensitivity in children. Allergol Immunopathol. 2017;45(1):40–7.
16. Kowalski ML, Asero R, Bavbek S, Blanca M, Blanca-Lopez N, Bochenek G, Brockow K, Campo P, Celik G, Cernadas J, Cortellini G, Gomes E, Nizankowska-Mogilnicka E, Romano A, Szczeklik A, Testi S, Torres MJ, Wohrl S, Makowska J. Classification and practical approach to the diagnosis and management of hypersensitivity to nonsteroidal anti-inflammatory drugs. Allergy. 2013;68(10):1219–32.
17. Topal E, Celiksoy MH, Catal F, Gamze Sayan Y, Sancak R. The value of the clinical history for the diagnosis of immediate nonsteroidal anti-inflammatory drug hypersensitivity and safe alternative drugs in children. Allergy Asthma Proc. 2016;37(1):57–63.

Chapter 47
Urticaria and Facial Angioedema

Elena Camelia Berghea

A boy was treated at the emergency department for two moderate episodes of acute urticaria and facial angioedema developing in context of fever and ibuprofen, in the past year. The onset of urticaria was prior to the administration of ibuprofen, but worsened 30–45 min after drug ingestion. There were no symptoms and no need for chronic treatment between episodes.

When the boy experienced a new episode of upper respiratory infection with fever, the primary care doctor recommended paracetamol as a safe alternative for children with NSAID hypersensitivity, in order to avoid a recurrence of drug induced/exacerbated urticaria and angioedema. Thirty minutes after oral intake of paracetamol, the patient developed a generalized pruritus, severe generalized urticaria and angioedema of lips and tongue. Emergency intervention with antihistamine drugs and systemic corticosteroids stopped the new episode of symptoms. Few days later at the regression of corticosteroids, wheals relapsed and since then the patient reports experiencing daily generalized uncontrolled urticaria for the last 8 month. His symptoms have persisted despite of the treatment with various antihistamine drugs, short courses of corticosteroids, avoidance of all NSAIDs and diet without salicylates and pseudo-allergens.

The patient's history was nonsignificant in terms of personal and familial atopy or allergic diseases. There was no connection between urticaria and food intake, nor was a history of urticaria induced by physical agents.

E. C. Berghea (✉)
Emergency Clinical Hospital for Children M.S. Curie, Bucharest, Romania

University of Medicine and Pharmacy Carol Davila, Bucharest, Romania

N. Rezaei (ed.), *Pediatric Allergy*, https://doi.org/10.1007/978-3-030-18282-3_47

Q1. At this moment we can take into consideration all below diagnoses, except:

A. Refractory chronic urticaria
B. Chronic spontaneous urticaria
C. Chronic inducible urticaria
D. Urticarial vasculitis
E. Autoimmune chronic urticaria

Answer: *The correct answer is **C**.*

On admission to our clinic, the patient had widespread macules and papules, wheals and erythema and palpebral angioedema. He had no dyspnea, and was afebrile. The individual lesions were basically round, ranging from 5 to 20 mm in diameter, some of them confluent. The rest of the examination was nonsignificant. Given the duration of symptoms our patients can now be classified as having chronic urticaria.

The underlying causes of chronic urticaria in children do not appear to differ from those seen in adults [1]. Most cases of chronic urticaria are considered idiopathic, formerly named as chronic idiopathic urticaria, and later, as chronic spontaneous urticaria (CSU). The EAACI/GA2LEN/EDF/WAO urticaria guideline recommends only very limited routine diagnostic measures in CSU, with an extended diagnostic programme to be used only where indicated, based on patient history and suspected cause [2]. Routine tests recommended by the current guidelines are: differential blood count and ESR or CRP, essential in children to eliminate juvenile idiopathic arthritis or hereditary auto-inflammatory syndromes. These can later be completed by extended diagnostic investigations.

Q2. Starting from the history of our patient, the least possible cause of chronic urticaria is?

A. Infection
B. Autoimmune disorder
C. NSAIDs hypersensitivity
D. IgE mediated allergy
E. All of them

Answer: *The correct answer is **D**.*

Results of secondary investigations were all within normal range, including anti-streptolysin antibody, serum levels of complement components C3 and C4, IgG, IgM, IgA, free thyroxin, TSH, anti-thyroglobulin antibodies, tryptase, infective panel including antibody titters for hepatitis C virus, toxoplasmosis, toxocariasis, Ascaris, other parasites, rubella, cytomegalovirus, herpes simplex virus, Epstein-Barr virus and finally *Helicobacter pylori* antigen in stool, stool culture, urine analysis and nasal and throat culture for *Streptococcus β-hemolyticus* and *Staphylococcus aureus* and finally chest and sinus X-rays.

The only significant test was serum total IgE that was slightly increased (140 IU/mL, reference range <60 IU/mL for patient age).

The specific IgE (sIgE) for grass, ragweed, *Parietaria*, *Dermatophagoides pteronyssinus*, *Dermatophagoides farinae*, *Alternaria*, dog and cat dandruff, cereals, egg, fish, nuts, peanuts, rice, cow milk, and soy were negative. Due to the severity of urticaria, it was not possible to stop the treatment in order to perform an accurate autologous serum skin test (ASST), meanwhile anti-FcεRI antibodies were negative and autoimmune urticaria was ruled out. Diagnostic pseudo-allergen free diet did not improve the urticaria outcomes and the quality of life of our patient. After extended investigations, more than what is usually recommended, we are confronting a little boy with chronic idiopathic/spontaneous urticaria.

Q3. Which of the following can be considered a therapeutic option for this case?

A. Increase the dose of antihistamine H1
B. Leukotriene modifiers
C. Cyclosporine
D. Systemic corticosteroids
E. All of the above

Answer: *The correct answer is* ***E.***

We decided to use only levocetirizine in higher doses and to add montelukast (4 mg/day) hoping that at tapering of corticosteroid therapy the patient will not re-experience symptoms. Due to previous failure to stop the prednisone, we decided to adopt a very slow tapering in the dose of corticosteroids. After endocrinology consult regarding the suppression of hypothalamic-pituitary-adrenal function axis, we recommended to parents to decrease the dose of prednisone with a half of tablet (2.5 mg) at 7 days for the first 2 weeks and then with a quarter of tablet (1.25 mg) at 5–7 day depending on whether the boy was symptomatic or not, until the complete stop of the prednisone. In about 10 weeks, the child was in good symptom control treated only with anti-H1 and montelukast.

In the earliest opportunity was performed drug provocation test (DPT), with paracetamol 15 mg/kg/total cumulative dose (TCD), aspirin 20 mg/kg/TCD, ibuprofen 10 mg/kg/TCD, at intervals of 1 week. DPT was positive for aspirin and ibuprofen, and negative for paracetamol.

Q4. Which option best describes the hypersensitivity reaction in this patient?

A. NSAIDs-exacerbated cutaneous disease
B. NSAIDs-induced urticaria/angioedema
C. Single-NSAID-induced urticaria/angioedema
D. None of them

Answer: *The correct answer is* ***A.***

Practical Points

- Chronic urticaria is less common in children than it is in adults [3]
- The underlying cause of chronic urticaria in children do not appear to differ from those seen in adults [4]
- The treatment algorithm recommended in children with chronic urticaria is the same like in adults
- NSAIDs hypersensitivity is common in pediatric population and may precede the onset of chronic spontaneous urticaria by years [5]
- Ibuprofen and paracetamol are among frequent causes of NSAID hypersensitivity in children
- Oral drug provocation test is the gold standard for diagnosis of oral hypersensitivity reactions and allow identification of a safe alternative NSAID [6]

References

1. Maurer M, Church MK, Goncalo M, Sussman G, Sanchez-Borges M. Management and treatment of chronic urticaria (CU). J Eur Acad Dermatol Venereol. 2015;29(Suppl 3):16–32.
2. Zuberbier T, Aberer W, Asero R, Bindslev-Jensen C, Brzoza Z, Canonica GW, Church MK, Ensina LF, Gimenez-Arnau A, Godse K, Goncalo M, Grattan C, Hebert J, Hide M, Kaplan A, Kapp A, Abdul Latiff AH, Mathelier-Fusade P, Metz M, Nast A, Saini SS, Sanchez-Borges M, Schmid-Grendelmeier P, Simons FE, Staubach P, Sussman G, Toubi E, Vena GA, Wedi B, Zhu XJ, Maurer M, European Academy of Allergy and Clinical Immunology; Global Allergy and Asthma European Network; European Dermatology Forum; World Allergy Organization. The EAACI/GA(2) LEN/EDF/WAO Guideline for the definition, classification, diagnosis, and management of urticaria: the 2013 revision and update. Allergy. 2014;69(7):868–87.
3. Sackesen C, Sekerel BE, Orhan F, Kocabas CN, Tuncer A, Adalioglu G. The etiology of different forms of urticaria in childhood. Pediatr Dermatol. 2004;21(2):102–8.
4. Sanchez-Borges M, Capriles-Behrens E, Caballero-Fonseca F. Hypersensitivity to non-steroidal anti-inflammatory drugs in childhood. Pediatr Allergy Immunol. 2004;15(4):376–80.
5. Asero R. Intolerance to nonsteroidal anti-inflammatory drugs might precede by years the onset of chronic urticaria. J Allergy Clin Immunol. 2003;111(5):1095–8.
6. Zambonino MA, Torres MJ, Muñoz C, Requena G, Mayorga C, Posadas T, Urda A, Blanca M, Corzo JL. Drug provocation tests in the diagnosis of hypersensitivity reactions to non-steroidal anti-inflammatory drugs in children. Pediatr Allergy Immunol. 2013;24(2):151–9.

Chapter 48
Hypotension and Erythema During Anesthesia

Silviya Mihaylova Novakova, Ivan Petkov Novakov, and Manuela Dimitrova Yoncheva

A 16-year-old girl was operated on for right-side lung hydatid cyst. Approximately 50 min after the beginning of the operation, hypotension, tachycardia and generalized erythema were observed. Serum tryptase was evaluated within 30 min after the reaction which was 5.21 μg/L, i.e. positive. The operation was halted and the patient was treated with epinephrine and methylprednisolone. In the patients past medical history, allergic asthma, well controlled with low-dose inhaled corticosteroids, and allergy to house dust mites were significant. She also had a history of allergy to cow's milk until 3 years of age. She had underwent appendectomy at 5 years old, without complication.

One month after complete recovery her baseline serum tryptase level was evaluated as 1.17 μg/L and skin prick test to rocuronium was positive.

Q1. Which statement is true about drug allergies?

A. They are dose-independent, noxious, unintended and unpredictable drug hypersensitivity reactions
B. Drug allergies are adverse reactions for which an immunological mechanism is responsible
C. They can occur at any time after the initial drug administration
D. All of the above

Answer: *The correct answer is* ***D***.

S. M. Novakova (✉)
Allergy Unit, Internal Consulting Department, University Hospital "St. George", Plovdiv, Bulgaria

I. P. Novakov
Department of Special Surgery, Medical University, Plovdiv, Bulgaria

M. D. Yoncheva
Internal Consulting Department, University Hospital "St. George", Plovdiv, Bulgaria

N. Rezaei (ed.), *Pediatric Allergy*, https://doi.org/10.1007/978-3-030-18282-3_48

Drug allergies are drug hypersensitivity reactions in which a definite immunological mechanism—either drug-specific antibody or T cell is demonstrated. They are unpredictable, dose-independent and can be life-threatening [1]. When allergy is the only suspected mechanism, drug hypersensitivity reaction is used as the preferred term. The drug-induced hypersensitivity reactions are classified as immediate and non-immediate. Immediate reactions are usually a result of IgE mediated activation of mast cells and typically occur within 1–6 h after the last drug administration. Non-immediate reactions are T-cell-mediated and may occur at any time from 1 h after initial drug administration up to several days [2].

Q2. What are the risk factors of anaphylaxis during anesthesia in the presented case?

A. History of atopy and allergic asthma
B. A history of food allergy
C. Personal history of previous operation
D. There are no risk factors in the presented case

Answer*: The correct answer is* ***D****.*

Although more common in women compared with men, perioperative anaphylaxis occurs equally in girls and boys. Patients who are atopic, i.e. have known allergic asthma, allergic rhinitis, or atopic dermatitis, or those who are allergic to drugs or products not being used during surgery, are not considered to have additional risk factors [3]. Food allergies have not been recognized as a risk factor, with the exception of allergy to some tropical fruits which have a cross allergy with latex [4]. Patients at risk for anaphylaxis during anesthesia are those who are allergic to the drugs likely to be used during the course of operation and for which the diagnosis has been established and those who have shown clinical signs suggesting an allergic reaction during previous anesthesia or exposure to latex [5].

Q3. Which statement is true regarding anaphylaxis to neuromuscular blocking agents (NMBAs)?

A. It is always due to an IgE-mediated allergic reaction
B. A previous history of specific drug exposure is necessary
C. IgE sensitization may persist for years
D. Cross-sensitivity between different NMBAs is uncommon.

Answer*: The correct answer is* ***C****.*

Allergic reactions to NMBAs are usually associated with preformed specific IgE. However, NMBA can also cause nonspecific mast cell release [6]. A previous history of exposure to NMBAs is not necessary as such history is found in fewer than 50% of patients with serious reactions. Cross-sensitivity between different NMBAs is relatively common, probably due to a shared quaternary ammonium epitope [5]. The IgE antibody response is not permanent over time and a decrease in antibody levels may occur from months to years after the event.

However, IgE sensitization may persist for years and lifelong avoidance is recommended [2].

Q4. What evaluation would you recommend in the presented case?

A. Total serum tryptase concentration should be measured between 1 and 4 h after the event with a repeated measurement after recovery.
B. The patient should undergo skin testing with all drugs or products administered during the surgery, carried out 4–6 weeks after the event.
C. Specific IgE to some NMBAs can be quantified at any time following reaction
D. All of the above

Answer: *The correct answer is* ***D***.

Any suspected hypersensitivity reaction during anesthesia must be extensively investigated. A total serum tryptase concentration can be measured between 1 and 4 h after the event and if it is elevated, a repeat measurement is recommended after recovery. High tryptase levels strongly suggest an immunological mechanism [6]. Skin test carried out 4–6 weeks after a reaction, combined with medical history is the generally accepted diagnostic method for any kind of IgE-mediated reaction [2]. Skin test should be performed for all drugs or products administered during the anesthesia. Sensitivity and predictive values of skin tests for NMBAs are high [2], and should be performed with standardized non-irritating test concentrations [7]. *In vitro* assay for drug-specific IgE is not available for most drugs [2]. Fortunately, specific IgE (sIgE) can be quantified at the time after the reaction.

Q5. Are there any preventive measures against anaphylactic reactions during anesthesia for the presented case?

A. Life-long avoidance of the culprit drug is the only measure
B. NMBAs which have a negative skin test are permitted
C. Premedication with glucocorticosteroids and H1-antihistamines can prevent drug allergy
D. Desensitization to NMBA
E. Answers A and B are correct

Answer: *The correct answers is* ***E***.

The patient (her parents) should be warned against future exposure to the culprit drug and all NMBAs, if possible. If it is mandatory to use NMBAs during anesthesia, an agent which has previously shown a negative skin test can be administered, accepting the risk that negative skin test does not guarantee that anaphylaxis will not occur [2, 3]. A preventive measure by pre-treatment with glucocorticosteroids and H1-antihistamines is useful mainly for non-allergic drug hypersensitivity reactions, and may not reliably prevent IgE-dependent anaphylaxis [2]. Desensitization to NMBAs is not feasible. Surgery protocols would take several hours and an anesthesiologist would need to be involved for airway support [6].

Practical Points

- Hypersensitivity reactions during anesthesia can be life-threatening
- In the absence of appropriate allergologist assessment and diagnosis, a subsequent re-exposure can result in serious consequences
- Serum tryptase level measured between 1 and 4 h after the reaction and skin prick test 4 to 6 weeks after the attack are confirmatory for an anaphylactic reaction

References

1. International drug monitoring: the role of national centres. Report of a WHO meeting. World Health Organ Tech Rep Ser. 1972;498:1–25.
2. Demoly P, Adkinson NF, Brockow K, Castells M, Chiriac AM, Greenberger PA, Khan DA, Lang DM, Park HS, Pichler W, Sanchez-Borges M, Shiohara T, Thong BY. International consensus on drug allergy. Allergy. 2014;69(4):420–37.
3. Mertes PM, Laxenaire MC, Lienhart A, Aberer W, Ring J, Pichler WJ, Demoly P. Reducing the risk of anaphylaxis during anaesthesia: guidelines for clinical practice. J Investig Allergol Clin Immunol. 2005;15(2):91–101.
4. Mertes PM, Demoly P, Malinovsky JM. Hypersensitivity reactions in the anesthesia setting/allergic reactions to anesthetics. Curr Opin Allergy Clin Immunol. 2012;12(4):361–8.
5. Harper NJ, Dixon T, Dugue P, Edgar DM, Fay A, Gooi HC, Herriot R, Hopkins P, Hunter JM, Mirakian R, Pumphrey RS, Seneviratne SL, Walls AF, Williams P, Wildsmith JA, Wood P, Nasser AS, Powell RK, Mirakhur R, Soar J. Suspected anaphylactic reactions associated with anaesthesia. Anaesthesia. 2009;64(2):199–211.
6. Hsu Blatman KS, Hepner DL. Current knowledge and management of hypersensitivity to perioperative drugs and radiocontrast media. J Allergy Clin Immunol Pract. 2017;5(3):587–92.
7. Brockow K, Garvey LH, Aberer W, Atanaskovic-Markovic M, Barbaud A, Bilo MB, Bircher A, Blanca M, Bonadonna B, Campi P, Castro E, Cernadas JR, Chiriac AM, Demoly P, Grosber M, Gooi J, Lombardo C, Mertes PM, Mosbech H, Nasser S, Pagani M, Ring J, Romano A, Scherer K, Schnyder B, Testi S, Torres M, Trautmann A, Terreehorst I. Skin test concentrations for systemically administered drugs -- an ENDA/EAACI Drug Allergy Interest Group position paper. Allergy. 2013;68(6):702–12.

Chapter 49
Deterioration After Emergency Treatment for Asthma Attack

Sakine Işık and Suna Asilsoy

A 2-year-old boy was admitted to our hospital with a history of asthma and two episodes of clinical deterioration during asthma attacks treatment in emergency room. In both episodes, he had experienced generalized urticaria, vomiting, respiratory distress and fainting after 5 min of inhalation of nebulized salbutamol for his asthma attack. Both times his symptoms had rapidly improved after intramuscular adrenalin injection. His physical examination and laboratory tests including skin prick test (SPT) for food and aeroallergen were normal. His chest radiography was also normal. He had no family history for atopy.

Q1. What is the most likely diagnosis?

A. Drug allergy
B. Latex allergy
C. Anaphylaxis
D. Vaso-vagal reactions
E. Answers A, B and C are correct

Answer*: The correct answer is* ***E****.*

Anaphylaxis is a severe, life-threatening, systemic allergic reaction that occurs rapidly after contact with the inducing substance. Common triggers of anaphylaxis include food, insect stings, drugs and latex [1, 2]. Symptoms of anaphylaxis may progress rapidly and involve multiple target organ systems including the skin, respiratory, gastrointestinal, and cardiovascular systems [1]. Several other conditions can present with symptoms similar to anaphylaxis, including vasovagal reactions and disorders that cause flushing of the skin, angioedema, and/or vocal cord dysfunction.

S. Işık (✉)
Department of Pediatric Allergy and Immunology, Süreyyapaşa Chest Diseases and Thoracic Surgery Training Hospital, Istanbul, Turkey

S. Asilsoy
Department of Pediatric Allergy and Immunology, Dokuz Eylul University, İzmir, Turkey

N. Rezaei (ed.), *Pediatric Allergy*, https://doi.org/10.1007/978-3-030-18282-3_49

Vasovagal reactions are quite common and should be differentiated from anaphylaxis. Pallor, diaphoresis, hypotension, bradycardia, and a lack of cutaneous manifestations such as urticaria, pruritus, angioedema, and flushing characterize vasovagal reactions [3]. Administration of any drug by any route can potentially cause anaphylaxis [2], yet the two most common medications causing anaphylaxis are antibiotics (beta-lactam) and NSAIDs [2]. The risk of drug-induced anaphylaxis (DIA) increases with age, and is most likely related to the increased use of multiple drugs. The role of atopy remains unclear as a risk factor for DIA [4].

Latex is a ubiquitously used substance to manufacture the objects most frequently associated with allergic reactions to gloves, condoms, balloons, and catheters. Latex allergy symptoms can be mild or severe and manifest as contact urticaria, rhinoconjunctivitis, asthma, and mucosal swelling. Systemic reactions consist of generalized urticaria and anaphylactic shock [5]. Latex allergy affects people who are frequently exposed to products made of natural rubber latex, such as healthcare workers. High risk groups include latex industry workers, and patients with a history of atopy or multiple surgical procedures [6]. At present, patient education, avoidance of contact with latex objects, and treatment with specific immunotherapy are the available treatments for latex-sensitized individuals [7].

We also, suspected latex allergy as of our patient experienced anaphylaxis after nebulized salbutamol inhalation. Nebulizer mask sets and gloves contain latex and they might cause anaphylaxis episodes in patients with latex allergy. Latex allergy was excluded through SPT.

Q2. Which one of the following is the most appropriate next step in the evaluation and management of this patient's condition?

A. Skin prick and intradermal tests for B2 adrenergic agonist
B. Skin prick test for latex
C. Drug provocation test
D. Serum histamine and tryptase level
E. Answers A and B.

Answer: *The correct answer is **E**.*

Asthma is major public health problem in many countries. The most commonly used asthma medications are the short-acting (inhaled) beta(-2) agonists (SABA) such as salbutamol (albuterol), first introduced more than 30 years ago, and for which there is now extensive clinical experience. Inhaled SABA can cause both pulmonary and extrapulmonary adverse effects including anaphylaxis [8], in which cross-reaction exists between different agents [9]. Our patient had two episodes of anaphylaxis after 5 min of nebulized salbutamol therapy during his asthma attacks in emergency room. In his history, he experienced similar symptoms at home when he took oral terbutaline. Therefore, beta-2 adrenergic agonist allergy was suspected.

Testing for medication and/or latex induced anaphylaxis is important for determining the etiology. SPTs are typically performed with the undiluted drug to evaluate possible DIA. If negative, intradermal test is performed sequentially with increasing concentrations of the drug, due to the potential risk of inducing systemic symptoms [10]. A positive SPT is defined by the size of the wheal, which should be at least 3 mm greater than that of the negative control [11]. This patient underwent SPTs for nebulized salbutamol which came back positive (Fig. 49.1). Even during SPTs he developed urticarial rashes on his body (Fig. 49.2).

Drug-provocation test (DPT) is the controlled administration of a drug to diagnose immune- or non-immune-mediated drug hypersensitivity and the last step for accurate recognition of drug-induced hypersensitivity reactions when previous diagnostic evaluations are negative or unavailable [12]. Due to a history of two previous anaphylaxis episodes and positive SPTs results for salbutamol, DPT with salbutamol was not performed in our patient.

Biological assessment, including plasma histamine and tryptase measurements, is an emerging diagnostic tool for anaphylaxis. The diagnostic accuracy of these assays is increased when histamine and tryptase measurements are combined [13]. Tryptase is a mast cell neutral serine protease and a preformed enzyme. An increase in total tryptase is highly suggestive of mast cell activation, as seen in anaphylaxis, but its absence does not preclude the diagnosis. In fact, elevated histamine and, less commonly, elevated tryptase levels are observed in almost 50% of patients presenting to the emergency room with acute allergic reactions [14]. Plasma histamine and tryptase levels remain elevated for only 15–60 min after onset of anaphylaxis [14].

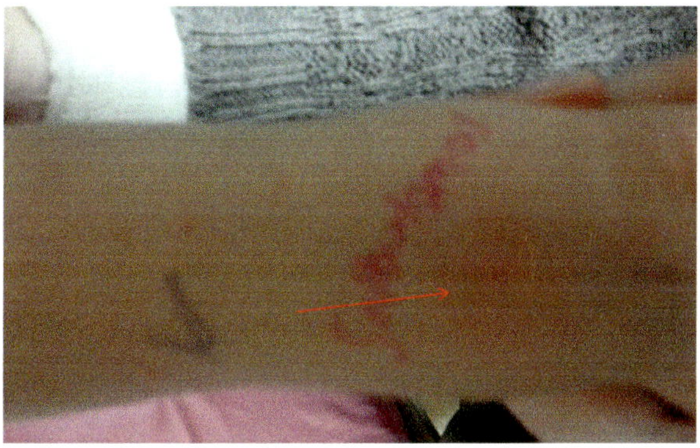

Fig. 49.1 Positive skin prick test with Salbutamol of a 2-year-old boy with asthma attack (red arrow)

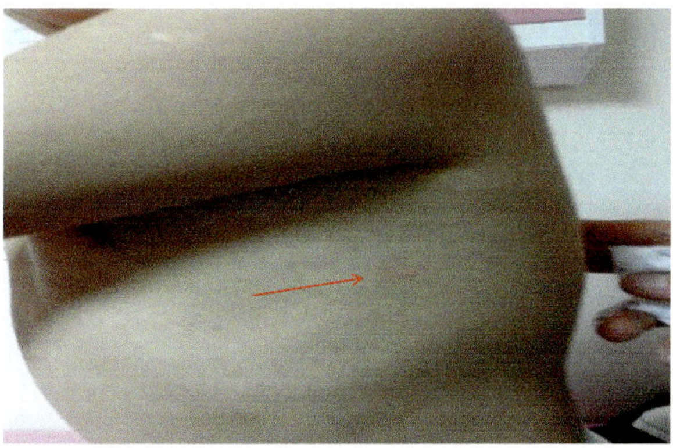

Fig. 49.2 Urticarial rash of a 2-year-old boy with asthma attack (red arrow)

Q3. On the basis of the clinical diagnosis, which one of the following would be the most appropriate recommendations for the patient's parents?

A. Avoidance for oral and inhaled B2 adrenergic therapy during asthma attacks
B. Education of parents about anaphylaxis
C. Regular assessment of pediatric allergy and immunology specialist
D. All of above

Answer: *The correct answer is* ***D***.

After discharge from the hospital, it is important for patients to be able to cope with possible future anaphylactic episodes. For this purpose, parents of patients with history of anaphylaxis should be trained about early recognition and medical treatment of anaphylaxis episodes before discharge from the emergency room.

Follow-up of patients with drug allergy by pediatric allergy and immunology specialist is also important, in order to coordinate additional outpatient testing, provide additional allergen avoidance counselling, develop a detailed emergency action plan for future reactions, and reinforce proper use of the adrenaline autoinjector, if needed.

Practical Points

- Anaphylaxis is a severe, life-threatening, systemic allergic reaction that occurs rapidly after contact with an inducing substance such as food, insect bite, drugs and latex
- Inhaled beta-2 receptor agonists can cause both pulmonary and extrapulmonary adverse effects including anaphylaxis
- Cross-reactivity can be seen between different skin prick test agents
- Skin prick test is typically performed with the undiluted drug, in suspicion of drug-induced anaphylaxis. If negative, intradermal test is performed sequentially with increasing concentrations of the drug to prevent the potential risk of inducing systemic reaction

References

1. Muraro A, Roberts G, Worm M, Bilo MB, Brockow K, Fernandez Rivas M, Santos AF, Zolkipli ZQ, Bellou A, Beyer K, Bindslev-Jensen C, Cardona V, Clark AT, Demoly P, Dubois AE, DunnGalvin A, Eigenmann P, Halken S, Harada L, Lack G, Jutel M, Niggemann B, Rueff F, Timmermans F, Vlieg-Boerstra BJ, Werfel T, Dhami S, Panesar S, Akdis CA, Sheikh A, Allergy EF, Anaphylaxis Guidelines Group. Anaphylaxis: guidelines from the European Academy of Allergy and Clinical Immunology. Allergy. 2014;69(8):1026–45.
2. Simons FE, Ebisawa M, Sanchez-Borges M, Thong BY, Worm M, Tanno LK, Lockey RF, El-Gamal YM, Brown SG, Park HS, Sheikh A. 2015 update of the evidence base: World Allergy Organization anaphylaxis guidelines. World Allergy Organ J. 2015;8(1):32.
3. Lieberman P, Nicklas RA, Randolph C, Oppenheimer J, Bernstein D, Bernstein J, Ellis A, Golden DB, Greenberger P, Kemp S, Khan D, Ledford D, Lieberman J, Metcalfe D, Nowak-

Wegrzyn A, Sicherer S, Wallace D, Blessing-Moore J, Lang D, Portnoy JM, Schuller D, Spector S, Tilles SA. Anaphylaxis--a practice parameter update 2015. Ann Allergy Asthma Immunol. 2015;115(5):341–84.
4. Alves B, Sheikh A. Age specific aetiology of anaphylaxis. Arch Dis Child. 2001;85(4):348.
5. Hamann CP, Rodgers PA, Sullivan KM. Prevalence of type I natural rubber latex allergy among dental hygienists. J Dent Hyg. 2005;79(2):7.
6. Nettis E, Di Leo E, Calogiuri G, Milani M, Delle Donne P, Ferrannini A, Vacca A. The safety of a novel sublingual rush induction phase for latex desensitization. Curr Med Res Opin. 2010;26(8):1855–9.
7. Cabanes N, Igea JM, de la Hoz B, Agustin P, Blanco C, Dominguez J, Lazaro M, Lleonart R, Mendez J, Nieto A, Rodriguez A, Rubia N, Tabar A, Beitia JM, Dieguez MC, Martinez-Cocera C, Quirce S, Committee of Latex Allergy; SEAIC. Latex allergy: position paper. J Investig Allergol Clin Immunol. 2012;22(5):313–30; quiz follow 30.
8. Windom HH, Burgess CD, Siebers RW, Purdie G, Pearce N, Crane J, Beasley R. The pulmonary and extrapulmonary effects of inhaled beta-agonists in patients with asthma. Clin Pharmacol Ther. 1990;48(3):296–301.
9. Bonniaud P, Favrolt N, Collet E, Dumas JP, Guilloux L, Pauli G, Camus P. Salbutamol, terbutaline and pirbuterol allergy in an asthmatic patient. Allergy. 2007;62(10):1219–20.
10. Brockow K, Garvey LH, Aberer W, Atanaskovic-Markovic M, Barbaud A, Bilo MB, Bircher A, Blanca M, Bonadonna B, Campi P, Castro E, Cernadas JR, Chiriac AM, Demoly P, Grosber M, Gooi J, Lombardo C, Mertes PM, Mosbech H, Nasser S, Pagani M, Ring J, Romano A, Scherer K, Schnyder B, Testi S, Torres M, Trautmann A, Terreehorst I, ENDA/EAACI Drug Allergy Interest Group. Skin test concentrations for systemically administered drugs -- an ENDA/EAACI Drug Allergy Interest Group position paper. Allergy. 2013;68(6):702–12.
11. Joint Task Force on Practice Parameters; American Academy of Allergy, Asthma and Immunology; American College of Allergy, Asthma and Immunology; Joint Council of Allergy, Asthma and Immunology. Drug allergy: an updated practice parameter. Ann Allergy Asthma Immunol. 2010;105(4):259–73.
12. Gonzalez de Olano D, Trujillo Trujillo MJ, Santos Magadan S, Menendez-Baltanas A, Gandolfo Cano M, Ariz Munoz S, Sanz Larruga ML, Gonzalez-Mancebo E. Anaphylaxis to salbutamol. J Investig Allergol Clin Immunol. 2008;18(2):139–40.
13. Mertes PM, Malinovsky JM, Jouffroy L, Working Group of the SFAR and SFA, Aberer W, Terreehorst I, Brockow K, Demoly P, ENDA; EAACI Interest Group on Drug Allergy. Reducing the risk of anaphylaxis during anesthesia: 2011 updated guidelines for clinical practice. J Investig Allergol Clin Immunol. 2011;21(6):442–53.
14. Lin RY, Schwartz LB, Curry A, Pesola GR, Knight RJ, Lee HS, Bakalchuk L, Tenenbaum C, Westfal RE. Histamine and tryptase levels in patients with acute allergic reactions: an emergency department-based study. J Allergy Clin Immunol. 2000;106(1 Pt 1):65–71.

Chapter 50
Viral Pneumonia and History of Short-Bowel Syndrome

Federica Porcaro, Maria Giovanna Paglietti, Antonella Diamanti, and Renato Cutrera

A 1-year-old male patient presented with fever, productive cough and dyspnea. On clinical examination he had pale face, nasal flaring and intercostal retraction. Physical examination revealed widespread crackles and radiographic findings suggestive of pneumonia. Laboratory data were not significant with the exception of nasopharyngeal aspirate that was positive for respiratory syncytial virus A (RSV-A) PCR. The child was affected by a polymalformative syndrome and his past medical history included necrotizing enterocolitis and cow's milk allergy.

Due to the respiratory distress, comorbidities and precariousness of clinical balance, antibiotic therapy with piperacillin/tazobactam was administered despite evidence for RSV infection. Moreover, because of the severity of bronchospasm, lactose free methylprednisolone (Urbason 40 mg, Sanofi-Aventis) was added to therapy. After 2 days of therapy without any side effect, hospital pharmacy sent methylprednisolone sodium succinate (Solu-Medrol 40 mg, Pfizer) instead of Urbason because of a temporary lack of availability. Within a few minutes of the first IV administration of steroid therapy, the patient presented wheezing and generalized urticaria that resolved after parenteral antihistamine. An allergic reaction to piperacillin/tazobactam was suspected and antibiotic therapy was discontinued. Steroid treatment was maintained, however, an anaphylactic reaction with giant urticaria, eyelid edema, tightened laryngospasm and severe dyspnea occurred within a few minutes of the second intravenous administration of 10 mg of methylprednisolone sodium succinate.

F. Porcaro (✉) · M. G. Paglietti · R. Cutrera
Respiratory Unit, Academic Department of Pediatrics, Bambino Gesù Children's Hospital, IRCCS, Rome, Italy
e-mail: federica.porcaro@opbg.net

A. Diamanti
Artificial Nutrition Unit-Gastroenterology, Hepatology and Nutrition Unit, Bambino Gesù Children's Hospital, Rome, Italy

N. Rezaei (ed.), *Pediatric Allergy*, https://doi.org/10.1007/978-3-030-18282-3_50

Q1. Which of the following is the most likely diagnosis?

A. Post-infective urticaria
B. Anaphylaxis due to accidental ingestion of cow's milk protein
C. Anaphylaxis due to intravenous administration of piperacillin/tazobactam
D. Anaphylaxis due to intravenous administration of methylprednisolone sodium succinate

Answer: *The correct answer is* ***D***.

On the basis of the clear clinical history, we hypothesized that Solu-Medrol 40 mg was the cause of allergic reaction.

Our patient had positive history for cow's milk allergy. Cow's milk proteins may be present in certain steroid preparations. Allergic reactions to IV methylprednisolone sodium succinate (Solu-Medrol 40 mg) in allergic cow's milk patients are already described in pediatric patients [1–3].

Intravenous Solu-Medrol has five parenteral formulations, but only 40 mg formulation contains lactose as an excipient as it is indicated in the drug technical document. Lactose in Solu-Medrol 40 mg vials might be contaminated by milk protein. This explains the allergic reaction to this steroid formulation and also immediate evolution of the symptoms due to parenteral administration route.

Q2. Which of the following is a risk factor for food sensitization?

A. Polymalformative syndrome
B. Short bowel syndrome
C. All of the above
D. None of the above

Answer: *The correct answer is* ***B***.

Our patient had a Short bowel syndrome (SBS) due to necrotizing enterocolitis surgically treated in the first period of life. SBS patients have higher risk for cow's milk allergy, compared to the general population [4]. They have low digestive capacity due to incomplete peptic digestion in early life, leaving protein remnants of the diet that could act as allergens. Studies on the use of antacid drugs have clearly linked impairment of gastric function with sensitization against oral proteins and drugs [5].

Gastroenterological surgery leading to SBS is associated with a high incidence of food allergy: gastrointestinal atresia, Hirschsprung disease, congenital diaphragmatic hernia, perforation of the ileum, necrotizing enterocolitis, exomphalos [6] and hepatic transplantation surgery [7] have been linked to cow's milk allergy. It is possible that a dysfunction of the gastrointestinal tract resulting from primary diseases, surgical invasion, small bowel bacterial overgrowth and/or mucosal atrophy caused by extended fasting before and after surgery, all play a role in cow's milk allergy inception. Furthermore, increased intestinal permeability to luminal contents relates to immune dysfunction derived from loss of gut-associated lymphoid tissue after small bowel resections [7, 8].

Q3. Which one of the following is the most appropriate diagnostic workup to diagnose the described condition?

A. Skin prick test with culprit allergen
B. Intradermal skin test with culprit allergen
C. Provocation test with culprit allergen
D. All the above

Answer*: The correct answer is* ***D****.*

In accordance with the European Network on Drug Allergy (ENDA) recommendations, complete allergy workup consists of skin test (skin prick test and intradermal) as well as provocation test, after 4–6 weeks of suspected reaction.

According to the ENDA guidelines the highest concentration for prick test to methylprednisolone is 20 mg/mL and for intradermal test only 2 mg/mL. Drug-provocation test (DPT) remains the "gold standard" to establish or exclude the diagnosis of drug-induced hypersensitivity reaction [9].

Practical Points

- Patients with a history of short bowel syndrome have a higher risk for cow's milk allergy
- Intravenous drug preparations might contain lactose as an excipient, which might have contaminated with milk protein

References

1. Gasparini F, Lingenhohl K, Stoehr N, Flor PJ, Heinrich M, Vranesic I, Biollaz M, Allgeier H, Heckendorn R, Urwyler S, Varney MA, Johnson EC, Hess SD, Rao SP, Sacaan AI, Santori EM, Velicelebi G, Kuhn R. 2-Methyl-6-(phenylethynyl)-pyridine (MPEP), a potent, selective and systemically active mGlu5 receptor antagonist. Neuropharmacology. 1999;38(10):1493–503.
2. Savvatianos S, Giavi S, Stefanaki E, Siragakis G, Manousakis E, Papadopoulos NG. Cow's milk allergy as a cause of anaphylaxis to systemic corticosteroids. Allergy. 2011;66(7):983–5.
3. Nahum A, Garty BZ, Marcus N, Shoenfeld T, Levy Y. Severe hypersensitivity reactions to corticosteroids in children. Pediatr Emerg Care. 2009;25(5):339–41.
4. Diamanti A, Fiocchi AG, Capriati T, Panetta F, Pucci N, Bellucci F, Torre G. Cow's milk allergy and neonatal short bowel syndrome: comorbidity or true association? Eur J Clin Nutr. 2015;69(1):102–6.
5. Pali-Scholl I, Jensen-Jarolim E. Anti-acid medication as a risk factor for food allergy. Allergy. 2011;66(4):469–77.
6. Miyazawa T, Itabashi K, Imai T. Retrospective multicenter survey on food-related symptoms suggestive of cow's milk allergy in NICU neonates. Allergol Int. 2013;62(1):85–90.
7. Wisniewski J, Lieberman J, Nowak-Wegrzyn A, Kerkar N, Arnon R, Iyer K, Miloh T. De novo food sensitization and eosinophilic gastrointestinal disease in children post-liver transplantation. Clin Transpl. 2012;26(4):E365–71.

8. Vanderhoof JA, Grandjean CJ, Burkley KT, Antonson DL. Effect of casein versus casein hydrolysate on mucosal adaptation following massive bowel resection in infant rats. J Pediatr Gastroenterol Nutr. 1984;3(2):262–7.
9. Brockow K, Garvey LH, Aberer W, Atanaskovic-Markovic M, Barbaud A, Bilo MB, Bircher A, Blanca M, Bonadonna B, Campi P, Castro E, Cernadas JR, Chiriac AM, Demoly P, Grosber M, Gooi J, Lombardo C, Mertes PM, Mosbech H, Nasser S, Pagani M, Ring J, Romano A, Scherer K, Schnyder B, Testi S, Torres M, Trautmann A, Terreehorst I. Skin test concentrations for systemically administered drugs -- an ENDA/EAACI Drug Allergy Interest Group position paper. Allergy. 2013;68(6):702–12.

Chapter 51
Collapse and Angioedema at the Emergency Department

Iva Topalusic, Irena Ivkovic-Jurekovic, Martin Cuk, and Marta Navratil

A 13-year-old boy with a history of cow's milk allergy and asthma was brought to our Pediatric Emergency Department due to anaphylactic reaction after ingestion of milk containing meal. Half an hour before admission to our clinic, and immediately after ingestion of pasta with cheese, the boy developed bronchospasm and acute urticaria with angioedema. Due to his previously known milk allergy and history of anaphylactic reaction, he used adrenaline autoinjector and all the symptoms resolved. At our Emergency Department, the boy was administered 40 mg of methylprednisolone (Solu-medrol 40 mg® Pfizer) intramuscularly. Immediately after methylprednisolone injection was administered, the boy collapsed and developed angioedema, generalised urticaria and wheezing. He was given another dose of adrenaline intramuscularly and a rapid crystalloid infusion. Hydrocortisone (Solu-Cortef 100 mg® Pfizer) 200 mg intravenously was then administered with oral antihistamines without any side effects. He was discharged the next day and left for his home country, therefore no additional allergic diagnostics was performed.

Q1. What is the differential diagnosis in this patient?

A. He developed a biphasic anaphylactic reaction caused by cow's milk proteins from his lunch
B. The boy developed anaphylactic reaction caused by the drug (methylprednisolone)

I. Topalusic (✉)
Children's Hospital Zagreb, Zagreb, Croatia

I. Ivkovic-Jurekovic · M. Navratil
Children's Hospital Zagreb, Zagreb, Croatia

Faculty of Medicine, University of Osijek, Osijek, Croatia

M. Cuk
Nephrology Department, Children's Hospital Zagreb, Zagreb, Croatia

N. Rezaei (ed.), *Pediatric Allergy*, https://doi.org/10.1007/978-3-030-18282-3_51

C. He had pseudoallergic reaction to additives from drugs that he received
D. All of the above

Answer: *The correct answer is **B**.*

Patient's signs and symptoms fulfill clinical criteria for anaphylactic reaction. Symptoms and signs of anaphylaxis occur within 2 h of exposure to the allergen, usually within 30 min for food allergy, and immediately after intravenous drug administration [1]. The fact that the boy developed symptoms immediately after IV methylprednisolone supports the clinical idea that the causing allergen was the drug.

Q2. What should be the best immediate approach in the described clinical situation in the Emergency Department?

A. Apply adrenaline intramuscularly, rapid crystalloid infusion, antihistamines intravenously and check patients drug history
B. Apply epinephrine and another injection of methylprednisolone
C. Apply adrenaline intravenously, rapid crystalloid infusion, antihistamines intravenously, other type of corticosteroid intravenously (for example hydrocortisone)
D. All of the above

Answer: *The correct answer is **A**.*

Anaphylaxis is a clinical emergency, and all healthcare professionals should be familiar with its management. According to contemporary guidelines, the culprit allergen should be immediately removed and adrenaline should be given by intramuscular injection into the mid-outer thigh as the first line treatment. Intravenous fluids should be administered to patients with cardiovascular instability (boluses of 20 mL/kg). Systemic antihistamines are commonly used in anaphylaxis but have only been demonstrated to relieve cutaneous symptoms. Methylprednisolone should not be applied in this patient, as it was the case of anaphylactic reaction. Generally, corticosteroids are used to prevent protracted anaphylaxis symptoms and biphasic reactions [1].

Q3. Which one of the following could be a cause of the anaphylactic reaction if the boy had an allergic reaction to the drug (methylprednisolone)?

A. Both molecule of methylprednisolone and/or a drug excipient
B. Corticosteroids can not cause allergic reactions because they have an anti-inflammatory effect
C. Drug excipients can not cause allergic reactions
D. All of the above

Answer: *The correct answer is **A**.*

Despite the extensive use of corticosteroids in clinical practice, systemic allergic reactions have rarely been reported. Immediate allergic reactions after oral or parenteral administration of corticosteroids have frequently been described in patients with asthma or NSAID intolerance [2–6]. Causative agents of allergic reactions can include steroid molecules or an excipient. It has been described in literature that

Solu-medrol 40 mg® Pfizer contains lactose as an excipient. In 2009 and 2011, two cases of anaphylactic reaction have been reported. Both children had a history of cow's milk allergy and both reacted to methylprednisolone lactose containing preparation. Using high-sensitivity ELISA, the authors managed to detect traces of casein and b-lactoglobulin in all samples of the product, proving their hypothesis of milk allergen contamination [7, 8]. Due to our patient's milk allergy with high concentration of specific IgE (sIgE) antibodies, we hypothesise that the causative agents were milk proteins contaminating lactose, as described in the literature. Our patient had no reaction to a steroid from the same group steroid (Group A, hydrocortisone). This, added to the fact that cross-reactivity is common in adverse drug reactions, supports our hypothesis.

Q4. On the basis of clinical knowledge, which is the recommended diagnostic algorithm to resolve the diagnostic dilemma?

A. Oral provocative drug test
B. To explore whether the medicine contains cow' s milk proteins
C. Basophil activation test
D. All of the above

Answer*: The correct answer is* ***B****.*

The diagnosis would be confirmed if we could explore whether the medicine contains cow's milk proteins. If yes, skin prick test with lactose-containing methylprednisolone preparation and methylprednisolone without lactose would have been recommended. If negative, intradermal test is recommended. Immediate allergic reactions can be detected by prick tests and early intradermal test. If the prick test is negative, then intradermal tests at progressively higher concentrations are carried out [3]. It is expected in our patient to have a positive skin reaction to lactose-containing methylprednisolone preparation. Only a few authors have been able to demonstrate the presence of specific IgE antibodies to corticosteroids [9–12]. Oral or other provocative tests with methylprednisolone should not be performed in this patient due to the history of life threatening anaphylactic reaction.

Q5. On the basis of the clinical diagnosis, which one of the following would be the most appropriate recommendation for the patient?

A. The patient should undergo hypo-sensitization to the medicine that he experienced a reaction
B. The patient should get an identification card with the recommendation on epinephrine autoinjector. He must not receive drugs containing lactose
C. He must not receive corticosteroids
D. None of the above

Answer*: The correct answer is* ***B****.*

The guidelines of the European Academy for Allergology and Clinical Immunology (EAACI) recommend to prescribe adrenaline autoinjector in patients with previous anaphylaxis with food, latex, aeroallergens, such as animals, or other unavoidable triggers [1]. The patient should get an identification card with the recommendations of strict avoidance of cow's milk allergens and epinephrine autoinjector. He must not receive drugs containing lactose. Hypo-sensitization to drugs is recommended only when there is no alternative drug for a patient (for example enzyme replacement therapy) [8].

Practical Points

- Adverse drug reactions might rise as a result of reaction to the drug molecule or any of the excipients
- Allergic reactions caused by corticosteroids have rarely been reported
- Due to the possible contamination with cow's milk proteins, lactose used as an excipient to drugs could be a iatrogenic cause of anaphylaxis in patients allergic to cow's milk proteins
- Patients allergic to cow's milk proteins should be treated with lactose free preparations only

References

1. Muraro A, Roberts G, Worm M, Bilo MB, Brockow K, Fernandez Rivas M, Santos AF, Zolkipli ZQ, Bellou A, Beyer K, Bindslev-Jensen C, Cardona V, Clark AT, Demoly P, Dubois AE, DunnGalvin A, Eigenmann P, Halken S, Harada L, Lack G, Jutel M, Niggemann B, Rueff F, Timmermans F, Vlieg-Boerstra BJ, Werfel T, Dhami S, Panesar S, Akdis CA, Sheikh A. Anaphylaxis: guidelines from the European Academy of Allergy and Clinical Immunology. Allergy. 2014;69(8):1026–45.
2. Matura M, Goossens A. Contact allergy to corticosteroids. Allergy. 2000;55(8):698–704.
3. Baeck M, Marot L, Nicolas JF, Pilette C, Tennstedt D, Goossens A. Allergic hypersensitivity to topical and systemic corticosteroids: a review. Allergy. 2009;64(7):978–94.
4. Atanaskovic-Markovic M, Gavrovic-Jankulovic M, Jankovic S, Blagojevic G, Cirkovic-Velickovic T, Milojevic I, Simic D, Nestorovic B. Immediate allergic reaction to methylprednisolone with tolerance of other corticosteroids. Srp Arh Celok Lek. 2012;140(3–4):233–5.
5. Aranda A, Mayorga C, Ariza A, Dona I, Blanca-Lopez N, Canto G, Blanca M, Torres MJ. IgE-mediated hypersensitivity reactions to methylprednisolone. Allergy. 2010;65(11):1376–80.
6. Compalati E, Guerra L, Rogkakou A, Zanella C, Scordamaglia A, Passalacqua G. Angioedema after administration of methylprednisolone to treat drug allergy. Allergy. 2007;62(11):1346–8.
7. Eda A, Sugai K, Shioya H, Fujitsuka A, Ito S, Iwata T, Funabiki T. Acute allergic reaction due to milk proteins contaminating lactose added to corticosteroid for injection. Allergol Int. 2009;58(1):137–9.
8. Savvatianos S, Giavi S, Stefanaki E, Siragakis G, Manousakis E, Papadopoulos NG. Cow's milk allergens as an infrequent cause of anaphylaxis to systemic corticosteroids. Clin Transl Allergy. 2011;1(Suppl 1):P18.
9. Isaksson M, Bruze M. Allergic contact dermatitis in response to budesonide reactivated by inhalation of the allergen. J Am Acad Dermatol. 2002;46(6):880–5.
10. Burgdorff T, Venemalm L, Vogt T, Landthaler M, Stolz W. IgE-mediated anaphylactic reaction induced by succinate ester of methylprednisolone. Ann Allergy Asthma Immunol. 2002;89(4):425–8.
11. Pryse-Phillips WE, Chandra RK, Rose B. Anaphylactoid reaction to methylprednisolone pulsed therapy for multiple sclerosis. Neurology. 1984;34(8):1119–21.
12. Rasanen L, Tarvainen K, Makinen-Kiljunen S. Urticaria to hydrocortisone. Allergy. 2001;56(4):352–3.

Chapter 52
Acute Reaction to Pentavalent Vaccine

Darko Richter

A 23-month-old male toddler was brought to the primary pediatrician for his first "diphtheria-tetanus-5-component acellular pertussis-inactivated polio-*Haemophilus influenzae* type b" (DTaP5-IPV-Hib) booster. Previously, he had BCG at birth, *Haemophilus influenzae* type b vaccine (Hib) at 2 months, inactivated *polio* vaccine (IPV) and diphtheria-tetanus-3-component acellular pertussis vaccine (DTaP3) at 3 months, and oral *polio* vaccine (OPV), Hib and DTaP3 at 5 and 6 months. His parents left the clinic without having waited the recommended 30 min as is usual for any parenteral therapy. At the first stop-light, they noticed in the rear-mirror that the child developed diffuse facial redness, started coughing, his lips became swollen and his head was drooping. They immediately returned to the clinic. When undressed generalized urticaria was present and he looked all swollen. He was given adrenaline 0.2 mg and methylprednisolone 40 mg IM. The time lag from vaccination to adrenalin was 25 min. He recovered and half an hour later was transported to the nearest hospital where he was monitored and discharged on loratadine.

Q1. The reaction to vaccination in this child is best diagnosed as:

A. Acute generalized urticaria
B. Hypotonic-hyporesponsive episode
C. Anaphylaxis
D. Convulsions

Answer: *The correct answer is* ***C***.

Reactions occurring within moments to 30 min of vaccination that include multiple symptoms of immediate-type hypersensitivity strongly suggest anaphylaxis [1] (Table 52.1).

D. Richter (✉)
Outpatient and Emergency Service, Department of Pediatrics, University Hospital Center, Zagreb, Croatia
e-mail: darko.richter@kbc-zagreb.hr

N. Rezaei (ed.), *Pediatric Allergy*, https://doi.org/10.1007/978-3-030-18282-3_52

Table 52.1 Clinical symptoms of anaphylaxis

Symptom category	Clinical manifestation	Remarks
Mucocutaneous	Itching, flushing, urticaria, angioedema	–
Respiratory	Nasal and/or conjunctival congestion/watery discharge, stridor, wheezing, dyspnea	–
Cardiovascular	Hypotension	Systolic blood pressure: • <70 mmHg in infants 0–11 months • <[70 mmHg + (2 × Age)] for children 1–10 years • <90 mmHg in 11–17 year-olds
Persistent gastrointestinal symptoms	Crampy abdominal pain, vomiting	Usually not applicable to parenteral allergen reactions

There are three combinations of the four symptom categories from Table 52.1 [1, 2] that are diagnostic for anaphylaxis:

1. The clinical diagnosis of anaphylaxis is assured when acute mucocutaneous symptoms concur with either one or both of the respiratory and cardiovascular symptom categories.
2. In the case of a probable exposure to an allergen for that person, the diagnosis can be made if any two of the four symptom categories concur.
3. Hypotension alone indicates anaphylaxis if there is exposure to a known allergen for that person.

Although we were not given all the details on physical examination, it is reasonable to deduce that the child manifested all the principal signs of anaphylaxis; mucocutaneous i.e. urticaria and angioedema, respiratory i.e. cough reflecting probable laryngeal or bronchial obstruction, cardiovascular i.e. head drooping and loss of tone reflecting arterial hypotension. He recovered after having received adrenaline.

Anaphylaxis to vaccines is rare. A recent estimate has put it at 1.3 per 1 million vaccine doses, 55% affecting children 0–17 years of age. More than 50% of anaphylactic reactions were due to trivalent influenza vaccine (TIV), the rest included common childhood combination vaccines or multiple vaccines given at the same visit (4-valent meningococcal vaccine, varicella, measles-mumps-rubella (MMR), hepatitis A virus, 4-valent human papilloma virus, DTaP, DTaP-IPV). Anaphylaxis may occur later than 30 min and up to 4 and more hours after vaccination [3].

Hypersensitivity can occur to any vaccine component. Hypersensitivity reactions occur mostly due to various vaccine additives [4]. Reactions should be evaluated by the clinical appearance and time elapsed since vaccine administration.

Q2. Which of the following measures should have been taken in the initial management of this patient?

A. He should have received intravenous antihistamine
B. He should have received a crystalline solution infusion
C. He should have had a blood sample drawn for evaluation of serum tryptase
D. He should have been fed with oral glucose solution

Answer: *The correct answer is* ***B***.

When the child was rushed back he was in a state of anaphylactic shock. Adrenaline was appropriately given and he recovered soon thereafter. Intravenous volume replacement at a dose of 10–20 mL/kg normal saline or 5% dextrose in water is also warranted. Intravenous antihistamine at this point is not universally recommended in an outpatient setting since it may lower the blood pressure. In emergent situations outside medical facilities, a oral antihistamine should promptly be given [5]. Another point of disagreement is the management in the hospital emergency department. He should not have been discharged but kept overnight for observation. At least 6% of patients with anaphylaxis experience a biphasic course within 24 h even if re-exposure to the offending allergen has not occurred [6]. Increased serum tryptase measured within 2 h of the acute reaction corroborates the diagnosis of anaphylaxis but is not essential in the urgent outpatient setting. Patients with anaphylaxis are historically described to be hyperglycemic and giving glucose is not vital.

Q3. How can you be sure that the anaphylaxis was due to DTaP5-IPV-Hib?

A. Determine specific IgE to vaccine components
B. Perform graded dose vaccination with the same vaccine in hospital setting
C. Perform basophil activation test to vaccine and vaccine components
D. Perform skin testing with the vaccine

Answer: *The correct answer is* ***D***.

The mainstay of vaccine hypersensitivity diagnosis is skin testing. Identifying *in vitro* IgE to vaccine components is not universally available. As many as 50% of vaccinated children develop IgG_4 and IgE to microbial antigens in the vaccines as a normal part of humoral immune response [7, 8], however its clinical significance is uncertain. Basophil activation tests are generally insensitive and poorly standardized. Skin tests should be done in a time window of 3–12 weeks and at least 5 days after discontinuation of oral antihistamines.

Skin tests were performed with the same vaccine brand 5 weeks later. Skin prick test (SPT)with the undiluted vaccine was negative, and intradermal testing with the 1:100 dilution gave an early positive wheal reaction of 22 mm with pseudopods (positive histamine control was 4 mm) (Fig. 52.1).

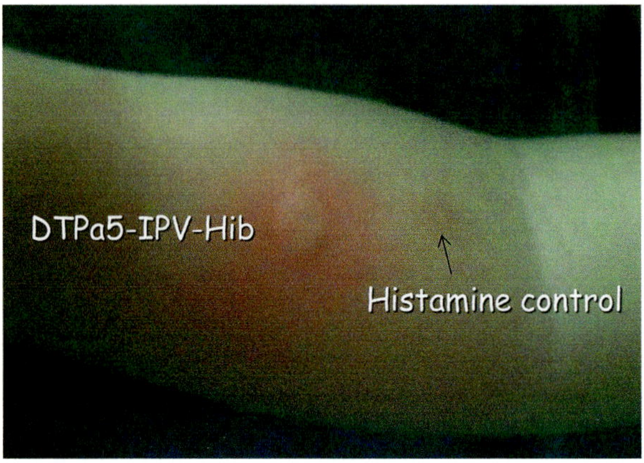

Fig. 52.1 Intradermal test with DTaP5-IPV-Hib vaccine diluted 1:100

Delayed reading at 24 h revealed circumferential redness of the forearm, edema and induration at the test site. In order to find out if a different vaccine brand is tolerated, DTaP3 + IPV + Hib was tested in parallel and gave an immediate positive intradermal reading of 10 mm.

Skin testing is the only practical way to verify if the vaccine was the cause of anaphylaxis. Positive (histamine) and negative (normal saline) prick controls are always performed. SPT with the undiluted vaccine is rarely positive, and intradermal test with 0.02 mL of vaccine diluted 1:100 is the mainstay of diagnosis. Skin tests are read at 15–20 min. A STP is considered positive if the wheal is at least 3 mm greater than the negative control, and the intradermal test is positive if at least 7 mm in diameter, or 3 mm greater than the positive histamine prick [9]. The size of the wheal is the mean value of the sum of the longest wheal diameter and the diameter perpendicular to it.

Q4. What should be done next?

A. Perform skin testing with lower valency vaccines: DTaP, DT, T
B. Nothing, since the child had already received four doses of DTaP, IPV/OPV, Hib
C. Continue only OPV at second booster
D. Continue DTaP in a graded dose protocol + OPV at second booster

Answer: *The correct answer is* ***A***.

The child was tested at a further visit with DTaP3, DT and T in the same way as previously described. He reacted with an immediate wheal of 12, 11 and 12 mm, respectively, and delayed reactions at 24 h. It was thus established that he was allergic to any vaccine containing the tetanus toxoid and further vaccination with vaccines containing tetanus toxoid was contraindicated.

He was found to have mild atopic dermatitis and the SPT to standard inhalant allergens was positive to house dust mite (2+). Total IgE was 220 IU/mL and specific IgE (sIgE) to *Dermatophagoides pteronyssinus* (house dust mite) 1.55 IU/mL (2+). Prick and sIgE were negative to cow's milk and egg-white.

Atopy is found in up to 85% of persons who had anaphylaxis to a vaccine [10]. However, given the rarity of anaphylaxis to vaccines, atopy and family history of allergy or asthma are not *per se* contraindications for immunization [10]. Clinical hypersensitivity to microbial antigens in vaccines is very rare. There have been individual reports of allergy to diphtheria and tetanus toxoids [11, 12] and to the genetically engineered diphtheria toxoid CRM197 used as a conjugating protein in pneumococcal conjugate vaccine [13].

However, almost any vaccine component can cause a hypersensitivity reaction [4, 14, 15]. When allergy to a vaccine is suspected, a full list of constituents should be obtained in order to plan a comprehensive diagnostic workup. Many of these constituents can be tested for sIgE.

Gelatin, a collagen of porcine or cow origin, is used as a stabilizer in many vaccines; with low content (up to 250 μg) in TIV and DTaP and with high content (up to 15 mg) in MMR, Varicella, rabies, Japanese encephalitis and yellow fever. Anaphylactic reactions have been noted to MMR, possibly following the priming with gelatin containing DTaP based vaccine.

Egg protein can be found in trace amounts (<1 ng) in MMR and some rabies vaccines. In influenza vaccines, both inactivated and live, the average ovalbumin content is about 350 ng per 0.5 mL dose, and the highest content is found in yellow fever vaccine. MMR and rabies vaccines can be administered to persons who tolerate eggs in food regardless of SPT or sIgE titers. The main risk is with yellow fever and TIV.

Casein can be found in trace amounts in DTaP based vaccines. Rare children with high cow-milk allergy (specific IgE >50 IU/mL) may experience an anaphylactic reaction to DTaP based vaccine.

Yeast (*Saccharomyces cerevisiae*) is found in HBV and HPV which are produced by recombinant DNA technology in *Saccharomyces cerevisiae* culture. The potential of yeast allergy in a child requires appropriate testing prior to vaccination with yeast containing vaccines.

Latex may cause allergic reactions if there is a latex vial stopper or there is a rubber plunger in the syringe.

Antibiotics (neomycin, polymyxin B, streptomycin) are often added in trace amounts to attenuated viral vaccines to keep them bacteriologically sterile. Like any other compound, these antibiotics can cause immediate hypersensitivity, but none has been linked to vaccine administration. If allergy to these drugs is known, the child should be referred to a specialist in allergy for testing and consultation prior to vaccination.

Preservatives (thiomersal and phenoxyethanol), and **adjuvants** (aluminum salts) may be found in various vaccines but have not been implicated in immediate-type hypersensitivity reactions. Contact dermatitis to these compounds does not constitute a contraindication to vaccination. Aluminum may cause indolent nodules at the injection site that can persist for months.

Dextran, a stabilizer in some freeze-dried vaccines (BCG, rotavirus 1), can cause severe immediate hypersensitivity reactions through specific IgG-complement-anaphylatoxin activation, even when administered in the neonatal period.

Q5. What if the child ever must get tetanus prevention?

A. Give tetanus toxoid in a graded dose protocol
B. Give fractionated tetanus toxoid
C. Administer tetanus immunoglobulin
D. Administer benzyl-penicillin

Answer: *The correct answer is* ***C***.

Having received four doses of tetanus toxoid in the first 2 years of life confers significant protection against tetanus until the scheduled booster with Tdap at age 4–6 years. Tetanus immunoglobulin should be administered as a prophylactic measure, i.e. a dirty, soiled wound in children in whom more than 5 years have elapsed since the last dose of vaccination. If the wound is minor and clean, the tolerated time lag may be up to 10 years. The tetanus immunoglobulin dose for children <7 years is 250 units IM, and 500 units IM for 7 years old and above [16].

If for some reason, it is impossible to administer tetanus immunoglobulin, and tetanus prevention is considered vital, a graded dose approach may be attempted in the intensive care setting. For example for a vaccine dose of 0.5 mL, administer graded doses in 15-min intervals: 0.05 of 1:10 dilution, followed by full strength graded doses of 0.05, 0.1, 0.15 and 0.2 mL [14, 15]. This is at once both desensitization and immunization.

In less risky situations, i.e. when the skin testing and *in vitro* IgE tests following a vaccine reaction are borderline or negative, the probability of a major hypersensitivity reaction is minimal. The undiluted vaccine may be administered by a fractionated protocol (1/10 + 9/10 of the dose separated by 30-min observation), under controlled conditions in a day-care or hospital setting, with at least another 30-min period of close monitoring [4, 15].

Practical Points

- Anaphylaxis to vaccines is rare; approximately once in one million doses
- Anaphylaxis usually occurs within the first 30 min after exposure, but sometimes it can take up to 4 h or longer
- Symptoms of anaphylaxis are polymorphic, but well systematized and should be readily recognized and carefully appreciated
- Anaphylaxis should be acutely treated with adrenaline, systemic corticosteroids, volume replacement, and antihistamines
- Twenty-four-hour hospital observation is indicated because a biphasic course is possible in anaphylaxis
- Diagnosis relies on skin testing with the culprit vaccine and its components, and where available, in vitro tests for the specific IgE to vaccine additives
- Anaphylaxis contraindicates further immunization with the culprit vaccine; in exceptional vital situations, a desensitization-immunization graded dose protocol may be attempted in an intensive care setting

References

1. Muraro A, Roberts G, Worm M, Bilo MB, Brockow K, Fernandez Rivas M, Santos AF, Zolkipli ZQ, Bellou A, Beyer K, Bindslev-Jensen C, Cardona V, Clark AT, Demoly P, Dubois AE, DunnGalvin A, Eigenmann P, Halken S, Harada L, Lack G, Jutel M, Niggemann B, Rueff F, Timmermans F, Vlieg-Boerstra BJ, Werfel T, Dhami S, Panesar S, Akdis CA, Sheikh A. Anaphylaxis: guidelines from the European Academy of Allergy and Clinical Immunology. Allergy. 2014;69(8):1026–45.
2. Muraro A, Roberts G, Clark A, et al. EAACI task force on anaphylaxis in children. The management of anaphylaxis in childhood: position paper of the European academy of allergology and clinical immunology. Allergy. 2007;62:857–71.
3. McNeil MM, Weintraub ES, Duffy J, Sukumaran L, Jacobsen SJ, Klein NP, et al. Risk of anaphylaxis after vaccination in children and adults. J Allergy Clin Immunol. 2015;137(3):868–78.
4. Wood RA. Allergic reactions to vaccines. Pediatr Allergy Immunol. 2013;24(6):521–6.
5. Sampson HA. Anaphylaxis and emergency treatment. Pediatrics. 2003;111(6 Pt 3):1601–8.
6. Lieberman P. Biphasic anaphylactic reactions. Ann Allergy Asthma Immunol. 2005;95(3):217–26; quiz 26, 58.
7. Edelman K, Malmstrom K, He Q, Savolainen J, Terho EO, Mertsola J. Local reactions and IgE antibodies to pertussis toxin after acellular diphtheria-tetanus-pertussis immunization. Eur J Pediatr. 1999;158(12):989–94.
8. Dannemann A, van Ree R, Kulig M, Bergmann RL, Bauer P, Forster J, Guggenmoos-Holzmann I, Aalberse RC, Wahn U. Specific IgE and IgG4 immune responses to tetanus and diphtheria toxoid in atopic and nonatopic children during the first two years of life. Int Arch Allergy Immunol. 1996;111(3):262–7.
9. Brockow K, Romano A, Blanca M, Ring J, Pichler W, Demoly P. General considerations for skin test procedures in the diagnosis of drug hypersensitivity. Allergy. 2002;57(1):45–51.
10. Nilsson L, Brockow K, Alm J, Cardona V, Caubet JC, Gomes E, Jenmalm MC, Lau S, Netterlid E, Schwarze J, Sheikh A, Storsaeter J, Skevaki C, Terreehorst I, Zanoni G. Vaccination and allergy: EAACI position paper, practical aspects. Pediatr Allergy Immunol. 2017;28(7):628–40.
11. Martin-Munoz MF, Pereira MJ, Posadas S, Sanchez-Sabate E, Blanca M, Alvarez J. Anaphylactic reaction to diphtheria-tetanus vaccine in a child: specific IgE/IgG determinations and cross-reactivity studies. Vaccine. 2002;20(27–28):3409–12.
12. Mayorga C, Torres MJ, Corzo JL, Alvarez J, Garcia JA, Rodriguez CA, Blanca M, Jurado A. Immediate allergy to tetanus toxoid vaccine: determination of immunoglobulin E and immunoglobulin G antibodies to allergenic proteins. Ann Allergy Asthma Immunol. 2003;90(2):238–43.
13. Arroabarren E, Anda M, Sanz ML. Anaphylaxis to pneumococcal vaccine; CRM(197): novel cause of vaccine allergy. Pediatr Allergy Immunol. 2016;27(4):433–7.
14. Caubet JC, Rudzeviciene O, Gomes E, Terreehorst I, Brockow K, Eigenmann PA. Managing a child with possible allergy to vaccine. Pediatr Allergy Immunol. 2014;25(4):394–403.
15. Richter D. Allergies to vaccines in children. Central Eur J Paediatr. 2017;13(1):24–9.
16. Chapman LE, Sullivent EE, Grohskopf LA, Beltrami EM, Perz JF, Kretsinger K, Panlilio AL, Thompson ND, Ehrenberg RL, Gensheimer KF, Duchin JS, Kilmarx PH, Hunt RC, Centers for Disease Control and Prevention (CDC). Recommendations for postexposure interventions to prevent infection with hepatitis B virus, hepatitis C virus, or human immunodeficiency virus, and tetanus in persons wounded during bombings and other mass-casualty events-United States, 2008: recommendations of the Centers for Disease Control and Prevention (CDC). MMWR Recommend Rep. 2008;57(Rr-6):1–21; quiz CE1–4.

Chapter 53
Allergy to Bus

Iraj Mohammadzadeh, Farzaneh Rahmani, and Nima Rezaei

A 17-year-old boy was referred to our allergy clinic with a complaint of severe generalized itching, skin lesions and mucosal ulcers, following a road trip with bus. He had experienced milder symptoms with wheal and flare and itching that lasted for a few hours to days after his previous bus trips in the same road. He did not explain any systemic reactions during his urticaria-like reactions. Interesting fact was that he did not experience any symptoms during inner city travels with bus.

On examination he had purpuric, livid macula all over his body which tended to confluent in places. We also noticed conjunctivitis, genital ulcers and stomatitis (Fig. 53.1). He had eosinophilia (920/μL) and elevated serum IgE levels.

Q1. Which of the following signs/symptoms would you expect to find in this patients and what would be your clinical diagnosis?

A. Targetoid lesions on palms → Fixed-drug eruption

I. Mohammadzadeh
Non-Communicable Pediatric Diseases Research Center, Babol University of Medical Sciences, Babol, Iran

F. Rahmani
Network of Immunity in Infection, Malignancy and Autoimmunity (NIIMA), Universal Scientific Education and Research Network (USERN), Tehran, Iran

NeuroImaging Network (NIN), Universal Scientific Education and Research Network (USERN), Tehran, Iran
e-mail: f-rahmani@alumnus.tums.ac.ir

N. Rezaei (✉)
Department of Immunology, School of Medicine, Research Center for Immunodeficiencies (RCID), Children's Medical Center, Tehran University of Medical Sciences (TUMS), Tehran, Iran

Network of Immunity in Infection, Malignancy and Autoimmunity (NIIMA), Universal Scientific Education and Research Network (USERN), Tehran, Iran
e-mail: rezaei_nima@tums.ac.ir

N. Rezaei (ed.), *Pediatric Allergy*, https://doi.org/10.1007/978-3-030-18282-3_53

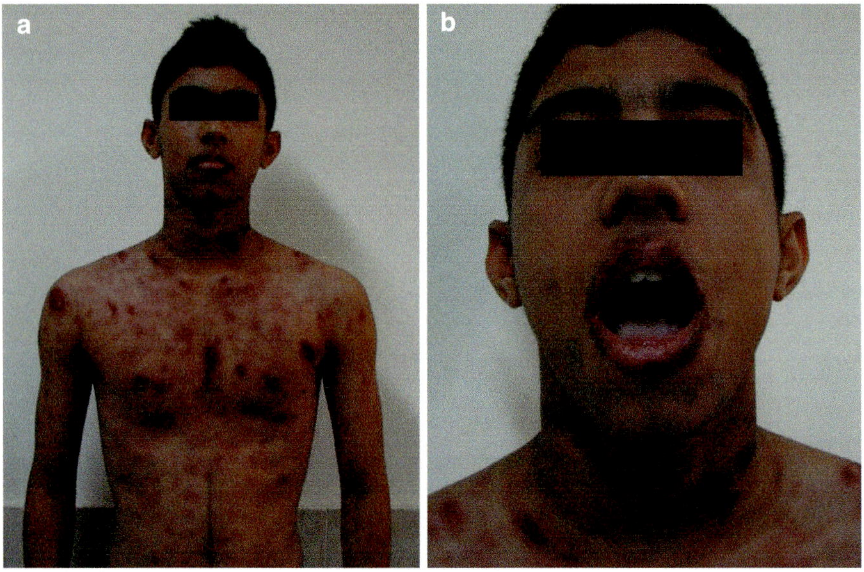

Fig. 53.1 Purpuric rash and livid macula all over the body (**a**) and oral mucosal ulcers (**b**), in a 17-year-old boy with allergy to bus

B. Targetoid lesions on chest → Erythema multiformis
C. Positive Nikolsky sign and sloughing on the upper arms and genitalia → Toxic epidermal necrolysis
D. Positive Nikolsky sign and sloughing on the dorsum of hands → Stevens-Johnson syndrome

Answer*: The correct answer is* ***D****.*

Presence of mucosal ulcers in mouth and genitalia, purple/livid-colored lesions and a history of previous cutaneous reactions in the same situation are in favour of a diagnosis of Stevens-Johnson syndrome (SJS). Positive Nikolsky sign would be suggestive for toxic epidermal necrolysis (TEN) and SJS. What helps us differentiate these two conditions is that, sloughing in less than 10% of body surface area (BSA) is in favour of SJS, while TEN usually involves more than 30% of BSA [1]. Moreover, lesions in TEN are mostly described as painful, rather than itching.

It should be noted that presence of erythema and itching or coalescent lesions should not be counted as positive Nikolsky sign. Nikolsky sign can be tested by insertion of a gentle lateral pressure to unaffected skin next to areas of sloughing. If the lesion extends to the unaffected area, with sloughing and epidermal necrosis, then the Nikolsky sign is considered positive [2].

Fixed drug eruption emerges as red to brown macules and plaques, without mucosal involvement. Lesions tend to disappear within 2–3 weeks after discontinuation of the culprit drug.

Typical target lesions are characteristic for erythema multiforme (EM), but are seen in SJS/TEN as well. Atypical, raised target lesions with purplish center can also be seen in SJS/TEN. Importantly, EM is often associated (up to 90%) with herpes simplex virus, while medications are the leading cause of SJS/TEN [3].

With a diagnosis of SJS made, we promptly started the boy on prednisolone 50 mg/day, while he was given supportive care and close observation to be able to detect signs of severity or progression of his condition. A comprehensive history was taken to identify the cause of SJS and to be able to disrupt exposure [4].

Q2. Which of the following options would be of more value to find a clue of the responsible cause of SJS in this boy?

A. History of seizure which had been under control with Carbamazepine since 10-years-old
B. Dry cough without fever that started a week ago that had been unresponsive to antihistamine
C. Taking Co-trimoxazole for a urinary tract infection for the preceding 3 days before symptoms
D. Taking ibuprofen for the headache he experienced during his bus trips

***Answer**: The correct answer is **D**.*

Medications are the leading cause of SJS, with allopurinol, aromatic anticonvalescents, i.e. phenobarbital, carbamazepine and lamotrigine, sulfonamides and NSAIDs being on top of the list. Symptoms usually occur within the first 8 weeks of exposure to the drug and lesions emerging after long periods of using the drug should not be attributed to drug-induced SJS/TEN [5]. *Mycoplasma pneumonia* infections is the next common cause of SJS, especially in the pediatric population. Atypical pneumonia with dry cough and mild fever is the most common pattern of *M. Pneumoniae* pneumonia. Meanwhile, mucosal lesions are more common in SJS due to mycoplasma infection than what is seen in this boy, and we expect the cutaneous lesions to be more sparse and the patient to be younger than the boy presented [6]. The boy did not have fever which is additionally against mycoplasma infection.

In up to one third of patients no cause is identified for SJS. The boy revealed no useful information is his history for the possible cause of SJS as he was healthy and had been on no medications, although he admitted that he had taken dimenhydrinate for motion sickness he experimented during trips. He was told to avoid using dimenhydrinate and simply became symptom-free during follow-ups.

Q3. All of the following statements is true about adverse drug reactions, <u>except</u>:

A. Immune mediated adverse drug reactions are almost always predictable
B. Non-immune mediated adverse drug reactions account for up to 80% of adverse drug reactions (ADR) to medications
C. Dimenhydrinate and other antihistamines are common causes of ADRs
D. Mucus membranes are affected in less than one third of patients with SJS due to dimenhydrinate

***Answer**: The correct answer is **B**.*

Non-immune mediated ADR are common and comprise more than 80% of all ADR and are usually predictable. Another 20% of all ADR are unpredictable and can be immune or non-immune mediated [7]. ADR to antihistamines can range from solar dermatitis to fixed drug eruptions, yet, alike other antihistamines, allergic reaction to dimenhydrinate is uncommon. SJS is known as an ADR of childhood and adolescent, yet SJS due to dimenhydrinate is reported to be least common between 10 and 19 years of age, due to low likelihood of previous exposures. Finally, mucosal involvement is almost a fixed feature—in more than 90% of patients—with SJS, making answer D, incorrect.

Dimenhydrinate is a combination of diphenhydramine and 8-chlorotheophylline. We performed skin patch testing which confirmed that the allergic reaction was due to diphenhydramine component. Cross-reactivity with other ethanolamine components was negative, reporting of the safety to use other antihistamine medications [4].

Practical Points

- Positive Nikolsky sign is suggestive for toxic epidermal necrolysis or Steven-Johnsons syndrome
- Medications are the leading cause of Steven-Johnsons syndrome with allopurinol, aromatic anti-convalescents, such as phenobarbital, carbamazepine and lamotrigine, as well as sulfonamides and NSAIDs being on top list

References

1. Dodiuk-Gad RP, Chung WH, Valeyrie-Allanore L, Shear NH. Stevens-Johnson syndrome and toxic epidermal necrolysis: an update. Am J Clin Dermatol. 2015;16(6):475–93.
2. Harr T, French LE. Toxic epidermal necrolysis and Stevens-Johnson syndrome. Orphanet J Rare Dis. 2010;5:39.
3. Schwartz RA, McDonough PH, Lee BW. Toxic epidermal necrolysis: Part I. Introduction, history, classification, clinical features, systemic manifestations, etiology, and immunopathogenesis. J Am Acad Dermatol. 2013;69(2):173.e1–13; quiz 85-6.
4. Mohammadzadeh I, Khaledi M, Rezaei N. Stevens-Johnson syndrome: report on a case with a strange complaint of allergy to bus. Acta Clin Croat. 2013;52(3):391–4.
5. Khalili B, Bahna SL. Pathogenesis and recent therapeutic trends in Stevens-Johnson syndrome and toxic epidermal necrolysis. Ann Allergy Asthma Immunol. 2006;97(3):272–80; quiz 81–3, 320.
6. Kunimi Y, Hirata Y, Aihara M, Yamane Y, Ikezawa Z. Statistical analysis of Stevens-Johnson syndrome caused by Mycoplasma pneumonia infection in Japan. Allergol Int. 2011;60(4):525–32.
7. Roujeau JC. Immune mechanisms in drug allergy. Allergology. 2006;55(1):27–33.

Chapter 54
Recurrent Loss of Consciousness

Hossein Esmaeilzadeh

A 17-year-old boy with a history of three episodes of loss of consciousness in the past year, was referred to allergy clinic for further workup. Two of the episodes had happened at school during rest time and one other 6 month later in a birthday party. He had dizziness, dyspnea and nausea just before losing consciousness with no rash and only mild itching. A simple biscuit that did not contain nuts or creams was ingested 10 min before attacks in school but he had had the same product without any reaction multiple times before.

On his admissions in the emergency department he had a blood pressure of 100–90/50–60 mmHg, and a pulse rate of 140 bpm, while temperature and respiratory rate were normal. Hydration, oxygen supplementation, antihistamine and cardiac monitoring were ordered each time. On our primary examination in the allergy clinic, no abnormal physical finding was observed. He stated that he felt well between episodes and had no history of any disease or medication use in his past medical history.

In our workup IgE titer was 40 IU/mL (reference range: 20–100 IU/mL) and skin prick test (SPT) was negative for milk, wheat and egg, aeroallergens and indoor allergens. Heart echocardiography and ECG were normal.

Q1. Which of the following is the most likely diagnosis?

A. Syncope
B. Anaphylaxis
C. Seizure
D. Vagus fainting

Answer: *The correct answer is* ***B****.*

H. Esmaeilzadeh (✉)
Allergy Research Center, Namazi Hospital, Shiraz University of Medical Sciences, Shiraz, Iran
e-mail: sesmaeilzadeh_ho@sums.ac.ir

N. Rezaei (ed.), *Pediatric Allergy*, https://doi.org/10.1007/978-3-030-18282-3_54

Q2. Which one of the following is the most appropriate next step in diagnosis?

A. Oral food challenge
B. ImmunoCAP Specific IgE
C. 24 h heart monitoring
D. Electroencephalograph

Answer: *The correct answer is* ***A****.*

According to anaphylaxis diagnosis criteria [1], patient have at least two organ involvement with exposure to a suspected allergen (biscuit) along with a decrease in blood pressure with increase heart rate, so vagal stimulation can be ruled out. There is no abnormal movement in favor of seizure. Gold-standard in food allergy diagnosis is oral food challenge (OFC) is gold standard in diagnosis of food allergy. Immunocap and SPT can reveal IgE sensitization to allergen.

OFC was done by milk and bread (wheat) that were negative and ImmunoCap of wheat was 0.3 U/mL (reference range < 0.1). Patient was finally challenged with biscuit that revealed no reaction to challenged food. The patient revealed same symptoms of anaphylactic attack after 5 min on running on a treadmill following ingestion of the biscuit. In repeated oral challenge with exercise 1 month later, anaphylaxis happened in response to wheat but there was no reaction by milk.

Q3. Which of the following is most likely the diagnosis?

A. Idiopathic anaphylaxis
B. Wheat non-IgE allergy
C. Exercise-induced anaphylaxis
D. Mastocytosis

Answer: *The correct answer is* ***C****.*

Exercise-induced anaphylaxis is an attack of anaphylaxis during exercise or within a few hour after ingesting of specific food [2]. Combination of a food item and exercise predispose the patient to anaphylaxis attack but the food item and exercise are tolerated separately. Wheat is the most common allergen in exercise-induced anaphylaxis [3]. Importantly, time between food ingestion and reaction that are less than 1 h means that reactions are IgE mediated [3]. There is no skin lesion in favor of mastocytosis.

Q4. On the basis of the clinical diagnosis, which of the following would be the most appropriate recommendation for patient?

A. Avoidance of wheat
B. Avoidance of exercise during 3–4 h after eating wheat
C. Daily antihistamine
D. Nothing

Answer: *The correct answer is* ***B****.*

Management of exercise-induced anaphylaxis is by avoidance of exercise for 3–4 h after ingestion of the culprit specific food for which there are specific IgE (sIgE). Patient should be informed and educated about injection of epinephrine during attacks and be instructed to stop exercise immediately by the onset of symptoms. Wheat or exercise separately do not cause any problem but both together make anaphylaxis.

Practical Points

- Exercise-induced anaphylaxis is defined as an anaphylactic attack during exercise or within a few hour after ingesting of specific food
- Food or exercise alone cannot produce an anaphylactic reaction
- Wheat is the most common allergen in exercise-induced anaphylaxis

References

1. Simons FER, Ardusso LRF, Bilò MB, El-Gamal YM, Ledford DK, Ring J, Sanchez-Borges M, Senna GE, Sheikh A, Thong BY. World Allergy Organization anaphylaxis guidelines: summary. J Allergy Clin Immunol. 2011;127(3):587–93.e22.
2. Feldweg AM. Food-dependent, exercise-induced anaphylaxis: diagnosis and management in the outpatient setting. J Allergy Clin Immunol Pract. 2017;5(2):283–8.
3. Romano A, Di Fonso M, Giuffreda F, Papa G, Artesani MC, Viola M, Venuti A, Palmieri V, Zeppilli P. Food-dependent exercise-induced anaphylaxis: clinical and laboratory findings in 54 subjects. Int Arch Allergy Immunol. 2001;125(3):264–72.

Chapter 55
Generalized Urticaria and Decreased Consciousness After Barbecue

Taher Cheraghi

On a hot sunny day, a 7-year-old boy goes on a picnic to a garden near the city with his family. They make barbecue, while the boy is stung by a yellow jacket bee. He feels warm on his face, has apparent flushing on his head and chest. His consciousness drops abruptly, and his breath is labored and short as he develops generalized urticaria all over his body. His family rush him to a local hospital, where his blood pressure is 65/40 mmHg, and he is tachypneic and tachycardic on admission. Generalized wheezing and stridor is audible in both lung fields.

Q1. Given the above scenario, what is the most likely diagnosis?

A. Asthma
B. Vasovagal syncope
C. Anaphylaxis
D. Foreign body aspiration

Answer: *The correct answer is* ***C.***

Clinical diagnostic criteria for anaphylaxis can be made using one of the three existing diagnostic set of criteria, based on the priori information about the responsible/possible allergen or the absence of it. When no suspected allergen exist or the patients is not previously identified as being allergic to the exposed substance, the diagnosis of anaphylaxis is based on involvement of cutaneous and mucous membranes and involvement of at least one of the respiratory or cardiovascular systems. The diagnosis is more easily confirmed, by involvement of only two out of four organ systems (cutaneous, respiratory, cardiovascular, gastrointestinal). When there is a history of exposure to a likely/common allergen—e.g. peanut—and even easier

T. Cheraghi (✉)
Department of Pediatrics, 17th Shahrivar Children's Hospital, School of Medicine, Guilan University of Medical Sciences, Rasht, Iran
e-mail: tcheraghi@gums.ac.ir

N. Rezaei (ed.), *Pediatric Allergy*, https://doi.org/10.1007/978-3-030-18282-3_55

when there is a history of exposure to a known allergen for that patient. In the latter setting, a decrease in blood pressure (hypotension) is enough to start treatment [1].

The authenticity of this definition and diagnostic criteria has been affirmed by many guidelines [2–5]. Involvement of more than two organ systems (cutaneous features, respiratory compromise as wheeze, collapse attack, and confusion) in our patient are all suggestive of anaphylaxis. In asthma we have wheezing but not cutaneous manifestations, hypotension, or profound change in consciousness. In vasovagal syncope, paleness, not flushing, often associates or heralds acute drop attack. History is often suggestive in foreign body aspiration and usually it is only the respiratory system that is involved [7, 8].

Q2. Which of the following organ systems is the most commonly involved in anaphylaxis?

A. Cardiovascular system
B. Central nervous system
C. Skin
D. Gastrointestinal tract

Answer: *The correct answer* ***C.***

Skin is the most common organ involved in anaphylaxis [1, 3]. Cutaneous signs and symptoms of anaphylaxis are: flushing, skin warmth sensation, pruritus, generalized urticarial or angioedema. Cutaneous manifestations may be absent in food-induced anaphylaxis and when anaphylaxis is associated with severe hypotension [1, 6, 8].

Q3. Which of the following medications is first priority for the treatment of anaphylaxis?

A. Antihistamines
B. Epinephrine
C. Methylprednisolone
D. Serum normal saline

Answer: *The correct answer is* ***B.***

Although other medications are usually used in anaphylaxis, the first choice of treatment of anaphylaxis is intramuscular (IM) epinephrine that is the only medication that reduces hospitalization and death [9]. Epinephrine should be administered with a dose of 0.01 mg/kg of 1 mg/mL vials and could be repeated every 5 min if necessary [1, 3, 5, 9]. Subcutaneous and inhaler use of epinephrine are not generally recommended.

Epinephrine is a potent alpha-1, beta-1 and beta-2 adrenergic. The alpha-1 agonist activity prevents airway edema, hypotension, and shock. As a beta-1 agonist it augments myocardial contractility and increases heart rate, and finally its beta-2 bronchodilator action leads to resolution of bronchospasm and reduction of release of mediators [3]. There is no absolute contraindication to the use of epinephrine in anaphylaxis [3, 9]. Epinephrine autoinjectors are preferred if available and are frequently under-prescribed and under-used [9], accounting for a proportion of out of hospital mortality due to anaphylaxis.

Q4. What are the second line treatment of anaphylaxis?

A. Removing the trigger and calling for help
B. Intravenous fluids, antihistamines, and glucocorticoids
C. Inhaled short acting beta agonists, correct position, high flow oxygen
D. All of the above

Answer: *The correct answer is* ***D.***

The above mentioned second line adjunctive treatments for anaphylaxis are life-saving [1, 7, 8, 10].

Q5. According to the presenting features of the following patients with anaphylaxis, all postures are appropriate for the pertinent patient, <u>except</u>:

A. Recovery position for an unconscious patient
B. Sitting up position for a patient with circulatory instability
C. Semi recumbent position on the left side for a pregnant patient with extremities elevated
D. Sitting up position for patients with respiratory distress

Answer: *The correct answer is* ***B.***

Most patients with anaphylaxis are comfortable at supine position with extremities elevated. If the patient has difficulty breathing when in supine position, a sitting up position is allowed, given the patient has no circulatory compromise, but standing position is never allowed. For pregnant woman with anaphylaxis, semirecumbent position on the left side is an appropriate position [2, 3, 7].

Q6. Which of the following medications do you administer first if the symptoms and signs of anaphylaxis are mild, such as urticaria associated with mild crampy abdominal pain?

A. Antihistamines
B. Corticosteroids
C. Epinephrine
D. Combination of antihistamines and corticosteroids

Answer: *The correct answer is* ***C.***

Antihistamines antagonize histamine at receptor level only. It has been shown that release of platelet activating factor (PAF), intensity of release of kinin and other anaphylactic mediators are associated with severe and potentially fatal reactions. The correlation between PAF and severity of anaphylaxis is more consistent than histamine or tryptase [11, 12]. Moreover, outcome of anaphylaxis is not predictable based on clinical course. Therefore, even with mild symptoms or single organ involvement, prompt and early use of epinephrine is recommended as a first priority [2].

Q7. Which of the following solutions is the fluid of choice for anaphylactic patients?

A. Lactated ringer
B. Dextrose 5%water

C. Normal saline
D. Albumin

Answer: *The correct answer is* ***C.***

Even after full dose injection of epinephrine, the patient might still be hypotensive or has orthostatic hypotension. Intravascular access should be provided and boluses of 20 mL/kg of body weight of normal saline should be infused over 5–10 min and this may be repeated as needed. Normal saline is the preferred fluid as Lactated Ringer may lead to metabolic alkalosis and Dextrose water shifts rapidly from intravascular to interstitial space. Colloids like albumin have no priority over normal saline in distributive shock like anaphylaxis and are more expensive [13]. The patient should be monitored and care should be taken to avoid volume overload [13].

Q8. Previous use of which of the following medications makes the anaphylaxis attack more severe?

A. Beta blockers
B. Angiotensin-converting enzyme inhibitors
C. Non-steroidal anti-inflammatory drugs
D. All of the above

Answer: *The correct answer is* ***D.***

Concurrent use of both beta-blockers and angiotensin-converting enzyme inhibitors makes anaphylaxis more severe than when they are using alone [3, 9]. Other factors intensify anaphylaxis by decreasing the threshold for anaphylaxis such as exercise, ethanol use, acute infections, stress, and perimenstrual status [9]. NSAIDs are among the most common causes of drug-induced anaphylaxis [14]. Presence of mastocytosis makes patients more prone to severe anaphylaxis [6].

Q9. Which of the following tests is most applicable and supportive of diagnosis of anaphylaxis?

A. Measurement of tryptase level
B. Measurement of histamine level
C. Measurement of N-methylhistamine level
D. Measurement of platelet-activating factor level

Answer: *The correct answer is* ***A.***

Serum level of tryptase is elevated in anaphylaxis and tryptase is more stable than other mediators of anaphylaxis, measureable in serum from 15 to 180 min after the onset of anaphylaxis. However, tryptase levels may not be increased in food-induced anaphylaxis and reliance on a single mediator to establish the diagnosis of anaphylaxis is not enough [1, 5, 6, 8].

Q10. The patient has recovered fully from the attack. How long would you observe the patient at the hospital before authorizing his release?

A. 1 h
B. 2 h

C. 3 h
D. 6 h

Answer: *The correct answer is* ***D.***

Patients presenting with anaphylaxis should be observed and monitored at the hospital for at least 6–8 h if they are respiratory compromised and 12–24 h when they are hypotensive on admission [1, 3].

Q11. Which of the following items would you recommend the patient and his family upon discharge?

A. Prescribe an autoinjector epinephrine for those at risk for recurrence and provide them with instruction of when and how to use it.
B. Provide advice sheet and train the patient and caregivers how to manage possible future attacks of anaphylaxis
C. Referral to an allergist/immunologist for personal risk reduction and when indicated: allergen specific immunotherapy
D. All of the above

Answer: *The correct answer is* ***D.***

When discharging the patient, you should instruct them about common signs and symptoms of anaphylaxis. They should be familiar with prompt recognition of anaphylaxis and take immediate actions including self/auto-injection of epinephrine, call for help, avoid exposure to responsible allergens, and follow allergist care. In addition their family members, friends, school teachers, and caregivers should be trained to help them in case of emergency.

Practical Points

- When no suspected allergen exists or the patients is not identified as being allergic to the exposed substance, the diagnosis of anaphylaxis is based on mucocutanous manifestations and at least one of the respiratory or cardiovascular systems
- When there is a history of exposure to a likely/common allergen, the diagnosis is confirmed by involvement of only two of the cutaneous, respiratory, cardiovascular, and gastrointestinal systems
- Following exposure to a known allergen for the patient a decrease in blood pressure (hypotension) is enough to start treatment
- Intravenous fluids, antihistamines, glucocorticoids and inhaled short-acting beta agonists, as well as high flow oxygen are second-line options for management of an anaphylactic reaction
- Previous use of beta blockers, angiotensin converting enzyme inhibitors, or non-steroidal anti-inflammatory drugs report of a more severe anaphylactic attack
- Provide the patient with anaphylactic attack with an autoinjector epinephrine and refer him/her to an allergist upon discharge from emergency department

References

1. Sampson HA, Munoz-Furlong A, Campbell RL, Adkinson NF Jr, Bock SA, Branum A, Brown SG, Camargo CA Jr, Cydulka R, Galli SJ, Gidudu J, Gruchalla RS, Harlor AD Jr, Hepner DL, Lewis LM, Lieberman PL, Metcalfe DD, O'Connor R, Muraro A, Rudman A, Schmitt C, Scherrer D, Simons FE, Thomas S, Wood JP, Decker WW. Second symposium on the definition and management of anaphylaxis: summary report--Second National Institute of Allergy and Infectious Disease/Food Allergy and Anaphylaxis Network symposium. J Allergy Clin Immunol. 2006;117(2):391–7.
2. Lieberman P, Nicklas RA, Randolph C, Oppenheimer J, Bernstein D, Bernstein J, Ellis A, Golden DB, Greenberger P, Kemp S, Khan D, Ledford D, Lieberman J, Metcalfe D, Nowak-Wegrzyn A, Sicherer S, Wallace D, Blessing-Moore J, Lang D, Portnoy JM, Schuller D, Spector S, Tilles SA. Anaphylaxis--a practice parameter update 2015. Ann Allergy Asthma Immunol. 2015;115(5):341–84.
3. Muraro A, Werfel T, Hoffmann-Sommergruber K, Roberts G, Beyer K, Bindslev-Jensen C, Cardona V, Dubois A, duToit G, Eigenmann P, Fernandez Rivas M, Halken S, Hickstein L, Host A, Knol E, Lack G, Marchisotto MJ, Niggemann B, Nwaru BI, Papadopoulos NG, Poulsen LK, Santos AF, Skypala I, Schoepfer A, Van Ree R, Venter C, Worm M, Vlieg-Boerstra B, Panesar S, de Silva D, Soares-Weiser K, Sheikh A, Ballmer-Weber BK, Nilsson C, de Jong NW, Akdis CA. EAACI food allergy and anaphylaxis guidelines: diagnosis and management of food allergy. Allergy. 2014;69(8):1008–25.
4. Simons FE, Ardusso LR, Bilo MB, Cardona V, Ebisawa M, El-Gamal YM, Lieberman P, Lockey RF, Muraro A, Roberts G, Sanchez-Borges M, Sheikh A, Shek LP, Wallace DV, Worm M. International consensus on (ICON) anaphylaxis. World Allergy Organ J. 2014;7(1):9.
5. Simons FE, Ebisawa M, Sanchez-Borges M, Thong BY, Worm M, Tanno LK, Lockey RF, El-Gamal YM, Brown SG, Park HS, Sheikh A. 2015 update of the evidence base: World Allergy Organization anaphylaxis guidelines. World Allergy Organ J. 2015;8(1):32.
6. Reber LL, Hernandez JD, Galli SJ. The pathophysiology of anaphylaxis. J Allergy Clin Immunol. 2017;140(2):335–48.
7. Stelle F, Simons R. Anaphylaxis: assessment and management. In: Leung Donald YM, Szefler SJ, Bonilla FA, Akdis CA, Sampson HA, editors. Pediatric Allergy, Principles and Practice. 3rd ed. Amsterdam: Elsevier; 2016.
8. Brown SGA. Anaphylaxis. In: Adkinson F, et al., editors. Middleton's allergy principles and practice. 8th ed. Amsterdam: Elsevier; 2013.
9. Craig T, Pursun EA, Bork K, Bowen T, Boysen H, Farkas H, Grumach A, Katelaris CH, Lockey R, Longhurst H, Lumry W, Magerl M, Martinez-Saguer I, Ritchie B, Nast A, Pawankar R, Zuraw B, Maurer M. [WAO guideline for the management of hereditary angioedema]. Arerugi. 2015;64(9):1215–1241.
10. Muraro A, Roberts G, Worm M, Bilò MB, Brockow K, Fernández Rivas M, Santos AF, Zolkipli ZQ, Bellou A, Beyer K, Bindslev-Jensen C, Cardona V, Clark AT, Demoly P, Dubois AEJ, DunnGalvin A, Eigenmann P, Halken S, Harada L, Lack G, Jutel M, Niggemann B, Ruëff F, Timmermans F, Vlieg-Boerstra BJ, Werfel T, Dhami S, Panesar S, Akdis CA, Sheikh A, the EFA, Anaphylaxis Guidelines Group. Anaphylaxis: guidelines from the European Academy of Allergy and Clinical Immunology. Allergy. 2014;69(8):1026–45.
11. Peters SP. Asthma phenotypes: nonallergic (intrinsic) asthma. J Allergy Clin Immunol Pract. 2014;2(6):650–2.
12. Schatz M, Rosenwasser L. The allergic asthma phenotype. J Allergy Clin Immunol Pract. 2014;2(6):645–8; quiz 9.
13. Campbell RL, Kelso JM, Walls RM, Randolph AG, Feldweg AM. Anaphylaxis: emergency treatment; 2018. www.uptodate.com
14. Aun MV, Blanca M, Garro LS, Ribeiro MR, Kalil J, Motta AA, Castells M, Giavina-Bianchi P. Nonsteroidal anti-inflammatory drugs are major causes of drug-induced anaphylaxis. J Allergy Clin Immunol Pract. 2014;2(4):414–20.

Chapter 56
Recurrent Abdominal Cramps, Diarrhea and Loss of Consciousness

Irena Ivkovic-Jurekovic and Marta Navratil

A 12-year-old girl was referred to our clinic with symptoms of anaphylaxis manifested with itchy skin, generalised flushing, nausea, abdominal cramps, diarrhea and loss of consciousness. Episodes were repeated up to five times monthly, requiring use of epinephrine, antihistamine and corticosteroids. The girl had symptoms of seasonal allergic rhinoconjunctivitis and had been hospitalized at the age of 12 years. Workup results showed sensitization to trees with positive skin prick test, elevated total IgE and specific IgE (sIgE) against birch and hazel. There were no data or sign of tick bite and no connection of symptoms with ingestion of mammalian food products or with exercise.

In her current workup, bone marrow aspiration was performed to rule out the diagnosis of systemic mastocytosis [1, 2]. Baseline serum tryptase level was within normal range (3.24 μg/L), but elevated during attacks up to 80.6 μg/L. Abdominal ultrasound was normal and pheochromocytoma and carcinoid syndrome were ruled out through measurements of catecholamines in 24-h urine, serum gastrin and 24-h levels of 5-hydroxyindoleacetic acid. Reaction to mammalian oligosaccharide α-gal was excluded based on medical history [3]. Prick-to-prick testing with fresh mammalian meat and oral challenge test were negative as well. The girl had positive autologous serum skin test (ASST) [4], but circulating auto-antibodies against IgE and against the Fc subunit of the high-affinity IgE receptor (FcεRIα) could not be detected, i.e. histamine-release test was negative [5]. The activity of histamine inactivating enzyme diamine oxidase (DAO) in plasma was reduced (very low, indicating high histamine intolerance) [6].

I. Ivkovic-Jurekovic (✉) · M. Navratil
Children's Hospital Zagreb, Zagreb, Croatia

Faculty of Dental Medicine and Helathcare, University of Osijek, Osijek, Croatia
e-mail: irena.ivkovic-jurekovic@kdb.hr

N. Rezaei (ed.), *Pediatric Allergy*, https://doi.org/10.1007/978-3-030-18282-3_56

Q1. Which of the following is the most likely diagnosis?

A. Hereditary angioedema
B. Histamine intolerance
C. Recurrent anaphylaxis
D. Idiopathic anaphylaxis

Answer: *The correct answer is* ***D.***

Absence of family history and responsiveness to antihistamine and epinephrine rule out the diagnosis of hereditary angioedema in this patient.

The patient had histamine intolerance along with recurrent anaphylaxis, thus histamine intolerance could not be solely responsible for all the symptoms she was experiencing.

The patient was having recurrent anaphylaxis, but the correct diagnosis is idiopathic anaphylaxis. The diagnosis of idiopathic anaphylaxis is made when a patient has signs and symptoms consistent with anaphylaxis, but no specific trigger can be identified, and other diseases have been ruled out. Patients experiencing six or more episodes of anaphylaxis per year or two or more episodes in 2 months may be classified as idiopathic frequent anaphylaxis [7, 8]. Our patient has fulfilled this criteria.

Q2. Imagine that her bone marrow aspiration had revealed presence of CD25-positive mast cells. What would be the most probable diagnosis?

A. Idiopathic mast cell activation syndrome
B. Systemic mastocytosis
C. Secondary mast cell activation syndrome
D. Idiopathic histaminergic angioedema

Answer: *The correct answer is* ***B.***

One of the minor diagnostic criteria for systemic mastocytosis is the presence of aberrant CD25 and/or CD2 expression on mast cells, which is a marker of mast cell clonality [1]. This marker is found neither in idiopathic mast cell activation syndrome nor in secondary mast cell activation nor in anaphylaxis.

Idiopathic histaminergic acquired angioedema is a common cause of recurrent angioedema without wheals. It is a mast cell mediated disease thought to belong to the same clinical entity as chronic urticaria [9]. The diagnosis is made when specific causes of immediate hypersensitivity reactions, associated autoimmune diseases, C1 esterase inhibitor deficiency and mutation in coagulation factor XII are excluded.

Q3. Which of the following differential diagnoses was considered an indication to perform ASST test in this patient?

A. Any allergic condition
B. Chronic urticaria

C. Acute urticaria
D. Recurrent angioedema

Answer: *The correct answer is **B.***

ASST is an *in vivo* test which assesses basophil histamine releasing activity of the serum. It has only moderate specificity as a marker for functional autoantibodies against IgE or the FcεR, detected by the basophil histamine release assay, but has high negative predictive value. False positive ASSTs have been reported in some subjects without chronic urticaria, including those with multiple drug intolerance, in patients with respiratory allergy and in healthy controls [4]. ASST has no diagnostic value in acute urticaria or recurrent angioedema.

Q4. On the basis of the patient's diagnosis, which of the following would be the most appropriate long-term management?

A. Antihistamine per need along with histamine-free diet
B. Low-dose oral corticosteroid
C. Epinephrine autoinjector per need
D. Antihistamine and corticosteroid daily for several months + histamine free diet

Answer: *The correct answer is **D.***

There are no standard treatment regimens for idiopathic frequent anaphylaxis and limited robust research has been conducted. Treatments are based on case series, observations, and expert opinion. The algorithm developed by Patterson and colleagues [10] has proved useful for the management of idiopathic anaphylaxis. Patients with frequent episodes require maintenance therapy, which includes 40–60 mg of prednisone daily and H1-antihistamine in the form of 10 mg cetirizine, 25–50 mg hydroxyzine, 25–50 mg diphenhydramine, or 180 mg fexofenadine [10, 11]. None of the other therapy possibilities, i.e. antihistamine per need, epinephrine per need or histamine-free diet are not sufficient to control symptoms. Low-dose oral corticosteroid alone, without antihistamine, is also not recommended.

Instructed how to use epinephrine autoinjector, upon advice our patient adopted a histamine-free diet. Due to the attack frequency, she was advised to take 120 mg of fexofenadine and 40 mg of methylprednisolone daily for 1 week [7, 8]. The same dose was then given on alternate days for 2 more weeks and was then further reduced by 5 mg every 2 weeks. The girl stopped having episodes after the first week of treatment, and remained symptom free for the next 8 months, while on antihistamine only. After that, three new episodes occurred during a 4-month period, and ketotifen 1 mg twice daily together with fexofenadine 120 mg daily was thus added to her regimen. The girl has been on this therapy for 11 months now and has been symptom free since then.

Practical Points

- Idiopathic anaphylaxis is a systemic syndrome of immediate hypersensitivity caused by release of mediators from mast cells and basophils with an unknown trigger
- Individual patients may have a different combination of symptoms but usually tend to have the same manifestations on repeated episodes
- The diagnosis of anaphylaxis is based on a thorough history and clinical examination and eliminating other known causes producing the same clinical picture
- Patients with idiopathic anaphylaxis must carry epinephrine and must be trained how to manage an acute attack

References

1. Akin C, Valent P, Metcalfe DD. Mast cell activation syndrome: proposed diagnostic criteria. J Allergy Clin Immunol. 2010;126(6):1099–104.e4.
2. Valent P, Akin C, Arock M, Brockow K, Butterfield JH, Carter MC, Castells M, Escribano L, Hartmann K, Lieberman P, Nedoszytko B, Orfao A, Schwartz LB, Sotlar K, Sperr WR, Triggiani M, Valenta R, Horny HP, Metcalfe DD. Definitions, criteria and global classification of mast cell disorders with special reference to mast cell activation syndromes: a consensus proposal. Int Arch Allergy Immunol. 2012;157(3):215–25.
3. Commins SP, Platts-Mills TA. Anaphylaxis syndromes related to a new mammalian cross-reactive carbohydrate determinant. J Allergy Clin Immunol. 2009;124(4):652–7.
4. Konstantinou GN, Asero R, Maurer M, Sabroe RA, Schmid-Grendelmeier P, Grattan CE. EAACI/GA(2)LEN task force consensus report: the autologous serum skin test in urticaria. Allergy. 2009;64(9):1256–68.
5. Platzer MH, Grattan CE, Poulsen LK, Skov PS. Validation of basophil histamine release against the autologous serum skin test and outcome of serum-induced basophil histamine release studies in a large population of chronic urticaria patients. Allergy. 2005;60(9):1152–6.
6. Mayer IMA, Wantke F, et al. Optimierter radioextraktionassay zur qunatitativen bestimmung der aktivität von diaminooxidase (DAO) in human serum und plasma. Allergologie. 2005;3:12–7.
7. Lenchner K, Grammer LC. A current review of idiopathic anaphylaxis. Curr Opin Allergy Clin Immunol. 2003;3(4):305–11.
8. Lieberman PL. Idiopathic anaphylaxis. Allergy Asthma Proc. 2014;35(1):17–23.
9. Cicardi M, Aberer W, Banerji A, Bas M, Bernstein JA, Bork K, Caballero T, Farkas H, Grumach A, Kaplan AP, Riedl MA, Triggiani M, Zanichelli A, Zuraw B, EAACI Hutpo. Classification, diagnosis, and approach to treatment for angioedema: consensus report from the Hereditary Angioedema International Working Group. Allergy. 2014;69(5):602–16.
10. Greenberger PA, Lieberman P. Idiopathic anaphylaxis. J Allergy Clin Immunol Pract. 2014;2(3):243–50; quiz 51.
11. Nwaru BI, Dhami S, Sheikh A. Idiopathic anaphylaxis. Curr Treat Options Allergy. 2017;4(3):312–9.

Chapter 57
Recurrent Hives After Sea Bathing

Eva Rebelo Gomes

A 15-year-old female patient presented to the allergy clinic reporting recurrent maculopapular skin lesions throughout the body surface with mild pruritus after sea bathing. The lesions resolved within 20–40 min after skin drying and re-warming. These complaints started by the age of 10. Over the last few months she also started having occasional episodes of facial angioedema and lip angioedema after ingestion of ice cream. Her past medical history revealed a previous diagnosis of asthma and rhinitis. She had a normal leukocyte count and ESR, while total serum IgE was moderately elevated and sensitization to house dust mites had been demonstrated in skin prick test (SPT). The family history was unremarkable except for a father with allergic rhinitis. The patient's physical examination was normal and she had no dermographism.

Q1. Which of the following tests will probably be more informative concerning diagnosis?

A. Skin prick tests with aeroallergens
B. Skin prick tests with food allergens
C. An ice cube test
D. An autologous serum skin test

Answer: *The correct answer is* ***C.***

Cold-induced urticaria is one subtype of inducible physical urticaria that is frequent among young patients with chronic urticaria and even higher in children residing in cold climates [1].

E. R. Gomes (✉)
Allergy and Clinical Immunology Service, Centro Hospitalar Universitário do Porto, Porto, Portugal
e-mail: u20945@chporto.min-saude.pt

N. Rezaei (ed.), *Pediatric Allergy*, https://doi.org/10.1007/978-3-030-18282-3_57

The diagnosis is based on clinical history. Urticarial lesions and angioedema occur within minutes after exposure to cold stimulus such as cold environment, aquatic activities and contact with cold objects or foods. A cold stimulation test as the ice cube test is the main tool for diagnosis of this condition although it can be negative in atypical cases [2]. The test is considered positive if an urticarial wheal develops after application of a cold stimulus (usually an ice cube in a plastic bag) on the forearm for 5 min. The wheal develops at 5–15 min during the re-warming phase and can stay for 30 min or longer. The pathogenic mechanisms underlying this condition are largely unknown. Temperature dependent IgE antibodies against skin antigens and mast cell activation inducing vascular changes are suggested to be involved [3]. The true role of mastocytes and histamine in the disease and the real contribution of cold stimulus are yet to be clarified [4, 5].

In this patient the diagnosis was confirmed by inducing an urticarial weal with an ice cube placed on the forearm for 5 min. As the skin warmed up, an urticarial lesion developed with a 40 mm mean diameter (Fig. 57.1)

Q2. Which of the following points must be clarified in the clinical history?

A. Previous history of infections and traveling
B. Family history of similar reactions
C. Use of medications/drugs
D. All of the above

Answer: *The correct answer is* ***D.***

Cold-induced urticaria it is an idiopathic condition [6] but an association with high serum cryoglobulins developed after a viral or bacterial infection (EBV, HIV, hepatitis, toxoplasmosis, syphilis, borreliosis) or with a lymphoproliferative disease is possible and should be investigated if the clinical history is not clear cut. In case of a suspicion for autoimmune disorders, based on personal or family history, additional tests such as dosing C3 and C4, anti-thyroid antibodies, antinuclear antibod-

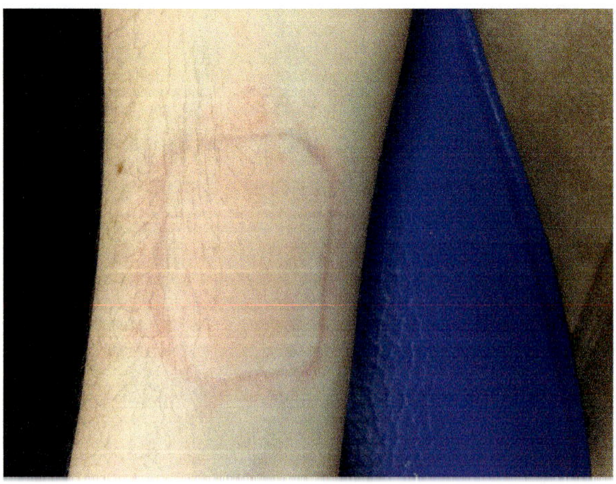

Fig. 57.1 Urticarial wheal after placing an ice cube on the forearm of the patient for 5 min. The girl had recurrent hives after sea bathing

ies and antineutrophil antibodies or an ASST can help. Familial cases have been reported, with symptoms often emerging in early childhood with symptoms such as joint pain, musculoskeletal symptoms and fever being present [7, 8]. Finally, there are reports of cold induced urticaria being associated with the intake of certain drugs such as benzodiazepines.

Q3. Which of the following would be the best treatment option at this time?

A. Second generation antihistamines at standard doses and avoidance of cold stimulus
B. First generation antihistamines and avoidance of cold stimulus
C. Monthly administration of omalizumab
D. Anti-leukotrienes and avoidance of cold stimulus

Answer: *The correct answer is* ***A.***

Avoidance of cold stimuli and high-risk activities such as swimming in cold water or ingesting ice cold beverage, or foods in the case of pharynx manifestations, are pillars of the management of the disease.

Second generation H1 antihistamines are the main agents for prophylactic therapy and have been shown to reduce the frequency and severity of episodes. Sometimes a higher than usual standard dose (up to four times) is necessary, as might be indicated in other forms of chronic urticaria, in order to control symptoms and guarantee the quality of life of the patient. Besides, extra doses of antihistamines can be used in a prophylactic manner if the patient is aware that she will be facing a colder than usual environment.

First generation antihistamines are not superior in controlling symptoms as they have a higher frequency of side effects as sedation and anticholinergic activities.

Omalizumab and leukotriene antagonists have been successfully used in a few cases but their use in this particular setting would be off label as they are only approved for chronic spontaneous urticaria. They can be considered an option if control is not achieved with high dose antihistamines.

The patient was treated with daily antihistamines (levocetirizine 10 mg/day) and was warned of the risk of generalized reactions with hypotension and lethal outcome that might rise by immersion in cold water.

Q4. What is the major concern in the follow-up of a patient like her?

A. Persistence of the disease in the majority of patients
B. Impact on quality of life and daily activities
C. Possible occurrence of a systemic reaction in one third of the patients
D. Appearance of other forms of urticaria in up to one half of the patients

Answer: *The correct answer is* ***C.***

The natural history of the disease is not known. The disease usually resolves spontaneously over 5–6 years in about 30% of the patients, thus a re-evaluation in 3–6 months is recommended [6, 9].

Mild forms of cold induced urticaria are usually well managed with the use of antihistamines and the education of patients in order to avoid cold stimuli. The physician needs to consider that avoidance of open air activities and aquatic sports can have an important impact in quality of life in young patients. Most patients achieve control under antihistamines and may need treatment only during cold months.

Systemic symptoms and anaphylaxis can develop in about one third of the patients specially triggered by extensive contact with low temperatures as in aquatic activities [10]. Patients with a previous anaphylactic episodes as well as patients with asthma, are at an increased risk for systemic reactions.

Patients should avoid cold drinks and foods as edema of the oropharynx can develop with possible asphyxiation. Precautions must also be taken in hospital settings as case reports of systemic reactions in operative rooms and following IV administration of cold solutions [11].

The association of cold induced urticaria with other forms of urticaria such as cholinergic urticaria and dermographism is possible and it can occur in about one in four cases [6].

In his her last medical appointment, the teen reported a new episode, this time with complaints of general malaise, generalized urticarial lesions and shortness of breath after a surfing lesson at sea during the winter and needed medical assistance. Patients at risk or not compliant with eviction measures should be instructed to carry and use an adrenaline autoinjector device, as we did for this patient.

Q5. Which other of the following could help in fine-tuning the management of this patient?

A. Threshold testing
B. Natural exposure test
C. Cold water bath test
D. Cold desensitization

Answer: *The correct answer is* ***A.***

The threshold test uses special electronic equipment (TempTest4.0) and allows determination of temperature threshold for an individual patient, which is the higher temperature to which the patient reacts. This threshold can be quite variable from patient to patient, and those with higher thresholds are at increased risk for a more severe disease.

The natural exposure test and the cold-water bath test are not recommended, especially in the cases of a previous anaphylaxis, unless there are still diagnostic doubts, as there is a considerable risk of inducing a systemic reaction.

Cold desensitization by repeated controlled exposure of the patients to cold through cold baths has been described as successful in some reports [12]. To maintain a non-reactive state a daily exposure to cold shower/bath is necessary. This gives an option for long term reaction avoidance in patients that routinely practice in cold environments such as surfers. Meanwhile, good compliance of the patient is mandatory and the use of this method is not commonly recommended.

Practical Points

- Cold-induced urticaria is an inducible physical type of chronic urticaria with higher frequency in children residing in cold climates
- Ice cube test would help to make the diagnosis and threshold testing would help tune the cold-avoidance measures in this patient
- Exclusion of an association with high serum cryoglobulins or lymphoproliferative disorders is warranted in all patients with cold-induced urticaria

References

1. Abajian M, Schoepke N, Altrichter S, Zuberbier T, Maurer M. Physical urticarias and cholinergic urticaria. Immunol Allergy Clin N Am. 2014;34(1):73–88.
2. Deza G, Brasileiro A, Bertolin-Colilla M, Curto-Barredo L, Pujol RM, Gimenez-Arnau AM. Acquired cold urticaria: clinical features, particular phenotypes, and disease course in a tertiary care center cohort. J Am Acad Dermatol. 2016;75(5):918–24.e2.
3. Meyer J, Gorbach AM, Liu WM, Medic N, Young M, Nelson C, Arceo S, Desai A, Metcalfe DD, Komarow HD. Mast cell dependent vascular changes associated with an acute response to cold immersion in primary contact urticaria. PLoS One. 2013;8(2):e56773.
4. Sabroe RA, Fiebiger E, Francis DM, Maurer D, Seed PT, Grattan CE, Black AK, Stingl G, Greaves MW, Barr RM. Classification of anti-FcepsilonRI and anti-IgE autoantibodies in chronic idiopathic urticaria and correlation with disease severity. J Allergy Clin Immunol. 2002;110(3):492–9.
5. Asero R, Tedeschi A, Lorini M. Histamine release in idiopathic cold urticaria. Allergy. 2002;57(12):1211–2.
6. Neittaanmaki H. Cold urticaria. Clinical findings in 220 patients. J Am Acad Dermatol. 1985;13(4):636–44.
7. Wanderer AA, Hoffman HM. The spectrum of acquired and familial cold-induced urticaria/urticaria-like syndromes. Immunol Allergy Clin N Am. 2004;24(2):259–86, vii.
8. Gandhi C, Healy C, Wanderer AA, Hoffman HM. Familial atypical cold urticaria: description of a new hereditary disease. J Allergy Clin Immunol. 2009;124(6):1245–50.
9. Katsarou-Katsari A, Makris M, Lagogianni E, Gregoriou S, Theoharides T, Kalogeromitros D. Clinical features and natural history of acquired cold urticaria in a tertiary referral hospital: a 10-year prospective study. J Eur Acad Dermatol Venereol. 2008;22(12):1405–11.
10. Alangari AA, Twarog FJ, Shih MC, Schneider LC. Clinical features and anaphylaxis in children with cold urticaria. Pediatrics. 2004;113(4):e313–7.
11. Park HJ, Park SY, Lee SH, Kim GH, Yang JE, Yoon SY, Kim SJ, Kwon HS, Cho YS, Moon HB, Kim TB. Cold-induced systemic reactions caused by infusion of intravenous fluid. Acta Derm Venereol. 2013;93(4):469–70.
12. von Mackensen YA, Sticherling M. Cold urticaria: tolerance induction with cold baths. Br J Dermatol. 2007;157(4):835–6.

Chapter 58
Bee Sting Reaction

Charmi Patel and Punita Ponda

An 18-year-old female with peanut and tree nut allergy, allergic rhinitis and intermittent asthma presented with a complaint of bee sting reaction a few weeks ago. She states that she was stung on her left arm by a bee while eating outdoors at camp. She immediately developed swelling on the arm and hives all over her body with respiratory distress. She was taken to the emergency room and was reportedly unconscious, where she was given IM epinephrine, IV diphenhydramine, nebulized albuterol and intravenous fluids with resolution of symptoms. When asked about the exact insect that stung her, she is unsure if it was a bee. Her family history is significant for atopy.

Physical examination revealed a well appearing female with boggy pale turbinates, suborbital bogginess and a normal lung examination. Skin prick test was negative to honey bee, yellow jacket, yellow hornet, white faced hornet and wasp. Intradermal testing was positive for yellow hornet, white faced hornet and wasp, but negative to honey bee and yellow jacket. Her honeybee specific IgE was <0.35 UA/mL.

Q1. Which of the following is the correct management of this patient?

A. Recommend venom immunotherapy (VIT)
B. Prescribe epinephrine autoinjector
C. Check baseline tryptase
D. Recommend measures to avoid future stings
E. All of the above

Answer: *The correct answer is* ***E.***

C. Patel
Division of Allergy and Immunology, Department of Medicine, Albany Medical Center, Albany Medical College, Albany, NY, USA

P. Ponda (✉)
Division of Allergy and Immunology, Cohen Children's Hospital of New York, Donald and Barbara Zucker School of Medicine at Hofstra/Northwell, Great Neck, NY, USA
e-mail: pponda@northwell.edu

N. Rezaei (ed.), *Pediatric Allergy*, https://doi.org/10.1007/978-3-030-18282-3_58

VIT decreases the risk of a future systemic reaction to <5% and reduces the severity of sting reactions during VIT [1]. Patients with severe anaphylactic reactions should be prescribed and instructed to carry a twin pack of epinephrine auto-injector. In patients with a history of severe anaphylaxis with any insect sting, a basal serum tryptase should be measured [1]. Her tryptase level was 6.2 ng/mL. Effective measures to avoid stings include avoid preparing, grilling or eating outdoors, avoid planting, avoiding drinking beverages outdoors or eliminating fallen fruit or pet feces, keeping trashcans covered, being aware of nests in bushes or when mowing lawn and wearing shoes when outdoors [1]. Measures like avoiding fragrances, bright colored clothing, insect repellents and running from insects, have been reported to be ineffective [1].

Q2. Patients with which of the following symptoms/conditions are not considered to have a low risk of hymenoptera reaction?

A. A history of only large local reactions to stings or of strictly cutaneous systemic reactions
B. Patients receiving maintenance VIT
C. Patients who have discontinued VIT after more than 5 years of treatment
D. Severe honeybee allergy

Answer: *The correct answer is* ***D.***

Patients with isolated large local reaction to stings or cutaneous systemic reactions, patients on maintenance VIT, and those who finished >5 years of VIT treatment are considered to have a low risk of hymenoptera reaction [1]. Near-fatal reactions to stings, systemic reactions during VIT due to an injection or a sting, severe honeybee allergy, elevated basal serum tryptase level, certain underlying medical conditions, or frequent unavoidable exposure are characteristics associated with a high risk of hymenoptera reaction [1].

Q3. Which of the following hymenoptera associations are correct?

A. Hornets build their nests in the ground and can be encountered during yard work.
B. Yellow jackets are extremely aggressive and build large nests in trees or shrubs.
C. Wasps usually leave a barbed stinger and attached venom sac in the skin after they sting.
D. A sterile pseudopustule is pathognomonic of a fire ant sting.

Answer: *The correct answer is* ***D.***

Yellow jackets build their nests in the ground and therefore are encountered during yard work, farming, and gardening [1]. Hornets are extremely aggressive and their nests are found in trees or shrubs [1]. Yellow jackets and hornets are scavengers i.e. are attracted to remaining of food and drinks are served outdoor [1]. Wasps build their nests in shrubs and under eaves of houses or barns [1]. Honeybees typically leave a barbed stinger in the skin. A sterile pseudopustule is pathognomonic of a fire ant sting [1, 2].

Q4. Which of the following shows a high cross-reactivity with yellow jacket venom?

A. Hornet
B. Paper wasp
C. Honeybee
D. Fire ant

Answer: *The correct answer is **A**.*

Extensive immunologic cross reactivity is noted between hornet and yellow jacket venoms (vespids). Cross-reactivity is less between Polistes wasp (paper wasp) and other vespid venoms, but still present [1]. It is even less between honeybee and vespid venoms [3–7]. Fire ant venom i.e. fire ant whole-body extract (WBE) has very limited cross reactivity with other stinging insect venoms [8, 9].

Q5. Which of the following is associated with increased serum tryptase levels in these patients?

A. More frequent and severe systemic reaction to VIT injections
B. Decreased failure rates of VIT
C. No change in relapse rates if VIT is discontinued
D. Shorter duration of VIT recommended

Answer: *The correct answer is **A**.*

Increased frequency and severity of systemic reactions to VIT, increased failure rates during VIT and increased relapse rates, including fatal reactions, if VIT is discontinued, all correlate with elevated baseline serum tryptase levels [1]. VIT should be considered for a prolonged period of time, even indefinitely, in patients with multiple risk factors including a history of severe reaction with syncope, hypotension, and severe respiratory distress, systemic reaction during VIT, honeybee allergy, and increased basal serum tryptase levels [1].

Q6. When is the appropriate time frame for stopping VIT in this patient to maximize the reduction in the risk of systemic reaction?

A. <3 years
B. 3–5 years
C. 7–9 years
D. Indefinitely

Answer: *The correct answer is **D**.*

Patients with a history of severe anaphylaxis defined as severe airway obstruction, shock, or loss of consciousness appear to remain at risk for a severe systemic reaction after 5 years of VIT treatment [1, 2]. Patients should be urged to continue VIT for a prolonged time or indefinitely if they have the following risk factors [1, 2]:

- Very severe reaction before VIT (syncope, hypotension, severe respiratory distress)
- Systemic reaction during VIT
- Honeybee allergy
- Increased basal serum tryptase

- Other high-risk factors for recurrent or severe sting reactions
  - Underlying cardiovascular or respiratory conditions
  - Select antihypertensive medications
  - Frequent exposure such as bee keepers
  - Limitation of activity due to anxiety of accidental stings

Practical Points

- A severe reaction with hymenoptera hypersensitivity mandates carrying epinephrine autoinjectors in any patient
- If initial skin testing is negative in a patient with systemic reaction, further testing should be pursued with *in vitro* testing and repeating skin testing a few weeks later
- Venom immunotherapy is extremely effective in reducing future sting reactions
- Venom immunotherapy should be recommended to patients with systemic reactions, large local reactions with frequent exposure, impaired quality of life, or underlying medical conditions such as mast cell disorder
- Basal serum tryptase is important in assessment of the risk for future reactions, failure rates of venom immunotherapy and risk of relapse post-immunotherapy cessation

References

1. Golden DB, Demain J, Freeman T, Graft D, Tankersley M, Tracy J, Blessing-Moore J, Bernstein D, Dinakar C, Greenhawt M, Khan D, Lang D, Nicklas R, Oppenheimer J, Portnoy J, Randolph C, Schuller D, Wallace D. Stinging insect hypersensitivity: a practice parameter update 2016. Ann Allergy Asthma Immunol. 2017;118(1):28–54.
2. Cox L, Nelson H, Lockey R, Calabria C, Chacko T, Finegold I, Nelson M, Weber R, Bernstein DI, Blessing-Moore J, Khan DA, Lang DM, Nicklas RA, Oppenheimer J, Portnoy JM, Randolph C, Schuller DE, Spector SL, Tilles S, Wallace D. Allergen immunotherapy: a practice parameter third update. J Allergy Clin Immunol. 2011;127(1):S1–S55.
3. Hoffman DR. Allergens in Hymenoptera venom XXV: the amino acid sequences of antigen 5 molecules and the structural basis of antigenic cross-reactivity. J Allergy Clin Immunol. 1993;92(5):707–16.
4. King TP, Joslyn A, Kochoumian L. Antigenic cross-reactivity of venom proteins from hornets, wasps, and yellow jackets. J Allergy Clin Immunol. 1985;75(5):621–8.
5. Reisman RE, Mueller U, Wypych J, Elliott W, Arbesman CE. Comparison of the allergenicity and antigenicity of yellow jacket and hornet venoms. J Allergy Clin Immunol. 1982;69(3):268–74.
6. Reisman RE, Wypych JI, Mueller UR, Grant JA. Comparison of the allergenicity and antigenicity of Polistes venom and other vespid venoms. J Allergy Clin Immunol. 1982;70(4):281–7.
7. Reisman RE, Müller UR, Wypych JI, Lazell MI. Studies of coexisting honeybee and vespid-venom sensitivity. J Allergy Clin Immunol. 1984;73(2):246–52.
8. Hoffman D, Dove DE, Moffitt JE, Stafford CT. Allergens in Hymenoptera venom. XXI. Cross-reactivity and multiple reactivity between fire ant venom and bee and wasp venoms. J Allergy Clin Immunol. 1988;82(5 Pt 1):828–34.
9. Rhoades RB, Kalof D, Bloom F, Wittig HJ. Cross reacting antigens between imported fire ant and other Hymenoptera species. Ann Allergy Asthma Immunol. 1978;40:100–4.

Chapter 59
Lip Angioedema Following Hepatitis B Vaccination

Darko Richter

A 12-year-old girl was referred by the local epidemiologist to consider a possible vaccine reaction to hepatitis B vaccine (Engerix™). Four hours after she had received the first dose of pediatric Engerix™, while at home, she complained of a prickling sensation in the lower lip and her mother had noted slight lip edema. Next she woke up at 4:30 in the morning complaining of pain in the mouth and inability to move the lip. It was more swollen than in the evening, but with no prominent itching. However, everything disappeared at about 8:00 o'clock. When she returned from school she reported that several children at school had pain and tenderness at the injection site and paresthesia in the arm, but nobody had lip swelling. This was the first time she had a lip swelling and she was not aware of any allergies to vaccines, food or inhalant allergens.

In her past medical history she said that as a preschool child, she used to get transitory wheals on exposure to cold air. She has Hashimoto autoimmune thyroiditis since 6 years old. Lately her TSH was increased (5.3 IU/mL (reference range 0.40–4.20)), and thyroxine replacement therapy was considered. Mother, too, has Hashimoto disease. The epidemiologist felt that mild and transient angioedema of the lower lip was temporally related to hepatitis B immunization and could not have been predicted on the basis of history.

Q1. What would be your primary diagnostic step?

A. Measure C1-esterase-inhibitor, complement fraction 3 and 4
B. Skin testing with the vaccine
C. Prick test and specific IgE to *Saccharomyces cerevisiae*
D. Thyroid ultrasound

Answer: *The correct answer is* ***B.***

D. Richter (✉)
Outpatient and Emergency Service, Department of Pediatrics, University Hospital Center, Zagreb, Croatia
e-mail: darko.richter@kbc-zagreb.hr

N. Rezaei (ed.), *Pediatric Allergy*, https://doi.org/10.1007/978-3-030-18282-3_59

Although the allergic reactions to vaccines were believed to occur mostly within minutes to 1 h, larger cohorts have revealed that only 25% of patients presented within the first hour, and 55% presented within 1–4 h, while the rest appeared later in the day of vaccination [1].

Skin testing may give the answer if there is a causal link, e.g. temporal correlation, between the vaccine and an adverse event [2]. Skin tests were performed with the same vaccine brand 4 weeks later. Both the skin prick test with the undiluted vaccine and the intradermal test with the 0.2 mL of 1:100 dilution gave negative results (positive histamine control 5 mm) [3, 4]. At the same time, a standard inhalant allergen panel was tested by prick method which returned a strong positive reaction (4+) to the mold *Alternaria alternata*. Since the HBsAg is produced using the recombinant DNA technology by the yeast *Saccharomyces cerevisiae*, testing was extended to the baker's yeast (i.e. *Saccharomyces cerevisiae*) by commercial prick and by the prick-prick method using the kitchen yeast and was also negative.

In theory, C1-esterase-inhibitor could be considered, although the probability is very slim, given the absence of family history of hereditary angioneurotic edema and the appearance of hives at early childhood in this girl, which point away from hereditary angioedema [5, 6].

A more plausible path to go would be to look for data supporting chronic urticaria (CU) since the girl has Hashimoto autoimmune thyroiditis. On average ≥10% (range 0–28%) of patients with chronic urticaria exhibit a positive autoimmune IgG serology to the thyroid gland (anti-thyroglobulin:anti-TG and anti-thyroid peroxidase:anti-TPO) [7]. Chronic urticaria can be precipitated by a number of physical stimuli, and the girl did exhibit cold-induced urticaria around the age she was diagnosed with autoimmune thyroiditis.

Q2. The scheme now shifts to the work-up of CU. What would you suggest as the next step?

A. Epstein-Barr virus and cytomegalovirus serology
B. Standard inhalant allergen testing and food preservative testing
C. Standard food allergen testing and food preservative testing
D. Anti-thyroid antibodies, antinuclear antibodies, and standard inhalant allergen testing

Answer: *The correct answer is* ***D.***

CU is characterized by wheals, erythema and mild to moderate itching that appears transiently or persists for up to 24 h, and recur or last for 6 weeks or more [8]. CU is not an extension of acute allergic urticaria, yet IgE-mediated allergy can contribute to its obstinate course and persistence. A central role is attributed to dermal mast cells and mediator release, as mast cells are ten times denser in skin of these patients compared to a normal one [9].The precipitating stimuli may include various bacterial and viral infections, pressure, stroking (dermographism), water immersion (aquagenic urticaria), solar ultraviolet radiation, cold exposure, increase in central body temperature (as in fever, physical effort, sweating: cholinergic urticaria) [10]. The workup may include search for: (1) infectious diseases (e.g.

Helicobacter pylori, *Yersinia enterocolitica*, and hepatitis B), (2) type I allergy reactions, (3) autoantibodies, (4) thyroid hormones, (5) physical tests, (6) a trial of preservative-free diet for 3 weeks, (7) elevated baseline tryptase levels and (8) skin biopsy for suspected rheumatic vasculitis (wheals persisting >24 h) [11]. If nothing can be found, the condition is termed chronic spontaneous urticaria (CSU). If there is autoimmunity, it is called chronic autoimmune urticaria.

An autoimmune etiology makes up for about 30% of all case of chronic urticaria cases [12]. Chronic autoimmune urticaria is presumed to be mediated by IgG autoantibodies that cross-link the Fc subunits of adjacent high-affinity IgE receptor in the IgE-FcεRI complex [13]. The autoimmune nature can be indirectly shown by autologous serum skin test (ASST), and basophil and/or histamine release test (HR-urticaria test). The ASST is a usual intradermal test performed with 50 μL of patient's own serum, with normal saline, as a negative, and histamine 10 μg/mL, as a positive control. When the wheal is at least 1.5 mm greater than the negative control, the results are considered positive [14]. The HR-urticaria test is performed in a number of specialized laboratories and is basically the *in vitro* variety of ASST. Donor basophils (usually from blood drawn from a healthy parent or from a blood donor or health worker) are incubated with the patient's serum, and the histamine released in comparison to a healthy control is measured [15].

Q3. Would you now go on with the second and third doses of Engerix™ in this girl?

A. No, this can cause a flare up of chronic autoimmune urticaria
B. Yes, there is no causal relation of angioedema to Engerix™
C. No, there is a risk of significant angioedema on repeat immunization
D. No, there is no need to incur further risk as one dose of Engerix™ is at least partially protective

Answer: *The correct answer is* ***B.***

The girl was found to have atopy, but no allergy to Engerix™ nor the baker's yeast (*Saccharomyces cerevisiae*). Autoimmunity to the thyroid was confirmed, although without hypothyroidism. The autoimmune nature of her chronic urticaria was established by the HR-urticaria test. ASST is a less sensitive test and was negative in this girl. Therefore, it appeared that this girl had a flare-up of her chronic autoimmune urticaria when she returned home, possibly facilitated by allergy to mold. Post marketing surveillance of Engerix™ mentions the occurrence of angioedema as an "adverse reaction"(i.e. more firmly related to the vaccine than a temporally related "adverse event" [2]) at an unknown, very low rate [16]. It is therefore important to dissect each case and separate coincidental adverse events from causally related reactions.

Immunizations in children have been repeatedly shown not to cause atopy [17], nor autoimmunity [18]. One instance of unresolved suspicion of inactivated influenza vaccine triggering narcolepsy was related to GSK's Pandemrix™ in 2009/2010, with significant epidemiological associations, but not unequivocally causally proven, nor noted with other influenza vaccines that season [19, 20]. One should, however, beware of situations in which the individual has a history of chronic diseases that might be worsened or exacerbated by immunization: multiple sclerosis by influenza vaccine (with the risk of natural infection far outnumbering the immunization related risk, i.e. natural infection approximately 30%, influenza vaccine 5%) [21], Guillain-Barré syndrome by anthrax, influenza and diphtheria-tetanus toxoid containing vaccines, and low platelet count (ever) by measles-mumps-rubella containing vaccines. For other possible associations/contraindications one should look up the updated CDC database “Who Should NOT Get Vaccinated with these Vaccines?” [22]. Conversely, some diseases can cause significant reactions to specific vaccines: e.g. the occurrence of large local necrotic BCG reactions in children with Kawasaki disease [23].

The girl was scheduled to receive the second Engerix™ dose in a day-care hospital setting. She was monitored for 4 h after the injection, and then by a telephone check-up with the parents 24 h later. There was no adverse event seen/reported. She went on to have her third dose of Engerix™ with her school epidemiologist and did not report any further adverse events.

In summary, this girl had angioedema of the lower lip temporally related to the first dose of Engerix™. The workup disclosed atopy and chronic autoimmunity against the thyroid, but no causal link to Engerix™ nor *Saccharomyces cerevisiae*. Initial workup allowed to proceed with immunization with a negligible risk of an adverse event. This was an example of the coincidental occurrence of allergy-like symptoms and immunization that were causally unrelated.

Practical Points

- Temporal association of an adverse event to immunization should not automatically be considered to constitute a causal relation
- If the events are not causally related, the continuation of immunization is advised
- Atopy and autoimmunity are not associated with history of immunization
- Comorbid disorders like multiple sclerosis, Guillain-Barré syndrome and thrombocytopenia may constitute relative or absolute contraindications to specific vaccines

References

1. McNeil MM, Weintraub ES, Duffy J, Sukumaran L, Jacobsen SJ, Klein NP, Hambidge SJ, Lee GM, Jackson LA, Irving SA, King JP, Kharbanda EO, Bednarczyk RA, DeStefano F. Risk of anaphylaxis after vaccination in children and adults. J Allergy Clin Immunol. 2016;137(3):868–78.
2. Barton L, Cobert M. Manual of drug safety and pharmacovigilance. Sudbury, MA: Jones and Bartlett; 2007.
3. Brockow K, Romano A, Blanca M, Ring J, Pichler W, Demoly P. General considerations for skin test procedures in the diagnosis of drug hypersensitivity. Allergy. 2002;57(1):45–51.

4. Caubet J-C, Rudzeviciene O, Gomes E, Terreehorst I, Brockow K, Eigenmann PA. Managing a child with possible allergy to vaccine. Pediatr Allergy Immunol. 2014;25(4):394–403.
5. Kaplan AP, Greaves MW. Angioedema. J Am Acad Dermatol. 2005;53(3):373–88; quiz 89–92.
6. Cicardi M, Aberer W, Banerji A, Bas M, Bernstein JA, Bork K, Caballero T, Farkas H, Grumach A, Kaplan AP, Riedl MA, Triggiani M, Zanichelli A, Zuraw B. Classification, diagnosis, and approach to treatment for angioedema: consensus report from the Hereditary Angioedema International Working Group. Allergy. 2014;69(5):602–16.
7. Kolkhir P, Metz M, Altrichter S, Maurer M. Comorbidity of chronic spontaneous urticaria and autoimmune thyroid diseases: a systematic review. Allergy. 2017;72(10):1440–60.
8. Joint Task Force on Practice Parameters. The diagnosis and management of urticaria: a practice parameter. Part I: Acute urticaria/angioedema. Part II: Chronic urticaria/angioedema. Ann Allergy Asthma Immunol. 2000;85(6 Pt 2):521–44.
9. Benoist C, Mathis D. Mast cells in autoimmune disease. Nature. 2002;420(6917):875–8.
10. Dodig S, Richter D. Chronic autoimmune urticaria in children. Acta Dermatovenerol Croatica. 2008;16(2):65–71.
11. Zuberbier T, Bindslev-Jensen C, Canonica W, Grattan CE, Greaves MW, Henz BM, Kapp A, Kozel MM, Maurer M, Merk HF, Schafer T, Simon D, Vena GA, Wedi B. EAACI/GA2LEN/EDF guideline: definition, classification and diagnosis of urticaria. Allergy. 2006;61(3):316–20.
12. Sabroe RA, Seed PT, Francis DM, Barr RM, Black AK, Greaves MW. Chronic idiopathic urticaria: comparison of the clinical features of patients with and without anti-FcepsilonRI or anti-IgE autoantibodies. J Am Acad Dermatol. 1999;40(3):443–50.
13. Vonakis BM, Saini SS. Basophils and mast cells in chronic idiopathic urticaria. Curr Allergy Asthma Rep. 2005;5(4):270–6.
14. Kilic G, Guler N, Suleyman A, Tamay Z. Chronic urticaria and autoimmunity in children. Pediatr Allergy Immunol. 2010;21(5):837–42.
15. Platzer MH, Grattan CE, Poulsen LK, Skov PS. Validation of basophil histamine release against the autologous serum skin test and outcome of serum-induced basophil histamine release studies in a large population of chronic urticaria patients. Allergy. 2005;60(9):1152–6.
16. Engerix B. 20 micrograms/1ml Suspension for injection in pre-filled syringe. Brentford, UK: GlaxoSmithKline; 2017.
17. Anderson HR, Poloniecki JD, Strachan DP, Beasley R, Bjorksten B, Asher MI. Immunization and symptoms of atopic disease in children: results from the International Study of Asthma and Allergies in Childhood. Am J Public Health. 2001;91(7):1126–9.
18. Heijstek MW, Ott de Bruin LM, Borrow R, van der Klis F, Kone-Paut I, Fasth A, Minden K, Ravelli A, Abinun M, Pileggi G, Borte M, Bijl M, Wulffraat NM. Vaccination in paediatric patients with auto-immune rheumatic diseases: a systemic literature review for the European League against Rheumatism evidence-based recommendations. Autoimmun Rev. 2011;11(2):112–22.
19. Partinen M, Saarenpaa-Heikkila O, Ilveskoski I, Hublin C, Linna M, Olsen P, Nokelainen P, Alen R, Wallden T, Espo M, Rusanen H, Olme J, Satila H, Arikka H, Kaipainen P, Julkunen I, Kirjavainen T. Increased incidence and clinical picture of childhood narcolepsy following the 2009 H1N1 pandemic vaccination campaign in Finland. PLoS One. 2012;7(3):e33723.
20. Han F, Lin L, Warby SC, Faraco J, Li J, Dong SX, An P, Zhao L, Wang LH, Li QY, Yan H, Gao ZC, Yuan Y, Strohl KP, Mignot E. Narcolepsy onset is seasonal and increased following the 2009 H1N1 pandemic in China. Ann Neurol. 2011;70(3):410–7.
21. De Keyser J, Zwanikken C, Boon M. Effects of influenza vaccination and influenza illness on exacerbations in multiple sclerosis. J Neurol Sci. 1998;159(1):51–3.
22. CDC. Who should NOT get vaccinated with these vaccines. Accessed 5 Dec 2017.
23. Bijl M, Agmon-Levin N, Dayer JM, Israeli E, Gatto M, Shoenfeld Y. Vaccination of patients with auto-immune inflammatory rheumatic diseases requires careful benefit-risk assessment. Autoimmun Rev. 2012;11(8):572–6.

Chapter 60
Extensive Rash and Swollen Eyelids Following Eating Peanut Cookie

Nima Rezaei

A 14-month old girl was referred to our center with an extensive rash developed around her mouth that spread to her chest and swollen eyelids. She was well without any history of any allergic reaction. The parents mentioned that her problems started a few minutes ago after she was given a few bites of peanut butter cookie.

Q1. What is the probable diagnosis in this case?

A. Atopic dermatitis
B. Celiac disease
C. Anaphylaxis
D. Inflammatory bowel disease

Answer: *The correct answer is* ***C.***

Food allergy is an adverse immune response to food proteins [1]. Peanut allergy seems to be the most common form of food allergy and is seen in almost 2% of all children [2–4]. Foods are the most common reason for anaphylaxis in children [5, 6].

Q2. The following statements are true regarding peanut allergy, except:

A. Atopy is a risk factor in peanut allergy
B. IgM has the main role in anaphylaxis to peanut antigens

N. Rezaei (✉)
Department of Immunology, School of Medicine, Research Center for Immunodeficiencies (RCID), Children's Medical Center, Tehran University of Medical Sciences (TUMS), Tehran, Iran

Network of Immunity in Infection, Malignancy and Autoimmunity (NIIMA), Universal Scientific Education and Research Network (USERN), Tehran, Iran
e-mail: rezaei_nima@tums.ac.ir

N. Rezaei (ed.), *Pediatric Allergy*, https://doi.org/10.1007/978-3-030-18282-3_60

C. Peanut allergy is an example of immediate hypersensitivity
D. The child should avoid tree nuts in addition to peanut

Answer: *The correct answer is **B.***

Q3. Which type of hypersensitivity is responsible for peanut allergy?

A. Type I
B. Type II
C. Type III
D. Type IV

Answer: *The correct answer is **A.***

Food allergy and anaphylaxis are examples of type I hypersensitivity reactions, also known as immediate hypersensitivity. T-helper 2 cells and IgE are major role players in this type of hypersensitivity, leading to release of histamine and other mediators from mast cells and basophils.

Q4. In type I hypersensitivity, all of the following cells have a contribution, except:

A. B cells
B. Antigen presenting cells
C. Mast cells
D. Neutrophils

Answer: *The correct answer is **D.***

Q5. All of the following sentences are correct in type I hypersensitivity, except:

A. Activated T helper cells produce cytokines, which stimulate B cells to proliferate and differentiate into plasma cells capable of producing IgE
B. IgE molecules attach to mast cells through their constant region
C. Two bound IgE molecules on a mast cell must react with a specific antigen for the mast cell to degranulate
D. Histamine released by mast cells leads to capillary dilation and airway constriction on first exposure to allergen

Answer: *The correct answer is **D.***

The mechanism of type I hypersensitivity starts from exposure to an allergen which is presented to naïve T cells by antigen presenting cells which in turn stimulate Th2 responses. Th2 cells further stimulate B cells to proliferate and differentiate into plasma cells capable of producing IgE. IgE binding to the Fcε receptors on mast cells, cross-linking of the IgE and the Fcε receptors by the allergen, and activation of mast cells, results in release of mediators in second exposure and hypersensitivity response.

Practical Points

- Food allergy and anaphylaxis are examples of type I hypersensitivity, also known as immediate hypersensitivity
- Peanut allergy seems to be the most common food allergy
- Food-induced anaphylaxis seems to be the most common reason for anaphylaxis in children

References

1. Anvari S, Miller J, Yeh CY, Davis CM. IgE-mediated food allergy. Clin Rev Allergy Immunol. 2018. doi: https://doi.org/10.1007/s12016-018-8710-3.
2. Dyer AA, Rivkina V, Perumal D, Smeltzer BM, Smith BM, Gupta RS. Epidemiology of childhood peanut allergy. Allergy Asthma Proc. 2015;36(1):58–64.
3. Gupta RS, Springston EE, Warrier MR, Smith B, Kumar R, Pongracic J, Holl JL. The prevalence, severity, and distribution of childhood food allergy in the United States. Pediatrics. 2011;128(1):e9–17.
4. Samady W, Trainor J, Smith B, Gupta R. Food-induced anaphylaxis in infants and children. Ann Allergy Asthma Immunol. 2018;121(3):360–5.
5. Lieberman P, Camargo CA Jr, Bohlke K, Jick H, Miller RL, Sheikh A, Simons FE. Epidemiology of anaphylaxis: findings of the American College of Allergy, Asthma and Immunology Epidemiology of Anaphylaxis Working Group. Ann Allergy Asthma Immunol. 2006;97(5):596–602.
6. Parrish CP, Kim H. Food-induced anaphylaxis: an update. Curr Allergy Asthma Rep. 2018;18(8):41.

Index

N. Rezaei (ed.), *Pediatric Allergy*, https://doi.org/10.1007/978-3-030-18282-3

D

K

L

M

N

R

Printed by Printforce, the Netherlands